ASBESTOS-RELATED DISEASE

ASBESTOS-RELATED DISEASE

Leslie Preger, M.B., Ch.B., D. Obst., R.C.O.G., F.R.C.R., F.F.R. (R.C.S.I.)

Clinical Professor of Radiology,
University of California, School of Medicine,
San Francisco, California

Associate Clinical Professor of Radiology,
University of California Davis,
Davis, California

Assistant Chief of Radiology,
French Hospital,
San Francisco, California

with

Donald T. Arai, M.D.
Paul Kotin, M.D.
Hans Weill, M.D.
Jack Werchick, J.D.

Foreword by Robert G. Fraser, M.D., F.R.C.P. (C)
Professor of Diagnostic Radiology,
University of Alabama,
Birmingham, Alabama

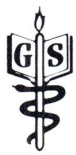

Grune & Stratton
A Subsidiary of Harcourt Brace Jovanovich, Publishers
New York   San Francisco   London

Library of Congress Cataloging in Publication Data
Main entry under title:

Asbestos related diseases.

    Bibliography: p.
    Includes index.
    1. Asbestosis—Diagnosis. 2. Lungs—Radiography.
3. Asbestos—Toxicology. 4. Diagnosis, Differential. I. Preger,
Leslie. [DNLM: 1. Asbestos—Poisoning. 2. Asbestosis—
Radiography. WF654 P923a]
RC775.A8A83   616.2'44   78-8760
ISBN 0-8089-1083-3

© 1978 by Grune & Stratton, Inc. All rights reserved. No part of this publication may be reproduced or transmitted in any form or by any means, electronic or mechanical, including photocopy, recording, or any information storage and retrieval system, without permission in writing from the publisher.

Grune & Stratton, Inc.
111 Fifth Avenue
New York, New York 10003

Distributed in the United Kingdom by
Academic Press, Inc. (London) Ltd.
24/28 Oval Road, London NW 1

Library of Congress Catalog Number 78-8760
International Standard Book Number 0-8089-1083-3

Printed in the United States of America

CONTENTS

FOREWORD   vi

PREFACE   viii

CONTRIBUTORS   x
  Robert G. Fraser

1 CLINICAL PROBLEMS IN ASBESTOS-RELATED DISEASES   1
  Donald T. Arai and Hans Weill

2 ORGAN INVOLVEMENT IN ASBESTOS-RELATED DISEASE   29
  Leslie Preger
  SECTION 1 PLEURAL PLAQUES   29
  SECTION 2 PULMONARY FIBROSIS   82
  SECTION 3 PLEURAL EFFUSIONS   113
  SECTION 4 PLEURAL AND PERITONEAL MESOTHELIOMA   121
  SECTION 5 LUNG CANCER   174
  SECTION 6 EXTRATHORACIC EFFECTS OF ASBESTOS   205
  SECTION 7 HYPERTROPHIC PULMONARY
             OSTEOARTHROPATHY   220

3 ILO U/C 1971 INTERNATIONAL CLASSIFICATION OF RADIOGRAPHS OF THE PNEUMOCONIOSES   227
  Leslie Preger

4 THE INDUSTRIAL MEDICAL OFFICER AND CORPORATE RESPONSIBILITY   239
  Paul Kotin

5 MEDICOLEGAL ASPECTS   247
  Jack Werchick

INDEX   263

FOREWORD

The relative incidence of respiratory diseases has changed considerably over the last quarter century. In some diseases, such as tuberculosis and bronchiectasis, a decreased frequency reflects improved public health measures and therapeutic innovations. In others, man himself has been responsible for varying the spectrum of respiratory disease as a result of his irresponsible insistence upon increasing the amount and variety of atmospheric pollutants. A great number of lung diseases derive from chemical aerosols and dust particles in our polluted atmosphere, and the increasing attention being paid to these environmental hazards by government agencies in recent years bears clear testimony to their impact on society as a whole. Although the "black lung" program has gained considerable notoriety in this regard, it is probable that the inhalation of coal dust and silica by the population at large is less hazardous than the inhalation of asbestos fibers. The use of asbestos in industry has increased enormously during this century: world production jumped from 500 tons in 1900 to 3 million tons in 1968 and an estimated 5 million tons in 1974. The prevalence of this mineral throughout the world is indicated by the frequency with which "asbestos bodies" (more properly called ferruginous bodies) are found in routine necropsies, the incidence ranging from 1 percent in rural Italy to 60 percent in New York City. Such findings indicate that exposure to asbestos dust is worldwide in distribution, and although the major sources of exposure are the primary occupations of mining and processing of asbestos and secondary occupations such as the manufacturing of textiles and insulation, there is irrefutable evidence that individuals living in the vicinity of a mine, mill, or factory associated with heavy asbestos dust pollution develop thoracic manifestations of asbestosis. The disease can, in fact, develop in persons who repeatedly handle the clothes of asbestos workers.

These statements do little more than scratch the surface of a highly complex group of conditions identified as asbestos-related disease. Although there are still many gaps in our knowledge of asbestosis and its complications, the past three decades or so have seen the appearance of a voluminous literature on the subject, a diligent search of which would undoubtedly reveal much of the truth. What Leslie Preger and his colleagues have accomplished in this eminently readable monograph is to save us the trouble of that search by bringing together a vast amount of previously scattered information that they have recorded in a systematic and easily accessible form. One of the major attractions of the book is the close attention paid to a correlation of the epidemiologic, pathogenetic, pathological, roentgenologic, and clinical manifestations of asbestos-related disease, a correlation that places the whole problem in proper perspective. The fact that the subject has become too vast for any one individual to master is implicit in the decision to acquire the expertise of a number of authorities in the field, specifically in the areas of clinical aspects (Professor Hans Weill and Dr. Arai from Tulane University, New Orleans), medicolegal aspects (Mr. Jack Werchick, an international authority on professional negligence and medical malpractice), and industrial considerations (Dr. Paul Kotin of Johns Manville). This approach brings under one cover a far more authoritative treatment of each of the various facets of the subject than would otherwise be possible.

As might be anticipated in a book dealing with a disease whose initial recognition and subsequent evaluation are primarily roentgenologic, a considerable amount of material is radiologically oriented. The illustrations are uniformly of high quality and reveal changes that are often subtle and extremely difficult to reproduce. The inclusion of a number of computed tomographic scans has provided a new dimension in illustration, particularly in the areas of pleural plaque formation and mesothelioma. Where appropriate, reference has been made to the use of ultrasonography and scintiphotography in the elucidation of various facets of the disease. The references are comprehensive, if not exhaustive.

This monograph consists of a comprehensive dissertation on the protean manifestations of a complex, fascinating disease. It answers a multitude of questions but goes further than that by posing questions to which answers are not yet apparent and which thus serve as a point of departure for further investigations. The completed work stands as tangible evidence of splendid cooperation between the several contributing authorities, and all are to be congratulated for an outstanding final product.

Robert G. Fraser, M.D., F.R.C.P.(C)
Professor of Diagnostic Radiology
University of Alabama
Birmingham, Alabama

PREFACE

Asbestos causes much distress both medically, because of its deleterious effects, and emotionally, because of the publicity given in the media regarding hazards associated with its use. The purpose of this book is to help identify asbestos-related disease and to provide a guide to physicians who must reassure the "worried well" who have been exposed to asbestos but who are free from asbestos-related disease.

Much has been written on asbestos in the past, but such material frequently appears in journals not usually read by general physicians and clinical radiologists. Computer searches of this material have allowed collation of many of these reports. Excellent current texts on occupational diseases are available, but their discussion of asbestos-related disease must, of necessity, be relatively limited, and a more extensive discussion seems justifiable. In addition, these texts do not describe recent innovations in imaging. Since the initial diagnosis and subsequent assessment of asbestos-related disease are frequently arrived at by radiographic techniques, a fuller discussion is warranted.

Chapter 1 makes use of the problem-orientated approach in discussing the clinical aspects. Subsequent chapters cover epidemiologic, pathological, and radiological data. The chapter on medicolegal aspects indicates the problems that radiologists in particular, but also physicians in general, may face while treating patients with these diseases. The role of industrial medical officers in the control of known hazards and the search for those as yet unknown is described in Chapter 4.

The radiographic material was collected during the course of routine clinical radiologic practice, not from a survey of those currently exposed to asbestos. Almost all types of physicians see such patients in their daily practice.

Preface

In nearly every instance the referring physician was unaware of the prior history of asbestos exposure until he or she was alerted by the radiologist's report and, in consequence, obtained a detailed occupational history. Many of these patients worked in shipyards in World War II and/or in housing construction soon afterward. A few are currently employed in work entailing exposure to asbestos. It is estimated that some 2 to 2.5 million persons now living in the United States once worked in war-time ship construction.

Adequate dust control measures in industries using asbestos are only recently being obtained. Because of the usually long, latent interval between exposure and the first signs of disease, patients with asbestos-related disease will remain a clinical problem until the end of the century; others who have been exposed but who have no evidence of disease, the "worried well," will need the benefit of careful assessment and reassurance. The contributors hope that this book will be of value in these regards.

Acknowledgments

French Hospital Medical Research and Education Foundation has provided most of the funds necessary for writing this volume. My editor at Grune & Stratton has been a most helpful advisor. Mrs. Sunne Thomas has been very effectively responsible in her secretarial duties. Gerald B. Levine, M.D., has given much helpful advice. The medical contributors have read each other's contributions, and I am most grateful for their constructive advice. Many colleagues have given me access to their radiographs.

CONTRIBUTORS

Donald T. Arai, M.D., is Assistant Professor of Medicine, Tulane University School of Medicine, New Orleans, Louisiana.

Paul Kotin, M.D., is Senior Vice-President, Department of Health, Safety, and Environment, Johns-Manville Corporation, Denver, Colorado; and Adjunct Professor of Pathology, University of Colorado.

Hans Weill, M.D., is Professor of Medicine, Tulane University School of Medicine, New Orleans, Louisiana.

Jack Werchick, J.D., is senior partner of Werchick and Werchick, Attorneys at Law, San Francisco; and Professor of Law, Hastings College of the Law, San Francisco, California.

ASBESTOS-RELATED DISEASE

1
CLINICAL PROBLEMS IN ASBESTOS-RELATED DISEASES

Donald T. Arai and Hans Weill

Asbestos production and utilization have increased dramatically since the 1900s, with an 80,000-fold increase from 1877 to 1967.[1] The development of new asbestos-containing products, increased utilization of existing products, and a period of inadequate asbestos dust control measures have led to increased opportunity for exposure and to more individuals with asbestos-related diseases. Individuals exposed to asbestos may present to their physician with knowledge of their exposure and fears of its consequences, but more commonly, a patient with definite evidence of disease is unaware of his exposure history or does not consider it relevant to his present complaint. The physician who encounters individuals presenting with a history of exposure must document and quantitate the exposure history, identify the type of asbestos, take appropriate diagnostic steps to establish the presence or absence of asbestos-related disease, reassure the worried well, and institute an appropriate treatment program for those patients with disease. In dealing with symptomatic patients, the physician must have a high degree of suspicion that the observed disease state is related to asbestos exposure if the correct diagnosis is to be reached. Once the association between asbestos exposure and disease is suspected, the physician is able to seek a history of exposure, look for other consequences of asbestos exposure, confirm the diagnosis, and provide appropriate treatment.

Conditions now accepted as resulting from asbestos exposure include pleural plaques, exudative pleural thickening, pleural effusion, asbestosis, lung cancer, pleural and peritoneal mesothelioma, and gastrointestinal cancer (stomach and colon). It is the purpose of this chapter to provide guidelines for the clinician in the diagnosis and management of patients with a history of asbestos exposure or with asbestos-related disease. The emphasis is on a practical approach, since not all physicians dealing with such patients have access to large hospitals with unlimited diagnostic capabilities and since simpler studies usually provide sufficient information to guide clinical decision making.

The chapter deals with the occupational history and the unique manifestations of asbestos exposure (pleural plaques, asbestosis, and mesothelioma) in greater detail than the more common lung and gastrointestinal carcinomas. We believe that this uneven distribution is warranted, since most physicians are familiar with these latter diseases. We have limited ourselves to a review of clinical and epidemiologic studies of humans in an effort to make the chapter relevant to clinicians.

EXPOSURE TO ASBESTOS

Since many patients with asbestos-related disease are unaware of their exposure to asbestos, the burden of establishing such exposure falls primarily upon the physician. The difficulty in establishing this history is demonstrated by the observation that an average of 3.3 medical histories were required before the exposure to asbestos was obtained in a group of patients with mesothelioma, where a strong suspicion of asbestos exposure should have existed on the part of the physicians.[2]

This difficulty in establishing the history of asbestos exposure is the result of several factors. Few physicians take complete occupational histories, and many are not aware of common sources of exposure. The patient may be unaware of the exposure either because he is not aware of the asbestos content of the materials he uses or because he does not use asbestos but is exposed by proximity to workers who do. The exposure often is remote, intermittent, or brief. Milne observed that at the time of diagnosis of mesothelioma, 66 percent of patients were no longer working in the occupation where exposure occurred.[3] Exposure may have occurred during the war years, a period that the patient and physician often do not consider in the occupational history. Exposure may not be related to occupational sources but, particularly in years past, may result from neighborhood air pollution near asbestos factories, from

Table 1-1
Occupational Sources of Asbestos Exposure

Industry	Occupation
Automobile repairs	Brake repairman, auto mechanic, body repairman
Construction	Insulation worker, spray insulator, carpenter, lagger, painter, tile layer, mason, demolition worker, janitorial worker, sheet metal and heating equipment workers, all other workers (plumber, welder, electrician)
Manufacturing of asbestos cement products, friction materials, insulation products, paper products, textiles	Bag opener, cutter and puncher of dried products, carder, spinner, weaver, other workers
Mining, milling, transportation	Driller, heavy equipment operator, truck driver, blender, bagger, packer, palletizer, car loader, crusher, dryer operator, laboratory technician, foreman, laborer, maintenance worker, mill operator
Shipbuilding or renovation	Sailmaker-lagger, lagger, sprayer, mason, painter, asbestos storeman, electrical fitter, welder, shipfitter, plumber, caulker, driller

unknowing inclusion of asbestos in house paint or in products used by handymen, or from household contact with asbestos-laden clothing.

Occupational Exposure

Because occupational sources of exposure constitute the most frequent, heaviest, and most clinically relevant exposures, the physician should start his search with the patient's work history. Table 1-1 lists common potential occupational sources of asbestos exposure. An individual patient can be exposed to asbestos in any of the occupations listed in Table 1-1 or, rarely, in unexpected occupations as described by Zielhuis (laundry worker and stagehand).[4] More cases will generally be found where large populations of workers are exposed to high levels of respirable asbestos fibers. It is therefore helpful to examine the number of workers involved in given industries, the amount of asbestos used by these industries, and the opportunity for asbestos fibers to become airborne.

In the United States in 1972, only 541 individuals were employed in all known active asbestos mines and mills.[5] Air samples taken at these sites indicate that the hazard is greater for mill workers. Because of the small number of individuals involved, these industries will not be a major source of

Table 1-2
Products That May Contain Asbestos

Acoustical products	Asbestos cement products (sheets, pipes, tiling)
Caulking material	Floor tiles
Friction materials (brake linings, clutch facings)	Gaskets
Insulation materials	Paints
Paper	Plastics
Roof coatings	Roofing felts
Shingles	Textiles

cases of asbestos-related disease. Although asbestiform rock deposits occur in 22 of the 50 states and miners or handlers of other mineral ores may be at risk, a hazard has not been demonstrated.

The United States' consumption of asbestos is four to five times greater than its production. Most individuals are exposed in the manufacturing industries utilizing asbestos or in trades that use asbestos-containing products. The construction industry accounts for about 75 percent of the asbestos used here, and 92 percent of this asbestos is firmly bound in the finished products, such as floor tiles, asbestos cement, roofing felts, and shingles.[5] The individuals at greatest risk from the manufacture of these products are those who handle the asbestos before it is bonded into the final product and those individuals whose handling of the product involves sawing, filing, sanding, clipping, or demolition of the dry material so that fibers may be liberated. The remaining 8 percent of the asbestos used by the construction industry is in powder form for insulation materials, asbestos cement powder or acoustic tiling, and these products provide a greater opportunity for asbestos fibers to become airborne.

Although shipyard use of insulation does not account for the great bulk of asbestos used, refitting processes involve the removal of old insulation in a closed environment. This has led to high levels of asbestos fibers in the atmosphere.

Our approach to the occupational history is to ask the patient if he knows of any previous contact with asbestos (or "fiber") or with asbestos-containing material such as insulation (excluding fibrous glass). The patient is then asked to list all jobs he has held since childhood and to indicate the years employed at each. If there are any years for which the patient does not account, he is asked to describe his activities during these years. Specific questions are asked about duties during the years of military service or the war years. If the exposure history is not confirmed at this point, the patient is then asked if he uses any of the materials listed in Table 1-2, either in vocational or avocational pursuits. Often these materials are not labeled as containing asbestos.

Nonoccupational Exposure

If no exposure to asbestos is found in a detailed occupational history, and if the physician is suspicious that the disease state is related to asbestos exposure, the possibility of exposure in a nonoccupational setting must be explored. This is particularly true for female patients. Occupational histories should be obtained for past and present household contacts. Anderson and co-workers have suggested that significant exposure occurs in household contacts, presumably because asbestos-laden clothing was worn and cleaned at home.[6]

The patient's areas of residence since childhood should be listed, and the presence or absence of nearby industrial plants (especially asbestos factories) should be determined. Newhouse and Thompson have noted that mesothelioma patients without occupational exposure more frequently lived within one-half mile of such factories than did members of the control population.[7]

A third source of nonoccupational exposure is use of the products listed in Table 1-2. Handymen who remodel their own homes or other homes during their leisure time may have significant exposure. Risk is greatest if the products are sanded, cut, or handled in other ways that will allow respirable asbestos fibers to be liberated.

In Turkey the occurrence of chrysotile-bearing rocks has led to a mixed occupational and nonoccupational exposure,[8] with equal numbers of women and men demonstrating pleural plaques. Evidently the women are exposed at home because of the frequent use of asbestos in paints.

Nonoccupational Environmental Exposure

Another source of asbestos exposure that has received widespread public attention must be mentioned here—asbestos air pollution in urban areas. Selikoff et al. were able to demonstrate asbestos fibers in the vicinity of construction sites and also at random sites of air collection in New York City.[9] Holt and Young sampled air in England (London and Rochdale), Germany (Bochum and Dusseldorf), Czechoslovakia (Prague and Pilsen), South Africa (Johannesburg), and Iceland (Reykjavik).[10] Only Rochdale has a large asbestos industry, but asbestos fibers were found in the air samples of all cities tested. These findings presumably explain the frequency with which ferruginous bodies are found in urban dwellers' lungs. No study to date has demonstrated an excess of asbestos-related disease in these individuals. The advisory committee report following the Lyon conference in 1972[11] expressed the opinion that there was no evidence of excess disease in the general public as a result of urban asbestos air pollution or a demonstrated risk from ingestion of fibers in water supplies.

In some cases, no history of exposure to asbestos will be found even after a detailed history is taken. If the patient has worked in a shipyard or industrial plant, however, one should not prematurely conclude that exposure has not taken place. Specific inquiry into all procedures involving the worker and a review of all products used at the site are necessary because of the widespread industrial applications of asbestos. This may require a visit to the plant to discuss possible sources of exposure with the plant industrial hygienist or medical officer.

DOSE–RESPONSE RELATIONSHIPS

Becklake has reviewed the evidence, based on epidemiologic studies, that a relationship exists between the level of exposure to asbestos (dose) and the biologic response of individuals exposed in terms of the development of fibrosis of the lung or pleura and cancer of the lung and pleura.[1] The dose has been estimated by years of exposure, years since first exposure, occupation, and estimated cumulative dust exposure in terms of particle or fiber counts in the environment or in pathological material. Despite problems with estimating dose, the bulk of the evidence favors a dose–response relationship for the development of asbestosis, pleural plaques, and lung cancer, thus strengthening the association between asbestos exposure and these diseases. An increased prevalence of gastrointestinal carcinoma has not been a uniform finding in all studies, indicating that the association between asbestos exposure and these neoplasms is a weaker one.

When a history of contact with asbestos is elicited, the physician should estimate the magnitude of exposure based on the onset of exposure, the number of years of exposure, the circumstances of exposure, any dust control measures the patient is aware of employing, and visible dust in the environment. The plant industrial hygienist may be of help in obtaining particle counts or fiber counts for the patient's environment. Table 1-3 lists factors favoring heavy asbestos exposure.

The amount of time elapsed since initial exposure is important for two reasons. Most of the consequences of asbestos exposure have a long latency period. Also, the level of exposure in the 1930–1950 period, before effective dust control measures were introduced or enforced, was often high. The number of years of exposure, combined with the measured or estimated asbestos fiber or dust particle levels, gives a general estimate of the magnitude of exposure, which is shown by epidemiologic studies to be related to the prevalence and extent of disease in the exposed population.

Although visible dust particles are much larger than particles of respirable size, there is a rough correlation between the visible dust levels and the concentration of invisible respirable particles. A variable portion of the visible and invisible dust will be composed of asbestos fibers, depending on the site

Table 1-3
Factors Suggesting Heavy Dust Exposure

Initial exposure before 1950s
Long history of exposure
Constant exposure to high dust levels
High visible dust levels where asbestos is used
No dust control measures or protective devices
Certain occupations
  Asbestos mill workers
  Asbestos textile factory workers (spinners, carders, weavers, disintegrators, openers)
  Insulation workers
  Sprayers using asbestos insulation slurries
  Laggers installing asbestos insulation
  Openers of bags of asbestos
  Demolition workers at sites where asbestos insulation exists
  Ship refitting

chosen, product composition, and how asbestos is handled. In spite of these limitations, visible dust can be used as a crude indication of previous exposure levels in environments where airborne asbestos fibers are known to have existed and where more specific measurements are unavailable.

Various epidemiologic studies have demonstrated that persons in the occupations listed in Table 1-3 have had heavy exposure and a significant excess of asbestos-related diseases. Even though dust control measures and protective equipment have been widely used in recent years, the majority of patients now being seen were exposed before these measures were introduced.

Of what value is this information on the severity of exposure to the physician concerned with an individual patient? If exposure levels have been high and prolonged, the physician will be more willing to attribute interstitial fibrosis to asbestosis than if exposure were brief and at a low level. In areas where the physician may see more than one individual from the same plant or industry, the discovery of one case will alert him to potential risk in other patients with similar occupations. Finally, the prognosis of the patient, along with recommendations concerning future employment, will be based on the physician's estimation of past exposure and how much future dust exposure will add to the total dust burden already encountered.

TYPES OF ASBESTOS AND THEIR BIOLOGIC EFFECTS

Asbestos is not a single substance. The major types of asbestos used commercially (chrysotile, crocidolite, amosite, and anthophyllite) have different physical and chemical characteristics and, as several studies indicate, different biologic effects. Although exposure to a single type of asbestos is rare, Enterline has demonstrated that crocidolite is the most dangerous carcinogen, while amosite and chrysotile occupy an intermediate position.[12] Gilson reviewed several studies on the occurrence of lung cancer and mesothelioma in workers exposed to different types of asbestos and reached a similar conclusion.[13] Finnish studies of workers in anthophyllite mines and mills suggest no increased incidence of mesothelioma.[14] In evaluating the fibrogenicity of various forms of asbestos, Weill and co-workers have shown that crocidolite may be more fibrogenic than other fiber types at similar cumulative dose of exposure.[15]

The physician should attempt to determine which types of asbestos the workers have encountered, since more frequent occurrence of lung cancer and mesothelioma is expected in workers exposed to crocidolite. However, this information is of less clinical importance than an estimate of the magnitude of exposure.

THRESHOLD EFFECT

As improved industrial hygiene standards for asbestos dust have been implemented in the past decades, the question concerning the presence of a threshold level of exposure remains. Is there a level of asbestos exposure below which no excess of cases of asbestos-related disease will be seen? Weill et al. have suggested that a threshold effect may exist for fibrosis in a group of asbestos cement workers,[16] but this remains to be documented by further epidemiologic studies. A threshold level for malignant effects has not been established for human exposure. This question is of great importance, because the establishment of this level would allow the implementation of maximum allowable dust level standards that would protect workers without excessive costs to the industry.

OBJECTIVE EVIDENCE OF ASBESTOS EXPOSURE

Various investigators have used clinical and pathological findings as indicators of asbestos exposure. Ferruginous bodies and pleural plaques have been demonstrated to be such indicators in epidemiologic studies. This discussion deals with ferruginous bodies as objective evidence of past asbestos exposure, since they are the most useful clinically.

What are ferruginous bodies? These yellow-brown structures are 20–200

Clinical Problems in Asbestos-related Diseases

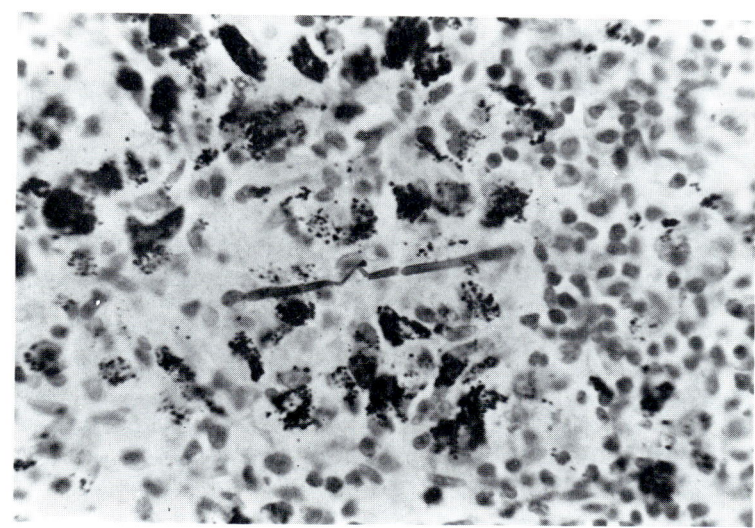

Fig. 1-1. *Ferruginous body in lymph node of a patient with pleural plaques. (Courtesy of Deba Sarma, M.D., New Orleans, Louisiana.)*

μ in length and 2–6 μ in width. Clubbed ends and a segmented appearance are apparent as shown in Figure 1-1. The coating consists of ferritin granules. Originally, it was thought that such bodies were specific for asbestos exposure and represented coated asbestos fibers; thus the term "asbestos bodies" was used to refer to these structures. Recent studies by Gross et al. have demonstrated that other inhaled fibers besides asbestos can produce such bodies (e.g., talc).[17] Thus, it has been proposed that the general term "ferruginous body" be used, rather than asbestos body, unless the central fiber has been identified as asbestos by special research techniques.

The clinician who receives a report that ferruginous bodies (or asbestos bodies) were noted in a specimen of sputum, lung, or other tissue must interpret this finding in light of the history of exposure to asbestos. If such a history is known, the presence of ferruginous bodies supports the history, and identification of the central fiber adds little information. Pooley has shown that ferruginous bodies found in lung tissue of known asbestos workers do have asbestos as the central fiber.[18] If no history of exposure has been obtained, the presence of ferruginous bodies in a patient with a disease resembling an asbestos-related disease should lead to an exhaustive review of the patient's occupational history and possible sources of nonoccupational exposure.

An increased prevalence of individuals with ferruginous bodies in lung tissue have been found in the following groups at autopsy:[19]

Urban dwellers
Males
Older individuals
Heavy manual laborers
Individuals living near docks or industrial areas
Workers in the shipping, electrical, transport, and engineering trades

However, the number seen (1–5 per 6.75 mm^3 of lung tissue) is much lower than the counts seen in patients with asbestosis, where counts of 1000 or more per 6.75 mm^3 can be expected.

Ferruginous bodies (coated fibers) do not make up the majority of fibers found in lung tissue but constitute 10 to 30 percent of fibers found.[1] The other 70 to 90 percent are uncoated and are not demonstrated by light microscopy. Fortunately, a count of ferruginous bodies remains a valid indicator of total fiber count, since the ratio of coated to uncoated fibers tends to be constant. Light microscopy is thus suitable for estimating total fiber counts for clinical purposes.

THE "WORRIED WELL"

As the general public has become more aware of the hazards of asbestos exposure, the clinician has been called upon more frequently to evaluate patients who have been exposed to asbestos but who have minimal or no symptoms. A complete medical history and physical examination with special attention directed toward the cardiorespiratory and gastrointestinal systems should be performed. A chest x-ray, pulmonary function studies of ventilatory capacity (forced expiratory volume at 1.0 second, forced vital capacity), lung volumes (total lung capacity and subdivisions), and pulmonary diffusing capacity (transfer factor, $D_{L_{CO}}$) will be helpful in the evaluation of the lungs. Stool examinations for occult blood and proctosigmoidoscopy should be performed. This evaluation should be sufficient to detect individuals with obvious manifestations of asbestos exposure—pleural plaques, asbestosis, lung cancer, mesothelioma, or gastrointestinal neoplasia.

What signs of early asbestos effect should be sought in individuals with no obvious evidence of disease? This discussion will focus on the early detection of asbestosis. On physical examination, basilar crepitations in two or more locations are the earliest signs. The earliest radiographic findings are small, irregular densities that favor both lung bases; if present in a profusion greater than 1/0 on the ILO U/C classification, the suspicion of early asbestos effect should be high. The presence of small irregular opacities increases with age and cigarette smoking without asbestos exposure,[20] however, so undue emphasis should not be placed on a low-grade profusion as an isolated finding in elderly cigarette smokers.

Various pulmonary function tests have been considered as being the most sensitive indicator of early asbestos effect on the lung. Pulmonary diffusing capacity has been shown in several studies to be abnormal in some asbestos workers before other functional, radiographic, or clinical abnormalities appear and is invariably reduced in advanced asbestosis. On the other hand, other investigators have demonstrated that the earliest adverse changes involve the airways, and they suggest that simple measurements of airway function (FEV_1, FFF_{25-75}) are the most useful guide to monitoring those exposed to asbestos dust.[16,21]

Many factors other than asbestos dust exposure affect both pulmonary diffusing capacity, e.g., infiltrative lung diseases, pulmonary vascular abnormalities, widespread pulmonary emphysema, cigarette smoking, technical problems with measurement in various abnormalities of airway function (e.g., bronchitis or asthma). Therefore, an isolated abnormality on either test in a given individual is not of specific diagnostic value. Caution should be used in interpreting mild reductions in total lung capacity, vital capacity, and FEV_1 (and in $D_{L_{CO}}$ to a lesser extent) in black asbestos workers, since Rossiter and Weill have demonstrated important ethnic differences in the relations of lung function to age and height, with blacks having smaller volumes or maximum flows by about 13 percent.[22] Repeated observations showing progressive decline unexplained by other disease processes, coupled with information concerning dust exposure, enhance the suspicion that these abnormalities are related to asbestos exposure. It is still not clear whether these functional abnormalities invariably lead to asbestosis and whether asbestosis would be prevented if exposure were to cease at this time.

Various authors have compared the value of clinical examination, radiographic studies, and pulmonary function studies in the detection of early asbestos effect on the lung, but in an individual case, any one of these methods may be the first to reveal abnormalities. Therefore, all three should be obtained, with repeated observations at a later date if the significance of detected abnormalities is unclear.

Individuals with no significant history of asbestos exposure and no evidence on pulmonary function studies or chest x-rays of early manifestations of asbestos-related disease should be reassured of this fact, and follow-up is based on their age and the presence of other medical conditions.

For those patients with a history of substantial exposure but without evidence of early asbestos effect, regularly scheduled visits spaced at 1- to 2-year intervals should be instituted. These patients should be reassured that no abnormalities have been found. If the patient is returning to the same work environment in which he was exposed, evaluation of the environment in terms of dust levels and control measures must be made to ensure minimum exposure in the future. Minimum exposure should mean less than two fibers per milliliter.

Individuals with findings on examination, chest x-ray, or pulmonary function studies that are consistent with early asbestos effect should be followed no less frequently than at 1-year intervals, especially if they are still working in the environment that caused their exposure. Evaluation of asbestos fiber levels in the environment must be made to ensure minimal future exposure. If the dust levels are uncontrolled, it may be necessary to recommend that the individual switch to a different job, even though it has not been demonstrated that removal from exposure will be followed by regression of the changes noted. However, if past exposure has been heavy and subsequent institution of dust control measures have reduced the likelihood of significant future exposure before the worker retires, the individual may be allowed to continue employment, since future exposure will contribute a small part of the total dose of fiber.

All workers in an environment where asbestos exposure occurs should be strongly encouraged to discontinue cigarette smoking for several health reasons. The smoking habit makes it more difficult to attribute early pulmonary function abnormalities to asbestos dust exposure. There is increased risk of emphysema or bronchitis, even without asbestos exposure, and the excess risk of developing lung cancer is essentially limited to smokers.

PLEURAL PLAQUES

The typical patient with hyaline pleural plaques as an isolated finding is a middle-aged or older male who presents with an "abnormal" chest x-ray, often detected as an incidental finding on routine examination or on examination for some other complaint. Respiratory symptoms are absent or are referable to coexistent respiratory disease. A history of exposure to asbestos can often be obtained. Although several reports have documented cases in which no asbestos exposure was apparent, the clinician should assume that these plaques are related to previous exposure to asbestos unless an exhaustive search for such exposure is unrevealing or another cause for pleural disease is uncovered. Navratil and Trippe demonstrated in Czechoslovakia that asbestos workers were 16 times more likely to have calcified pleural plaques than members of the general population.[23]

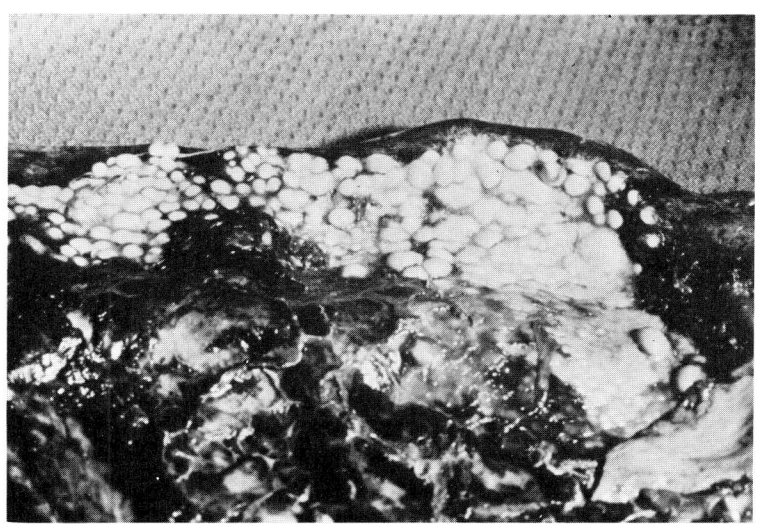

Fig. 1-2. *Gross appearance of pleural plaques at operation. (Courtesy of Deba Sarma, M.D., New Orleans, Louisiana.)*

Physical examination is usually normal; abnormalities detected usually reflect changes due to the presence of asbestos-related diseases, such as asbestosis, pleural effusion, lung cancer, or mesothelioma, or changes due to unrelated respiratory diseases.

The radiographic discription of these hyaline pleural plaques is covered in detail in Chapter 2, Section 1.

Pulmonary function tests can be expected to be normal unless the pleural plaques are extensive and thick. In these cases, mild restrictive abnormalities may be present. Other functional changes are best attributed to the presence of other respiratory diseases.

If the pleural location of the plaques has been established, a history of asbestos exposure has been obtained, and the clinical presentation is not suggestive of neoplasm, there is no pressing need for tissue removal for histological confirmation of the diagnosis. Should biopsy of these lesions be necessary because of an atypical clinical or radiographic picture, the gross and histological appearance will resemble that shown in Figures 1-2 and 1-3.

The main significance of the presence of pleural plaques in a patient with asbestos exposure is that there is an increased risk of developing other manifestations of asbestos-related disease. Fletcher demonstrated an increased incidence of both lung cancer and mesothelioma in 408 shipyard workers with pleural plaques, as opposed to shipyard workers without pleural plaques.[24]

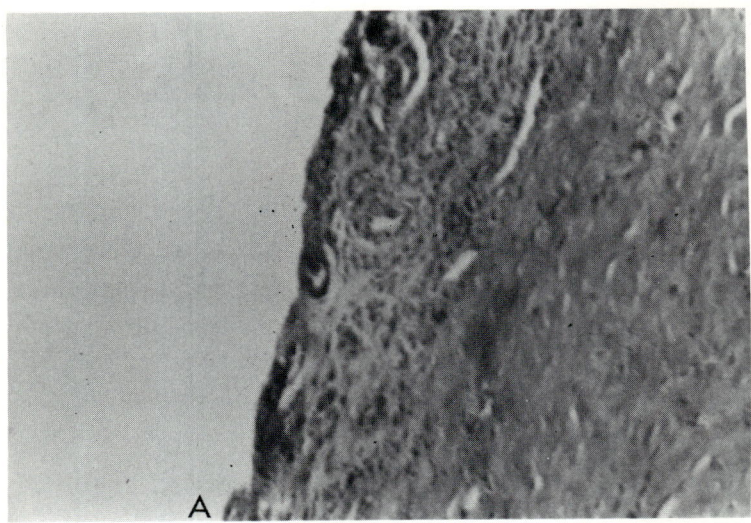

Fig. 1-3. *(A and B) Microscopic appearance of pleural plaque (see facing page). (Courtesy of Deba Sarma, M.D., New Orleans, Louisiana.)*

This is to be expected, since plaques and these neoplasms are both consequences of the same causal factor, asbestos exposure. A discussion with the patient concerning his increased risk of developing malignant disease may have beneficial consequences if it allows the individual to make an informed decision whether to continue working at his current job, if it leads to cessation of cigarette smoking, or if it leads to improved compliance with medical surveillance. The physician must judge whether these potential benefits are likely to occur or whether the result will be undue alarm, however.

A program of medical supervision including examination and chest x-rays should be outlined for the patient. Routine examination of sputum cytology or fiberoptic bronchoscopy in these patients should be considered experimental at present, until such time that specific data demonstrate that early detection resulting in improved survival is achievable through these means.

For the retired individual or one whose present job involves no exposure to asbestos, follow-up is similar to that outlined previously for individuals with significant exposure only. In contrast, the individual who is employed in a work situation where exposure to asbestos will continue should be advised to minimize further dust exposure. This advice should be tempered by the physician's evaluation of the level of past exposure and future exposure. If the past exposure has been extensive, but dust control measures have reduced future exposure to a minimum (the present TLV of two fibers per cubic

Clinical Problems in Asbestos-related Diseases

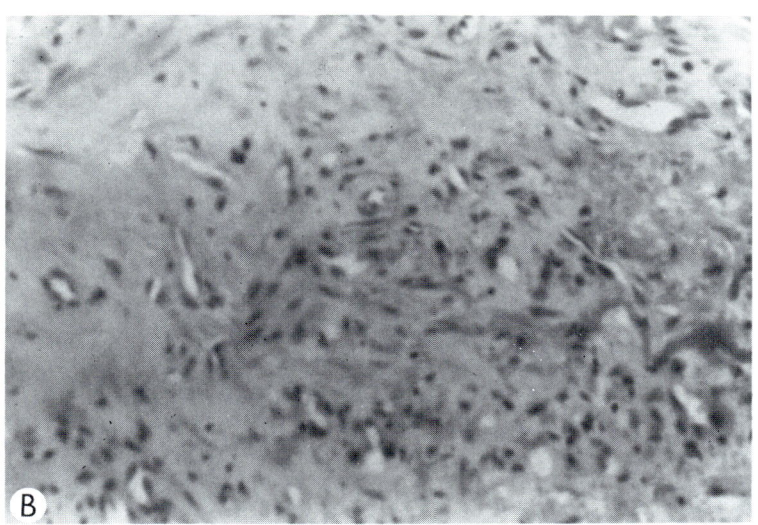

centimeter) or the time until retirement is short, the patient may elect to remain at his present job.

One less frequent variant of benign pleural thickening deserves separate mention because of the clinical confusion it causes. Navratil and Dobias[25] term this group "hyalinosis complicata" as opposed to "hyalinosis simplex" for individuals with pleural plaques as described in the preceding pages. Hyalinosis complicata is rarely seen in individuals with calcified pleural plaques.

Hyalinosis complicata, or exudative pleural rind as described by Mattson,[26] is characterized clinically by chest pain and dyspnea, with subsequent development of restrictive lung disease as the rule rather than the exception. Death is often due to the pleural lesions, either pleuropneumonia or, rarely, mesothelioma.

Histopathologically, the process is an acute exudative inflammatory one, with a coexistent exudative effusion in some cases. An extensive pachypleuritic reaction results, unlike those seen in other posteffusion adhesions. The reaction involves both the visceral and parietal pleura and obliterates the pleural space. It is not clear whether this reaction is specific for asbestos or whether it can occur in individuals without exposure to asbestos.

The differentiation between hyalinosis complicata and mesothelioma is a most difficult one, and individuals with this diagnosis should be followed closely for their lifetime before concluding that mesothelioma is not present.

ASBESTOS PLEURAL EFFUSION

Patients who present with asbestos pleural effusions represent a difficult diagnostic problem because of the lack of attention this manifestation of asbestos exposure has received. A recent report by Gaensler and Kaplan indicates that this effect of asbestos exposure may be more frequent than previously thought.[27]

The presenting complaint is usually pleuritic chest pain associated with a moderate pleural effusion. The effusion may be bilateral and tends to linger but eventually clears spontaneously. Recurrence is common on the same or opposite side. The onset of symptoms is usually insidious or chronic, but acute or subacute onsets are not rare. The duration of exposure has varied from 1 to 38 years, and the effusion may present during exposure or many years after exposure has ceased.

Physical examination usually reveals only signs of effusion, with dullness to percussion and decreased breath sounds, although in some cases with concomitant asbestosis, clubbing and basilar crepitant rales will be noted. There are no diagnostic characteristics to the fluid; it may be sterile and serous or a serosanguineous exudate. Results of cytological studies of the fluid are normal. The chest x-ray reveals the effusion but may also show some combination of asbestosis, hyaline or calcified pleural plaques, or an exudative rind.

Since the fluid has no diagnostic characteristics, the diagnosis must be based on suspicion because of the exposure history and on exclusion of all other causes of persistent pleural effusions such as congestive heart failure, malignancy, infection, connective tissue disorders, and pulmonary infarction. Thoracotomy with pleural and lung biopsy may be necessary to establish the diagnosis; the lung biopsy may reveal ferruginous bodies and/or asbestosis.

In patients in whom a thick exudative pleural rind is present or in whom the fluid recurs repeatedly on the same side, a suspicion of mesothelioma is raised, and such patients should be kept under regular surveillance. Treatment is aimed at symptomatic relief, along with reassurances that more dangerous causes of pleural effusion have not been found.

ASBESTOSIS

Asbestosis refers to the pneumoconiosis caused by inhalation of sufficient asbestos fibers to cause lung scarring and should be restricted to refer to the pathological alterations within the lung and visceral pleura but not the parietal pleura. To the clinician who is unaware of the occupational history, the patient with asbestosis presents as a case of interstitial fibrosis, a disorder with a multitude of causes, both occupational and nonoccupational. Because of the many causes of interstitial fibrosis, knowledge of the history of asbestos exposure is extremely important in raising the possibility of asbestos as the etiologic agent.

The patient with fully developed asbestosis presents with dyspnea, first noticed on exertion and later at rest. Cough, with or without sputum production, is likely to be troublesome with advanced disease. Cigarette smoking is widely accepted as a major cause of chronic bronchitis, but several authors suggest that asbestos dust may also influence the development of bronchitis. Chest pain is infrequent. As the disease progresses, ankle edema and other symptoms of cor pulmonale appear.

On physical examination the classically described findings are dry rales or crepitations in the basilar regions and clubbing. Basilar crepitations are also found in other diseases with diffuse fibrosis, however. The crepitations become more widespread as disease progresses. Rhonchi and wheezing are rarer auscultatory findings. Clubbing is a nonspecific finding, does not reflect the severity of fibrosis, and often is a subjective finding unless objective measurement of the hyponychial angle is obtained. Pedal edema, a right ventricular gallop and heave, and cyanosis appear late in the course.

Typical radiographic findings are no different from other forms of interstitial fibrosis but do favor the bases initially. If associated with pleural plaques, especially calcified pleural plaques, the picture is strongly suggestive of asbestosis.

Pulmonary function findings are those of restrictive lung disease due to interstitial fibrosis, with hypoxemia at rest which worsens with exercise, reduced lung volumes (total lung capacity, vital capacity, and inspiratory capacity), and a normal or slightly increased residual volume. Pulmonary diffusing capacity is reduced. Flow rates (forced expiratory volume at 1 second, FEV_1) are reduced in proportion to the reduction in vital capacity unless airway obstruction is present as well.

Antinuclear factor and rheumatoid factor tests may be positive but should not be interpreted as indicating rheumatoid arthritis or a collagen disease unless other clinical manifestations support these diagnoses. Sputum cytological studies will be positive for ferruginous bodies in approximately one-third of patients if repeated specimens are obtained.

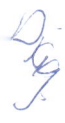

How does one establish the diagnosis of asbestosis? A definite history of exposure, coupled with dyspnea on exertion, basilar crepitations, radiographic changes compatible with interstitial fibrosis and calcified pleural plaques, and a restrictive ventilatory pattern on pulmonary function studies, establishes the diagnosis clinically. If any of these findings are absent, the diagnosis becomes less certain.

When should lung biopsy be undertaken? Lung biopsy is indicated if the exposure history is absent or minimal or if clinical features strongly suggest another diagnosis and the clinical status of the patient permits. At present, open lung biopsy is the preferred method of approach because of the small sample size obtained by transbronchial lung biopsy or transthoracic needle biopsy. The demonstration of interstitial fibrosis is not adequate for the diagnosis; ferruginous bodies should be identified to provide objective evidence that exposure was heavy. If no coated asbestos fibers are found, electron-microscopic studies are indicated to look for uncoated fibers.

Transbronchial lung biopsy via a fiberoptic bronchoscope, with examination of millipore-filtered tissue digestate for ferruginous bodies, has recently been described to give a high yield.[28] The series is too small to determine if this method will become a useful approach. If the findings are confirmed by a larger series with adequate controls and can differentiate between significant exposure and exposure described for urban dwellers, transbronchial lung biopsy would allow sampling of tissue in a less invasive fashion.

Other causes of interstitial fibrosis must be considered, since they can occur in individuals who have been exposed to asbestos. Of the collagen diseases, rheumatoid arthritis, scleroderma, and dermatomyositis are the most likely to have associated pulmonary fibrosis; less frequently, systemic lupus erythematosus is accompanied by diffuse lung involvement. Evidence of multisystem involvement with arthritis, esophageal dysfunction, sclerodactaly, or renal or cardiac dysfunction is not characteristic of asbestosis and suggests the presence of one of these diseases.

Sarcoidosis is another cause of interstitial fibrosis. The presence of granulomatous uveitis, hilar or generalized lymphadenopathy, granulomatous hepatitis, splenomegaly, hypercalcemia or hypercalcuria, central nervous system involvement, or erythema nodosum supports the diagnosis clinically. Lung biopsy early in the course frequently reveals noncaseating granulomas which are consistent with the diagnosis, although they are not diagnostic. In later stages of the disease, interstitial fibrosis without granulomas may be seen on lung biopsy, and the diagnosis is not obvious. Ferruginous bodies or uncoated asbestos fibers are absent or rare. Chronic beryllium disease can present a similar picture but is rarely encountered at present.

Patients with idiopathic diffuse interstitial fibrosis tend to have a more rapidly progressive course than those with asbestosis, but this is not invariable. Lung biopsy will reveal interstitial fibrosis, and the absence or rare occurrence of ferruginous bodies or uncoated asbestos fibers make asbestosis an unlikely diagnosis.

Lipid pneumonia with subsequent fibrosis favors the lower lobes. The history of chronic use of oily nose drops or mineral oil is often obtained if sought. Chronic gastrointestinal regurgitation associated with esophageal dysfunction, hiatal hernia, or neurological disorders can also cause chronic lower lobe pneumonitis and later fibrosis.

Other major mineral dust diseases of the lung—silicosis and coal workers' pneumoconiosis—will generally not be confused with asbestosis because they produce discrete nodules in the early stages and large coalescent masses in those cases where progressive massive fibrosis occurs.

Effective management of asbestosis requires the prevention of excessive exposure before disease occurs. For hypoxemic patients, attempts are made to improve oxygenation with home and portable oxygen. Prompt treatment of bacterial pulmonary infections is mandatory, and influenza vaccination prophylactically is indicated. Further exposure to silica or asbestos dust must be avoided. Cigarette smoking should be strongly discouraged. Any suggestion of neoplasm—hemoptysis, weight loss, or vague chest pains—should be investigated promptly, since death in recent series is more often related to cancer than to respiratory failure. Finally, the patient should be informed of the causal relationship between asbestos exposure and his disease.

LUNG CANCER

Presenting symptoms and signs of lung cancer in individuals exposed to asbestos are no different than those without exposure. The clinical picture is determined by the location of the tumor, the extent and location of metastases, and the presence of syndromes associated with bronchogenic cancer (superior vena cava syndrome, myopathy, neuropathy, ectopic hormone production, and polymyositis). A detailed description is beyond the scope of this chapter.

Evaluation of the patient follows the same pattern for any lung cancer—with the main objective being to obtain histological confirmation of the tumor by the least invasive means possible and to determine if the tumor is resectable. Preoperative evaluation to exclude coexistent asbestosis is important, since markedly reduced lung function may preclude surgery or even radiotherapy.

It is impossible to attribute the carcinoma to asbestos exposure in most cases, since the great majority of tumors occur in cigarette smokers.

PLEURAL MESOTHELIOMA

The most common presenting complaint in patients with pleural mesothelioma is chest or shoulder pain, which is found in 70 to 90 percent of cases and is vague in nature initially, with sharper pain as the tumor invades the chest wall. The pain tends to be less sharply pleuritic in nature than the chest pain associated with viral pleurisy, having an insidious onset and slow progression. The pain is not aggravated by breathing and chest wall motion but tends to be constant and eventually is severe enough to interfere with sleep and to require narcotic medication. Dyspnea is also a common presenting complaint and is related to the rapid accumulation of a massive pleural effusion. Dry cough is frequent. Constitutional symptoms such as weight loss, weakness, and fever are less frequent chief complaints but commonly accompany the presenting complaints as the tumor progresses.

A history of asbestos exposure, when present, heightens the suspicion of mesothelioma, but has been found in 15 to 90 percent of cases in various studies. Becklake reviewed ten studies with control subjects and noted a similar range of positive histories.[1] If the results of these ten controlled studies are summated, 52 percent of 829 mesothelioma cases had either a history of asbestos exposure or the presence of coated or uncoated fibers, as compared to 18 percent of 777 control subjects. Studies conducted in Canada and Italy, where chrysotile asbestos is the predominant variety mined and used, revealed the lowest percentage of positive work histories (26 percent and 18 percent respectively), with all other series ranging from 48 to 95 percent. Elmes and Simpson reviewed 327 cases, the largest series analyzed to date.[29] Of 277 cases where occupational histories had been taken, only 13 had no history of exposure and another 24 cases had probable exposure.

On the physical examination, dullness to percussion, decreased breath sounds, and other signs referable to pleural effusion are found in 80 to 90 percent of cases. Occasionally, basilar crepitations of associated asbestosis will be heard; clubbing in infrequent (9.5 percent in Elmes and Simpson's series.)

Erythrocyte sedimentation rates are generally increased, but this finding is nonspecific.

Pleural fluid or pleural thickening or both are invariably present on chest x-ray. The effusions tend to be massive and persistent. In a few cases, lower lung zone fibrosis compatible with asbestosis may be seen. More radiographic details are given in Chapter 2, Section 3.

Pulmonary function tests most commonly show restrictive lung disease, with low values for total lung capacity and vital capacity. These alterations may be due either to the thick pleural tumor or to associated asbestosis. When asbestosis is present, the transfer factor ($D_{L_{co}}$) is often reduced as well.

How does one establish the diagnosis of mesothelioma? Churg and coworkers[30] list the following criteria: (1) no primary tumor capable of serosal spread is present; (2) the tumor tends toward superficial growth along serosal planes with only shallow invasion; (3) metastases occur only to regional lymph nodes; and (4) the histological picture is one of epithelial-type cells (tubular, papillary, tubulopapillary, sheets, nests), or mesenchymal-type cells (sarcomatous), or mixed. Variable degrees of anaplasia are present. Histochemical stains (PAS-D, mucicarmine, and colloidal iron after hyaluronidase digestion) may aid in the diagnosis when epithelial-type cells predominate and resemble carcinoma.

Hasan et al. demonstrated the need for strict adherence to these criteria by reviewing cases diagnosed as mesothelioma over a 28-year period.[2] The diagnosis was confirmed in 8 of 9 patients with a history of asbestos exposure but was equivocal or excluded in 9 of 13 cases without history of exposure. Six of the equivocal or excluded cases were women. Thus the diagnosis of mesothelioma in women without a history of exposure should be accepted only if all criteria are fulfilled.

Using these criteria, it becomes apparent that a definitive diagnosis of mesothelioma rests heavily on postmortem findings to establish with certainty the absence of another primary tumor and the extent of direct invasion and metastatic spread. In addition, adequate tissue must be obtained to demonstrate the characteristic histological pattern. Churg recommends that any diagnosis made during life be considered "probable" mesothelioma.

The pleural fluid is an exudate and is often bloodstained or frankly bloody, but this is not invariable. In 50 percent or more of cases, the fluid is serous. In Elmes and Simpson's series, fluid could not be obtained in 23 percent.

The clinical picture described above is by no means pathognomic for mesothelioma; metastatic pleural deposits are much more frequent causes of a similar picture. Lung and breast carcinoma are frequent primary sources of tumor, along with ovarian and pancreatic carcinoma. Less frequently, adenocarcinomas from other body organs can spread to the pleural surface. Other causes of bloody pleural fluid, such as pulmonary infarction and post-pneumonic effusion, can usually be distinguished by the lack of significant pleural thickening, a different clinical presentation, and a strong tendency to show resolution with appropriate therapy and the passage of time. The differentiation between mesothelioma and benign exudative pleural thickening is much more difficult and may not be settled until postmortem examination. Tuberculous effusions can present a similar clinical picture.

How does one approach the diagnosis during life? Unfortunately, the standard approach of aspiration, fluid analysis and cytological studies, and needle biopsy of the pleura tends to be unrewarding. The pleural fluid findings are nonspecific. Several authors have emphasized the value of hyaluronic acid measurements on the fluid, but this test is not generally available and is not an adequate substitute for confirmation of the diagnosis by tissue sampling. Cytological studies on pleural fluid may identify malignant cells, but frequently the origin of these cells is uncertain or no malignant cells are found.

Usually the clinician must rely on pleural biopsy, either by needle, thorascopy, or thoracotomy. The latter procedure obviously will provide the largest amount of tissue for the pathologist and give the best opportunity for diagnosis, but it is not always the procedure of choice because of the distressing tendency of the mesothelioma to extend through the chest wall, following the track left by a needle or surgical procedure. Tumor spread appears to be more frequent after needle biopsy of the pleura than after simple aspiration with a small needle. Because of the diffuse nature of the tumor, pleural biopsy by needle should probably be attempted first. If adequate tissue for diagnosis is not obtained, consideration should be given to thorascopy or thoracotomy, depending on the preference of the surgeon involved. The physician must keep in mind that firmly establishing the diagnosis as mesothelioma will not lead to an effective program of treatment and that the discovery of metastatic carcinoma may allow chemotherapy to be given, but life expectancy is still short. Elmes and Simpson reviewed various attempts at therapy, including surgical excision, fluid aspiration only, local chemotherapy, systemic chemotherapy, and radiotherapy.[29] None of the programs were beneficial in terms of prolonging life, although pleurectomy resulted in less fluid accumulation and less need for repeated aspiration. However, the major drawback to more aggressive therapy is the observation that chemotherapy, radiotherapy, and surgery appear to be followed by the occurrence of widespread metastases and local extension through the chest wall in more than a few cases. DeLajartre reported on 31 operated cases but was only able to achieve total pleurectomy in one-fifth of the cases.[31]

Our approach to therapy, once the diagnosis is reasonably well established clinically, is to take a conservative approach, with pleural fluid aspiration as needed for symptomatic relief. This can mean frequent aspiration at first, but generally a decrease in the amount of fluid produced occurs.

Life expectancy averages about 1 year, with occasional patients living several years.

PERITONEAL MESOTHELIOMA

The early manifestations of mesothelioma of the peritoneal cavity are vague abdominal discomfort, loss of appetite, and constipation. Symptoms of intestinal obstruction tend to occur later but may be the presenting complaint if the patient delays seeking medical attention. Physical examination in the early stages of disease is unrevealing in many cases. As time passes, the presence of an abdominal mass and ascites become apparent. In contrast to cases of pleural mesothelioma, where the rapid accumulation of pleural fluid causes progressive dyspnea and obvious physical findings, patients with peritoneal mesothelioma may have no striking historical or physical findings.

Because the ascites does not often reach the massive proportions seen in more common diseases such as cirrhosis of the liver, aspiration of fluid is seldom attempted. Upper gastrointestinal tract series or barium enema may show a mass displacing gastrointestinal structures, without the constricting lesions seen in large or small bowel malignancies. Diagnosis is usually made by abdominal exploration, but even at surgery or subsequent autopsy the correct diagnosis is elusive. Peritoneoscopy is one method of sampling the fluid and visualizing the tumor in the least invasive fashion possible if mesothelioma is suspected. However, Elmes and Simpson found that only 6 of 37 cases were diagnosed before death, even after laporotomy.[29] The disease progresses more rapidly than does pleural mesothelioma, and death due to intestinal obstruction is common. No effective therapy is available, so treatment is supportive.

GASTROINTESTINAL CANCER

Carcinoma of the stomach and colon caused by asbestos exposure is identical to that not associated with asbestos exposure in terms of presenting symptoms and signs. The same diagnostic approach is employed. Careful preoperative pulmonary evaluation is necessary if surgery is contemplated because of the possibility of coexistent asbestosis. Pleural effusions in such patients should not be assumed to be due to metastatic carcinoma without attempts at histological confirmation by pleural fluid cell studies and pleural biopsy, since pleural effusions occur with asbestos exposure as well. This is most important if the pleura is the only apparent site of metastases.

IMMUNOLOGIC FINDINGS IN ASBESTOS WORKERS

Several observations in asbestos-exposed individuals remain unexplained. First, although the dose–response relationship described earlier applies to the development of mild-to-moderate fibrosis, this relationship is not apparent for progression from moderate-to-severe fibrosis. Second, asbestosis may present long after exposure has ceased and, likewise, may show progression after exposure has ceased. Third, if two workers are exposed to the same dose of asbestos, one may develop disease, while the other does not.

Ashcroft and Heppleston have suggested that nonspecific inflammatory processes may be the explanation for progression of disease.[32] One can speculate that the depression of viral interferon induction by asbestos fibers, demonstrated in vitro by Hahon and Eckert,[33] could cause slower recovery from viral infections. It is generally believed that interferon plays a nonimmunologic role in recovery from acute primary viral infections. Thus, persistent viral infections could be the cause of the nonspecific inflammation postulated by Ashcroft and Heppleston.[32]

In contrast, Turner-Warwick has suggested that host responses, mediated by antinuclear antibodies, act as self-perpetuating accelerators of fibrosis initiated by the asbestos fibers.[34] This hypothesis is based on observations by Pernis[35] that asbestos workers, especially those with abnormal chest roentgenograms, had an increased incidence of circulating rheumatoid factor and by Turner-Warwick and Parkes[36] that asbestos workers had a fourfold increase in the prevalence of antinuclear antibodies and rheumatoid factor. Turner-Warwick and Haslam found no increased incidence of lung-reactive autoantibodies.[37] Edge was unable to demonstrate an increased incidence of antinuclear antibodies and rheumatoid factor in 160 workers with pleural plaques,[38] but his group did not include workers with evidence of asbestosis. Toivanen also showed no increased incidence of positive ANA or rheumatoid factor tests in 66 Finnish asbestos workers,[39] but his group had exposure only to anthophyllite, and none of the workers had asbestosis. He concluded that the positive serological tests are the result of the asbestosis, not the cause.

Merchant and co-workers noted an increased incidence of HL-A-W27 antigen in 56 asbestos workers with known or suspected asbestosis.[40] The presence of W27 antigen seemed to correlate with more severe radiographic abnormalities. Since the W27 antigen has been linked with diseases such as ankylosing spondylitis, Reiter's syndrome, and acute anterior uveitis, which have immunological abnormalities, and since some immune response genes are believed to be closely linked to the HL-A system, the authors suggested that the presence of W27 might serve as a marker for individuals with increased susceptibility to tissue damage from asbestos.

Evans et al. were unable to confirm the finding of an increased incidence of HL-A-W27 antigen in a group of 37 patients with asbestosis or in a group of 37 patients with asbestos exposure when compared to a control group.[41] Subjects who were positive for HL-A-B12 tended to have advanced radiographic fibrosis, however. In addition, asbestos workers without pulmonary fibrosis had an unexpectedly high frequency of HL-A-BW5, suggesting that the presence of this antigen might protect against the development of pulmonary fibrosis.

Badr and El-Sewefy[42] demonstrated an association between asbestosis and individuals with blood group O, but this was not confirmed by Merchant et al.[40] The immunoelectrophoretic pattern from sera of 33 asbestos workers with unspecified signs of asbestos was studied by El-Sewefy and Hassan.[43] Decreases in the prealbumin and albumin fractions were noted, along with an increase in the glycoprotein, lipoprotein, transferrin, and IgG, IgM, and IgA fractions. These changes are not specific for asbestosis, since similar changes have been described in cases of silicosis, and are not related to the degree of fibrosis present.

In a study of blood lymphocytes in patients with pulmonary asbestosis, Kang and co-workers noted a decrease in the percentage of T cells present and a decrease in lymphocyte response to phytohemagglutinin in vitro.[44] The magnitude of these decreases paralleled the severity of the disease. Lymphocyte transformation studies appeared to be more sensitive than the T-cell to total lymphocytes ratio or skin tests. Only 7 cases were studied, however, and 4 had associated lung cancer or tuberculosis.

Kagan and co-workers have confirmed Kang's results in a larger series of patients with radiographic evidence of asbestosis.[45,46] In addition, a disproportionate number of patients demonstrated cutaneous anergy to recall antigens (streptokinase-streptodornase and *Candida albicans* allergenic extract but not tuberculin-purified protein derivative) and to 2, 4-dinitrochlorobenzene. Phytohemagglutinin-induced proliferative and cytotoxic assays provided in vitro evidence of impaired cellular immunity in the patient group. Several patients also had serum inhibitors of PHA-induced lymphocyte transformation. Studies of humoral immunity revealed significant elevation of salivary secretory IgA and serum IgA, IgG, IgM, and IgE, and frequent occurrence of non-organ-specific autoantibodies and cold-reactive lymphocytotoxins in the patient group. The authors concluded that an imbalance between cellular and humoral components of the immune response exists and suggested that this may play a role in the development of malignant diseases in patients with asbestosis.

The exact relationship between these findings and the development of pulmonary fibrosis or neoplasia is not clear. The major finding of clinical relevance is that a positive antinuclear antibody or rheumatoid factor test occurs frequently in a patient with asbestosis. Thus, undue emphasis should not be placed on these tests as signs of an underlying collagen disorder in the patient with asbestos exposure and interstitial fibrosis if other clinical manifestations of a collagen disease are lacking. At present, no study has identified individuals who should be excluded from work in the asbestos industry because of increased individual susceptibility to the effects of asbestos inhalation. Individuals with significant respiratory impairment from any cause, however, probably should be discouraged from seeking employment where significant exposure may result.

REFERENCES

1. Becklake MR: Asbestos-related diseases of the lung and other organs: Their epidemiology and implications for clinical practice. Am Rev Respir Dis 114:187–227, 1976
2. Hasan FM, Nash G, Kazemi H: The significance of asbestos exposure in the diagnosis of mesothelioma: A 28-year experience from a major urban hospital. Am Rev Respir Dis 115:761–768, 1977
3. Milne JEH: Thirty-two cases of mesothelioma in Victoria, Australia: A retrospective survey related to occupational asbestos exposure. Br J Ind Med 33:115–122, 1976
4. Zielhuis RL, Versteeg JPJ, Planteijdt HT: Pleural mesothelioma and exposure to asbestos: A retrospective case-control study in the Netherlands. Int Arch Occup Environ Health 36:1–18, 1975
5. Schutz LA, Bank W, Weems G: Airborne Asbestos Fiber Concentrations in Asbestos Mines and Mills in the United States. Technical Progress Report 72, US Department of Interior, June 1973
6. Anderson HA, Lilis R, Daum SM, et al: Household-contact asbestos neoplastic risk. Ann NY Acad Sci 271:311–323, 1976
7. Newhouse ML, Thompson H: Mesothelioma of pleura and peritoneum following exposure to asbestos in the London area. Br J Ind Med 22:261–269, 1965
8. Yazicioglu S: Pleural calcification associated with exposure to chrysotile asbestos in southeast Turkey. Chest 70:43–47, 1976
9. Selikoff IJ, Nicholson WJ, Langer AM: Asbestos air pollution. Arch Environ Health 25:1–13, 1972
10. Holt PF, Young DK: Asbestos fibres in the air of towns. Atmos Environ 7:481–483, 1973
11. Report of the Advisory Committee on Asbestos Cancers to the Director of the International Agency for Research on Cancer, in Bogoviski P, Gilson JC, Timbrell V, Wagner JC (eds): Biological Effects of Asbestos. Lyon, IARC Scientific Publications, No. 8, 1973, pp 341–346
12. Enterline PE, Henderson V: Type of asbestos and respiratory cancer in the asbestos industry. Arch Environ Health 27:312–317, 1973
13. Gilson JC: Asbestos cancer. Past and future hazards. Proc R Soc Med 66:395–403, 1973
14. Meurman LO, Kiviluoto R, Hakama M: Morbidity and mortality among the working population of anthophyllite asbestos miners in Finland. Br J Ind Med 31:105–112, 1974
15. Weill H, Rossiter CE, Waggenspack C, et al: Differences in lung effects

resulting from chrysotile and crocidolite exposure, in Walton WH (ed): Inhaled Particles IV. Oxford and New York, Pergamon Press, 1977 pp 789–798

16. Weill H, Ziskind MM, Waggenspack C, et al: Lung function consequences of dust exposure in asbestos cement manufacturing plants. Arch Environ Health 30:88–97, 1975
17. Gross P, deTreville RTP, Cralley LJ, et al: Pulmonary ferruginous bodies: Development in response to filamentous dust and methods of isolation and concentration. Arch Pathol 85:539–546, 1968
18. Pooley FD: Asbestos bodies, their formation, composition and character. Environ Res 5:363–379, 1972
19. Doniach I, Swettenham KV, Hathorn MKS: Prevalence of asbestos bodies in a necropsy series in East London: Association with disease, occupation, and domiciliary address. Br J Ind Med 32:16–30, 1975
20. Weiss W: Cigarette smoking and diffuse pulmonary fibrosis. Arch Environ Health 14:564–568, 1967
21. Becklake MR, Fournier-Massey G, Rossiter CE, et al: Lung function in chrysotile asbestos mine and mill workers in Quebec. Arch Environ Health 24:401–409, 1972
22. Rossiter CE, Weill H: Ethnic differences in lung function: Evidence for proportional differences. Int J Epidemiol 3:55–61, 1974
23. Navratil M, Trippe F: Prevalence of pleural calcification in persons exposed to asbestos dust, and in the general population in the same district. Environ Res 5:210–216, 1972
24. Fletcher DE: A mortality study of shipyard workers with pleural plaques. Br J Ind Med 29:142–155, 1972
25. Navratil M, Dobias J: Development of pleural hyalinosis in long term studies of persons exposed to asbestos dust. Environ Res 6:455–472, 1973
26. Mattson SB: Pleura-plaques and exposure to asbestos dust, in Studia Laboris et Salutis, Report No. 10, 1971, pp. 131–152
27. Gaensler EA, Kaplan AI: Asbestos pleural effusion. Ann Intern Med 74:178–191, 1971
28. Kane, PB, Goldman SL, Pillai BH, et al: Diagnosis of asbestosis by transbronchial biopsy: A method to facilitate demonstration of ferruginous bodies. Am Rev Respir Dis 115:689–694, 1977
29. Elmes PC, Simpson MJC: The clinical aspects of mesothelioma. Q J Med 179(45):427–449, 1976
30. Churg J, Rosen SH, Moolten S: Histological characteristics of mesothelioma associated with asbestos. Ann NY Acad Sci 132:614–622, 1965

31. DeLajartre M, DeLajartre AY, Michaud JL, et al: Diffuse pleural mesotheliomas: Preliminary study of 31 operated cases (French). Rev Fr Mal Respir 1 (5-6):697–710, 1973
32. Ashcroft T, Heppelston AG: The optical and electron microscopic determination of pulmonary asbestos fiber concentration and its relationship to human pathological reaction. J Clin Pathol 26:224–234, 1973
33. Hahon N, Eckert HL: Depression of viral interferon induction in cell monolayers by asbestos fibers. Environ Res 11:52–65, 1976
34. Turner-Warwick M: Immunological mechanisms in occupational disorders. Proc R Soc Med 66:927–930, 1973
35. Pernis B, Vigliani EC, Selikoff IJ: Rheumatoid factor in serum of individuals exposed to asbestos. Ann NY Acad Sci 132:112–120, 1965
36. Turner-Warwick M, Parkes WR: Circulating rheumatoid and antinuclear factors in asbestos workers. Br Med J 3:492–495, 1970
37. Turner-Warwick M, Haslam P: Antibodies in some chronic fibrosing lung diseases. Clin Allergy 1:83–95, 1971
38. Edge JR: Asbestos related diseases in Barrow-in-Furness. Environ Res 11:244–247, 1976
39. Toivanen A, Salmivalli M, Molnar G: Pulmonary asbestosis and autoimmunity. Br Med J 1:691–692, 1976
40. Merchant JA, Klouda PT, Soutar CA, et al: The HL-A system in asbestos workers. Br Med J 1:189–191, 1975
41. Evans CC, Lewinsohn HC, Evans JM: Frequency of HL-A antigens in asbestos workers with and without pulmonary fibrosis. Br Med J 1:603–605, 1977
42. Badr FM, El-Sewefy AZ: The association between asbestosis and ABO blood groups. Ann Occup Hyg 14:35–40, 1971
43. El-Sewefy AZ, Hassan F: Immunoelectrophoretic pattern changes in asbestosis. Ann Occup Hyg 14:25–28, 1971
44. Kang KY, Sera Y, Okochi T, et al: T. lymphocytes in asbestosis. N Engl J Med 291:735–736, 1974
45. Kagan E, Solomon A, Cochrane JC, et al: Immunological studies of patients with asbestosis. I. Studies of cell-mediated immunity. Clin Exp Immunol 28:261–267, 1977
46. Kagan E, Solomon A, Cochrane JC, et al: Immunologic studies in patients with asbestosis. II. Studies of circulating lymphoid cell numbers and humoral immunity. Clin Exp Immunol 28: 268–275, 1977

2
ORGAN INVOLVEMENT IN ASBESTOS-RELATED DISEASE: SECTION 1 PLEURAL PLAQUES

Leslie Preger

Plaques of the parietal pleura are associated with exposure to all types of asbestos fibers. The plaques are probably not harmful in themselves but are an objective sign of prior exposure. Their number usually increases with dose and elapsed time after exposure and so are more common in older patients; but there is no definite relation with total dust exposure.[1] A certain minimal exposure will ensure development of radiographically identifiable plaques, usually after an interval of more than 20 years; in some patients, plaques may appear after a shorter interval, this usually but not invariably implies a heavier exposure.

LOCATION

The parietal pleural plaques are multiple and lie against rigid areas such as the inner surface of the lower ribs, costovertebral angles, and central tendinous portion of the diaphragm. They may, if large, extend into the intercostal space and even penetrate the diaphragm by direct extension into the abdomen (see

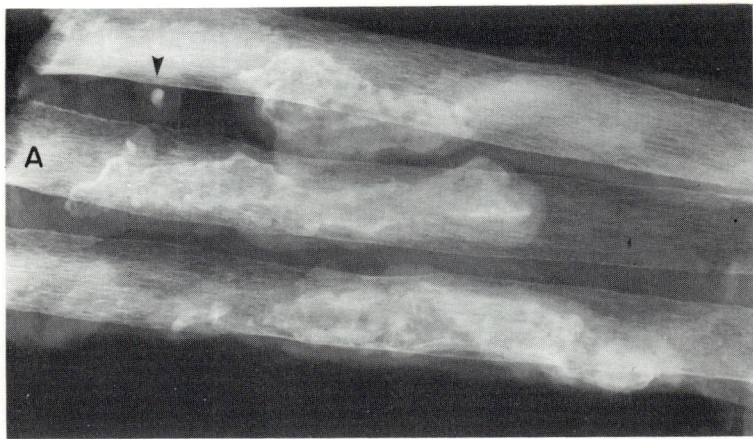

Fig. 2-1. *Autopsy specimen of rib. X-rayed in two planes (A and B). The plaques originate against the inner surface of the rib and extend with growth onto intercostal muscle. (B) Calcification is present in parts of pleura lying against inner surface of rib and in the intercostal spaces. The ease with which plaques may be stripped from ribs, despite their consistency akin to that of cartilage, is seen in B.*

Fig. 2-1). Sometimes they are seen posterior to the upper sternum, arising in the mediastinal pleura reflected over the aorta. The mediastinal pleura along the cardiac border is another less common site. In the case of the parietal pleura adjacent the aorta and left ventricle, both these segments may be construed as being against rigid areas, analogous to the locations near ribs and the tendinous portion of the diaphragm. Involvement of diaphragmatic and mediastinal pleura is usually a late event and not seen in absence of peripheral plaques. The plaques do not develop adjacent to the costal cartilages or against the ribs in the costophrenic angles or apical areas. Distribution is bilateral; occasionally the left side is slightly more involved, and the posterolateral aspects are nearly always the most involved.

GROSS APPEARANCE

The plaques are raised and are gray or yellowish-white. The surface may be flat or uneven, with a mammillated appearance. The edges may be abrupt, overhanging, or gently sloping. Their consistency is very hard, quite surprising to a radiologist accustomed to seeing them as "soft tissue" shadows on an x-ray. The thickness varies up to 1 cm. Their size and shape is variable, from tiny spots to many square centimeters, covering up four or five ribs and their

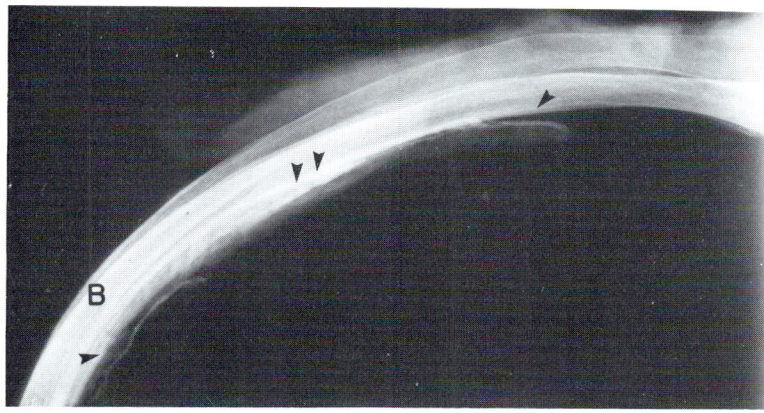

intercostal spaces. Their shapes may be punctate, oval, or irregular. When involvement has extended over an intercostal space, the earlier formed part lying against a rib is usually thicker than that over the intercostal space. They strip easily from the chest wall, as seen in Figure 2-1B.

MICROSCOPIC APPEARANCE

The plaques are extramesothelial structures in that they develop in connective tissue external to the mesothelial cells which usually remain as a surface covering for the plaque.[2] They are not associated with adhesions, but occasionally fibrinlike material may overlie the mesothelial cells.[1] The substance of the plaque consists of wavy interweaving bands of collagen fibers that lie parallel to the plaque surface. In early lesions, in their deeper growing part, there are some vessels and plump, nucleated fibroblasts and occasionally a slight infiltrate of lymphocytes and plasma cells. Older lesions are avascular, the fibrocytic nuclei are few, and the inflammatory cells are absent. The covering mesothelial cells may be difficult to identify. Since growth occurs from the deeper part of the plaque, it is there that the lesion is much more vascular and has nucleated fibroblasts and a cellular infiltrate.

Calcification

Calcified pleural plaques contain more asbestos fibers than noncalcified plaques, and the fibers are more numerous in the calcified zone than in the fibrous zone of these plaques[3] (see Fig. 2-2). Whether this is a causal factor is

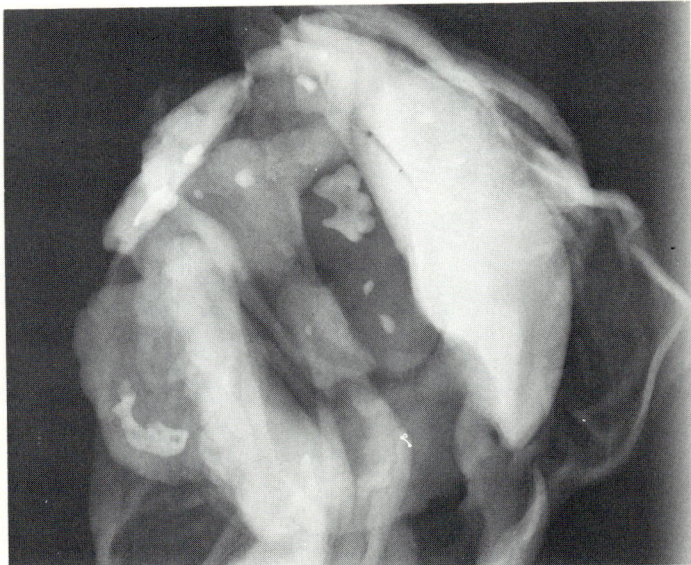

Fig. 2-2. *X-ray of excised portion of diaphragm to show calcified and noncalcified plaques of various shapes.*

not known. The incidence of calcification varies from area to area and may be caused by any type of asbestos fiber. Kiviluoto[4] found about a 40 percent incidence in persons working in or living near Finnish anthophyllite mines (see Fig. 2-3). Rom[5] found no pleural plaques, calcified or noncalcified, in a review of three independent radiological surveys of miners and their families in a Rhodesian asbestos-mining town. The older plaques may show dystrophic calcification in the more avascular central parts, and this is more common in older patients. Calcium deposits occur as fine granules that may coalesce into various shapes.[6] (see Fig. 2-4).

The calcified zone is in the central or deeper zone of the plaques, with a thick layer of noncalcified fibrohyaline tissue lying between it and the mesothelium. The calcium crystals, mainly acicular apatite crystals but with some whitlockite nodules, are aligned along the length of the collagen fibers. Chemical analysis shows that the phosphorous/calcium ratio in the calcified zones differs from natural calcium phosphates of the apatite or whitlockite type. Microscopic calcifications, however, which can be detected in the fibrous zone and which appear uncalcified on gross examination, have similar calcium/phosphorous ratios to naturally occurring apatite and whitlockite.

The amount of calcification is not related to the thickness of a plaque.[8] Diaphragmatic plaques in particular, but also those in the subaxillae, may

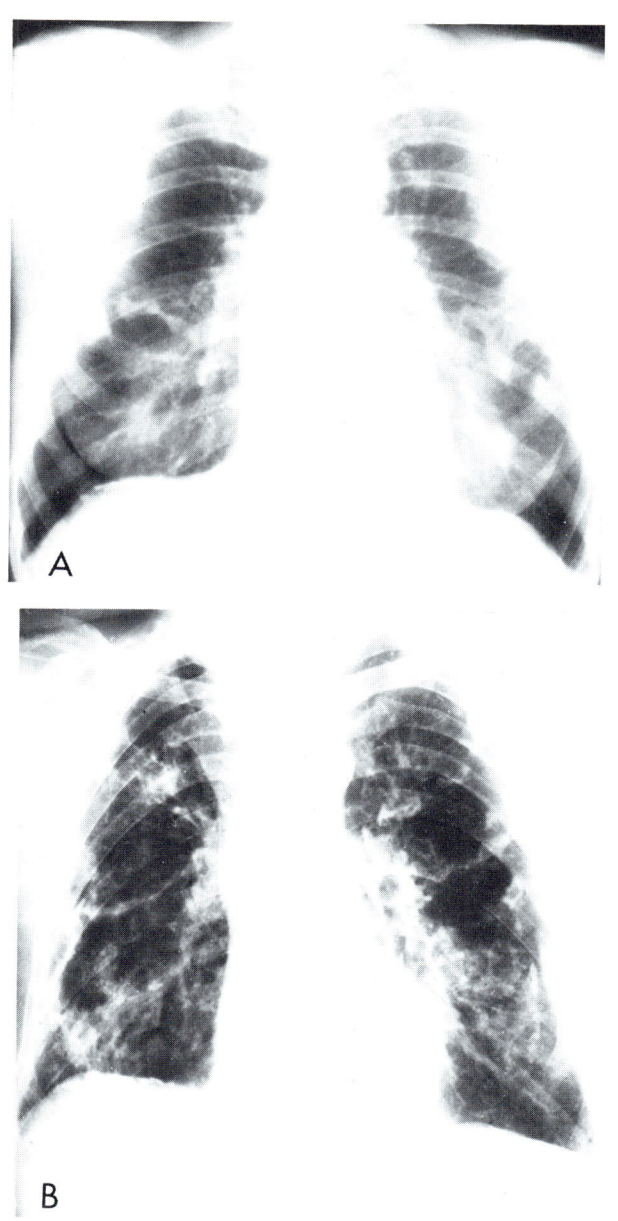

Fig. 2-3. *A. Environmental asbestos plaques. A woman living in the neighborhood of Finnish anthophyllite mines who has peripheral pleural plaques and diaphragmatic calcified plaques. There was no occupational exposure. (Courtesy of Prof. R. Kiviluoto.) B. Environmental exposure. Calcified geographical plaques and diaphragmatic calcification in a patient living near Finnish anthophyllite mines but who was not occupationally exposed. (Courtesy of Prof. R. Kiviluoto.)*

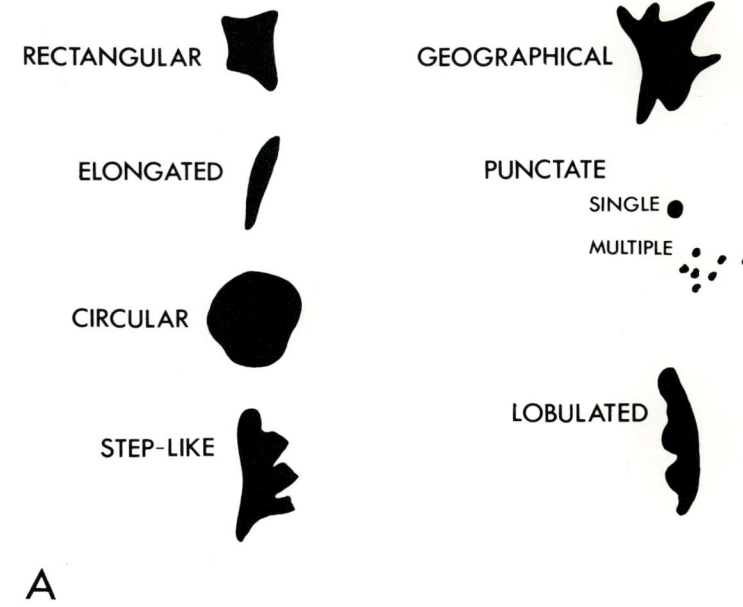

Fig. 2-4. *(A and B) Diagrammatic representation of plaque shapes (see facing page).*

attain large size and remain uncalcified (see Fig. 2-5). Calcification in diaphragmatic plaques is usually only linear in shape.

PRESENCE OF ASBESTOS PARTICLES IN PLEURAL PLAQUES

Earlier reports[8] did not reveal ferruginous bodies (coated asbestos fibers) in plaques. Later reports using ashed tissues[3,9] and electron diffraction techniques have demonstrated chrysotile fibers of very small size, length 0.1–2.0 μm and diameter 25–30 nm. They are only apparent when calcium deposits and collagen fibers have been removed by chemical techniques, the fibers being present 5 to 12 times more frequently in the calcified portion that in the fibrotic portion. Thus, asbestos may be difficult to detect in noncalcified fibrohyaline plaques, and such plaques, although commonly associated with asbestos exposure, are not specific to such exposure in that occasional plaques may be found at autopsies in which sophisticated techniques have not demonstrated

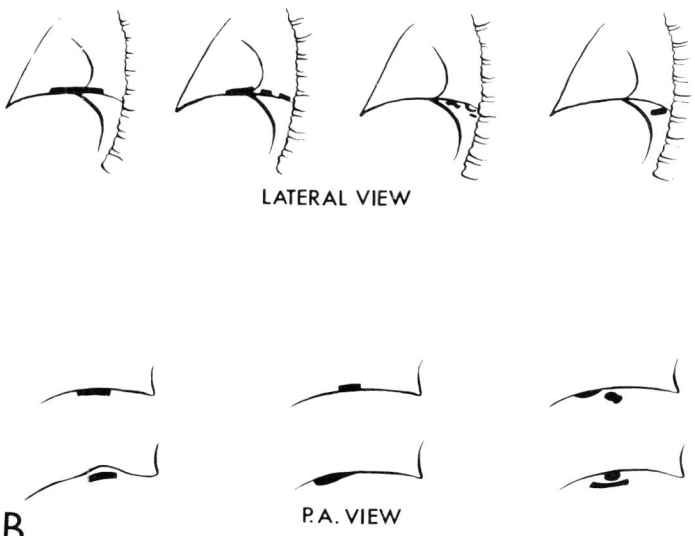

an asbestos fiber content and there is no known occupational environmental or leisure exposure.

PATHOGENESIS

The pathogenesis is unknown. Thomson[2] suggests that in an active patient with healthy lungs, inhaled asbestos fibers may move through lung parenchyma, breach the visceral pleura, and embed in the parietal pleura (see Fig. 2-6). The passage of asbestos fibers will be impeded if the fibers become coated with an iron–protein complex to become a ferruginous body (asbestos body), since these are wider and have blunter ends than uncoated asbestos fibers. Penetration of the pleura will be easier if adhesions are absent. Plaques are more common alongside the lower ribs and diaphragm because lung mechanics assure better ventilation of lower zones. Where upper zone plaques are present, a greater exposure or working or sleeping in the prone position may be a factor. When the fiber is held up against a rigid part (rib, tendinous portion of diaphragm, vertebra, aorta, left ventricle) plaque formation starts (see Fig. 2-7). The mesothelial cells do not contribute to development of the lesion but merely cover it, since development begins from the deeper part of the pleura; i.e., plaques are essentially extramesothelial. The fibrotic response is out of propor-

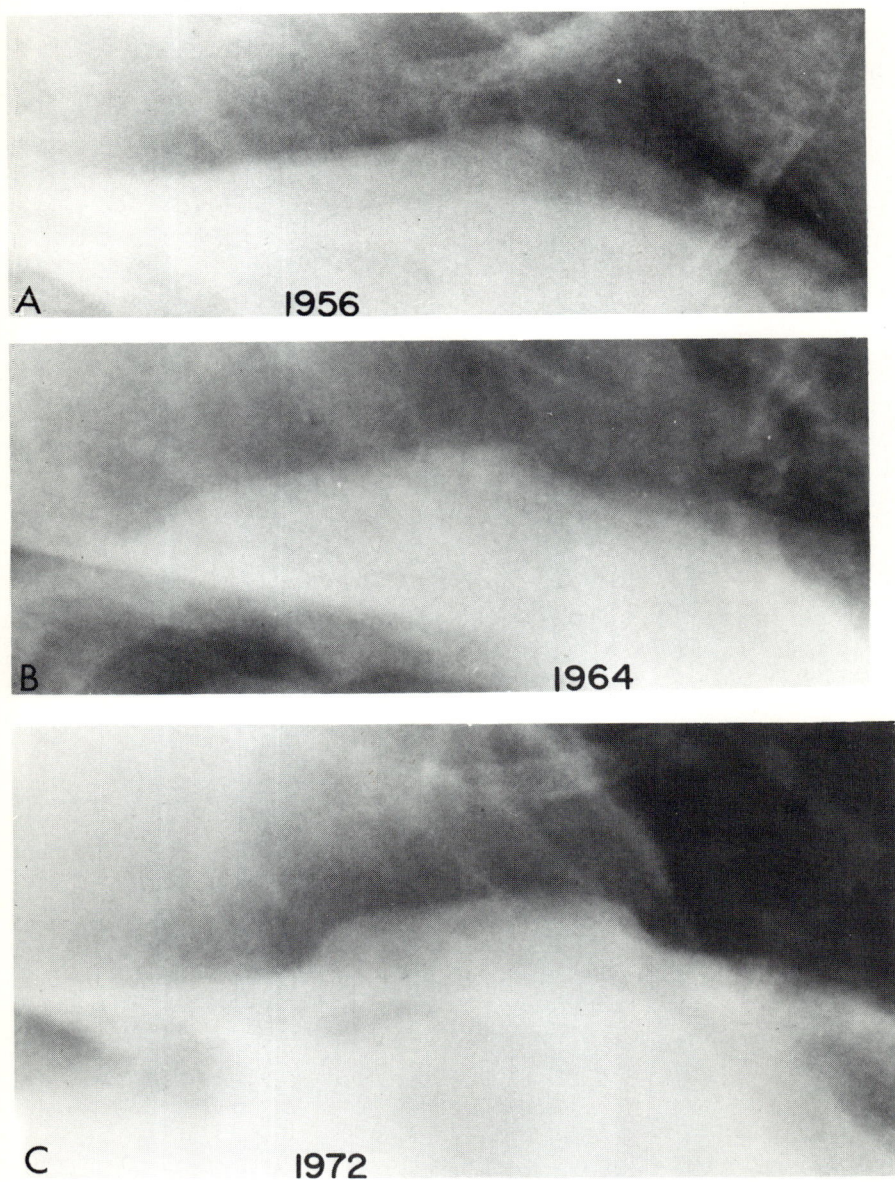

Fig. 2-5. Development of diaphragmatic plaque. PA view of left hemidiaphragm in 1956 (A), 1964 (B), and 1972 (C). In the earliest view, no abnormality is detected. A small plateau-shaped plaque is seen in 1964 and has become deeper in 1972. There was exposure to asbestos during work in World War II shipyards.

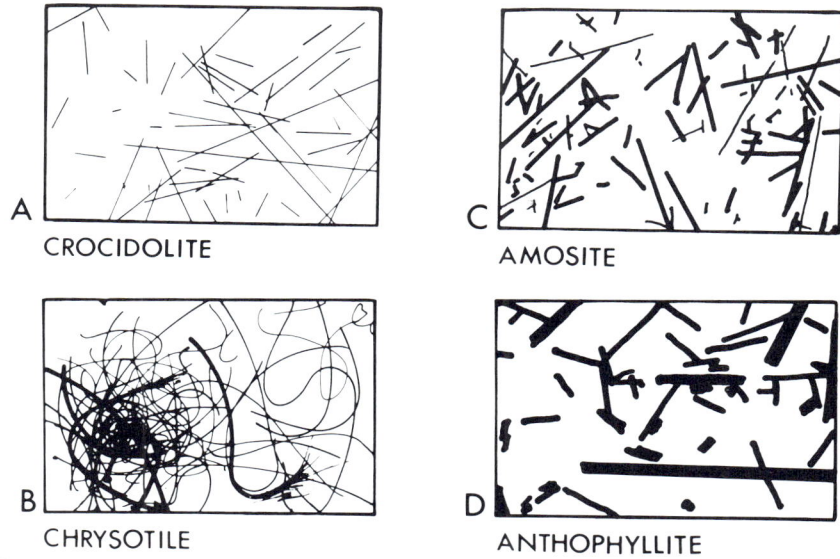

Fig. 2-6. *Asbestos fibers as seen under electronmicroscope (diagrammatic representation). Fiber shape plays a part in lung penetrability. The amphiboles (crocidolite, amosite, anthophyllite) are rectilinear and penetrate lung more efficiently than do the curly chrysotile fibers. Chrysotile fibers tend to fragment in the lung after a period of storage, and the short fragments produced may then behave more like the amphiboles. Amphibole fiber diameter is in increasing order—crocidolite, amosite, anthophyllite; the wider diameter fibers are more likely to be deposited in the proximal airways.*

tion to the few asbestos fibers found in the plaques, and this, together with the presence of lymphocytes and plasma cells in the early lesions, suggests a pleural sensitivity reaction for which there is some evidence (see below).

Other earlier hypotheses have stressed mechanical irritation or induction of minute hemorrhages by fibers and lymphatic rather than airway transport to the parietal pleura (see Fig. 2-8). Kiviluoto[4] has suggested that fibers project from the visceral pleura into parietal pleura to initiate an inflammatory response that subsequently organizes and fibroses. The absence of adhesions between the two pleural layers and the absence of surface inflammatory cells of parietal pleura (when present, they are deeply situated) make this explanation questionable. Meurman[8] thought that the sharp asbestos fibers might initiate subpleural hemorrhages that organize into plaques. The absence of adhesions again is not in keeping with this hypothesis. Instead of airway transport, earlier reports considered intracellular transport of asbestos particles within the lymphatics to the parietal pleura.[7,10] The hypothesis is based on the fact that plaques develop in areas of lymphatic drainage and on the possibility

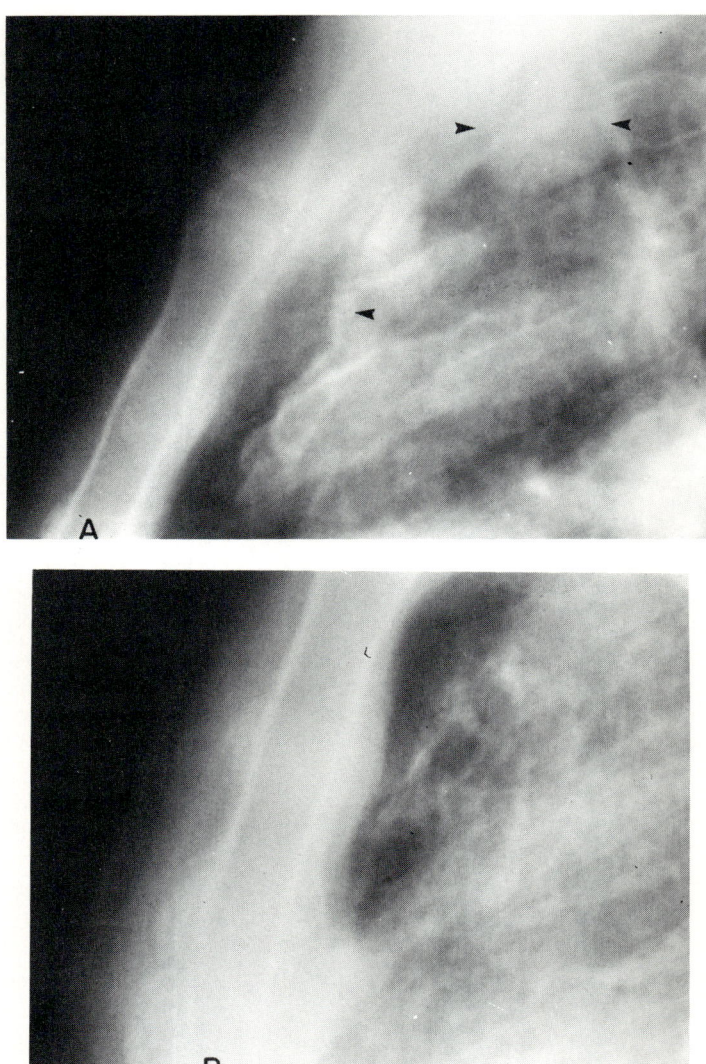

Fig. 2-7. *Retrosternal plaques. Calcified and noncalcified plaques are seen behind the sternum (A and B). The calcified plaques are in the mediastinal parietal pleural reflection over the aorta. This is a rigid area. In A, a circular mass (between arrowheads) simulates a lung mass. Involvement of mediastinal pleura is a late event and not seen in absence of peripheral subaxillary plaques.*

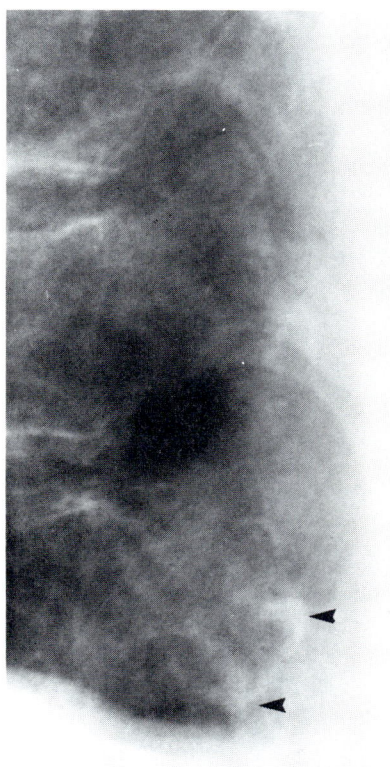

Fig. 2-8A. *Pathogenesis of plaques. Plaques are thought to originate when asbestos fibers have penetrated lung and pleura and are held up against rigid parts. Lateral view of chest shows plaques lying against bony costovertebral areas.*

A

of lymph stasis; the diaphragmatic muscle propels the particles toward the inactive central tendinous portion, while the intercostal muscles may move particles toward the ribs. To reach these sites, particles would have to reach hila of lungs before the mediastinal pleura. Since hilar and mediastinal lymph nodes are unaffected in asbestosis, and since the mediastinal parietal pleura is less involved than the subaxillary pleura, this theory is also questionable. The lower parietal pleurae, both costal and mediastinal, can absorb particulate matter, however; the visceral pleura cannot.[11] This fact may explain the site of plaques. There is experimental evidence that, in mice,[12] asbestos fibers injected subcutaneously migrate to submesothelial tissues in the chest and abdomen and that, in humans, asbestos fibers are found in many parts of the body e.g. brain, kidney, and liver. In view of these various hypotheses, the pathogenesis is still considered sub judice.

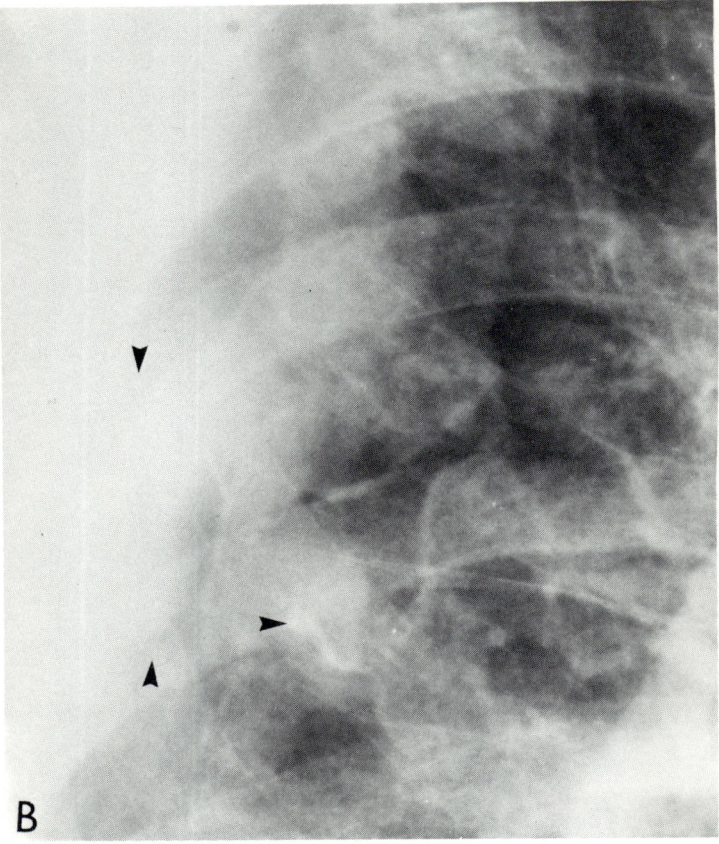

Fig. 2-8B. *Parietal pleural plaques are seen better when they extend medially and lie against air-filled lungs. The large lateral subaxillary plaques merge with the chest wall shadow. Most of the calcifications appear at the periphery of plaques and some traverse plaques (horizontal arrow).*

IMMUNOLOGY OF PATIENTS WITH ASBESTOS PLAQUES

A sensitivity reaction is suggested by the disparity between the size of the plaque and the few asbestos fibers found in them.[2] The incidence of circulating rheumatoid factor, antinuclear antibodies, and the level of gamma globulin is greater in asbestos workers with plaques than in those without plaques and in the nonexposed population.[13,14] The relation of immunologic factors in asbestos-related pulmonary fibrosis is described in Chapter 1.

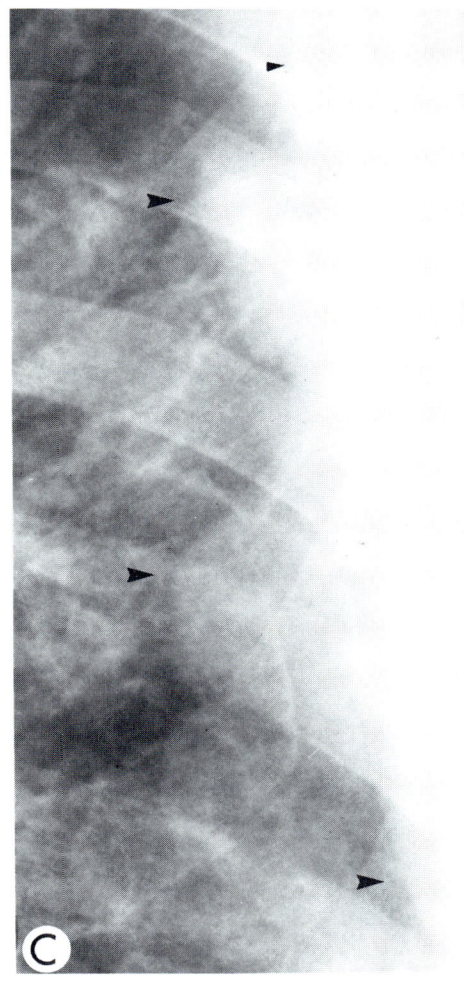

Fig. 2-8C. *Large parietal pleural plaques. Calcification is absent in these plaques, which extend medially in a lobular manner. Differentiation from a mesothelioma or metastatic pleural cancer would be difficult.*

EPIDEMIOLOGY

The prevalence of plaques has been assessed by necropsy examinations and x-ray surveys; the latter will show only a small portion of plaques noted at necropsy, the proportion varying with the sophistication of the x-ray techniques used. Exposure may be occupational, environmental, or leisure-related or may result from household (conjugal) contact. The incidence of plaques increases with age, i.e., with lapsed time since a minimal first exposure.[15] The pleural plaque incidence is considered dose-related by some, but this correlation is more apparent with mild to moderate pulmonary fibrosis. A 20-year interval between first exposure and radiographic recognition of plaques is common.[16a,16b] Persons below the age of 30 years who have plaques have usually had an environmental exposure, e.g., living in an asbestos-mining area or near a shipyard. The effect of age on incidence of calcified pleural plaques is described by Rom and Palmer.[5] A period of 20 to 29 years after first exposure gave an incidence of 10 percent; 30 to 39 years, 35 percent; and over 40 years, 58 percent. Pulmonary parenchymal ferruginous bodies are present in 86 percent of patients with bilateral plaques;[8] but autopsy reports on patients dying in large cities quote similar prevalence of ferruginous bodies in the general population.

All types of asbestos fibers may produce pleural plaques. Anthophyllite, mined in Finland, has been associated with a particularly high rate of 40 percent, but many of these were patients living near the mine and therefore subject to an environmental exposure at an early age (see Fig. 2-9).

Pleural plaques seen in radiographic surveys have been classified into three groups by Jones and Sheers[1]: (1) occupational groups, (2) environmental groups, and (3) nonexposed groups.

1. *Occupational exposure*

General asbestos workers in central Europe	5 percent incidence of plaques
New York asbestos insulators	38 percent incidence of plaques
United Kingdom shipyard workers	5 to 14 percent incidence of plaques
Quebec chrysotile mines and mills	0.5 to 9 percent incidence of plaques
Cypriot chrysotile mines and mills	6 percent incidence of plaques

The Quebec data varied from 0.5 to 9 percent incidence according to age, and the incidence at one mine was 13 times greater than that at an adjacent mine working chrysotile from the same geologic formation. The reason is unknown.[15] Pleural calcification in those exposed to talc and mica has been attributed to associated asbestos fibers.

2. *Environmental factors.* Pleural plaques may occur in those living near anthophyllite, crocidolite, amosite, and chrysotile mines although they are not occupationally exposed. Similarly, those living near factories using

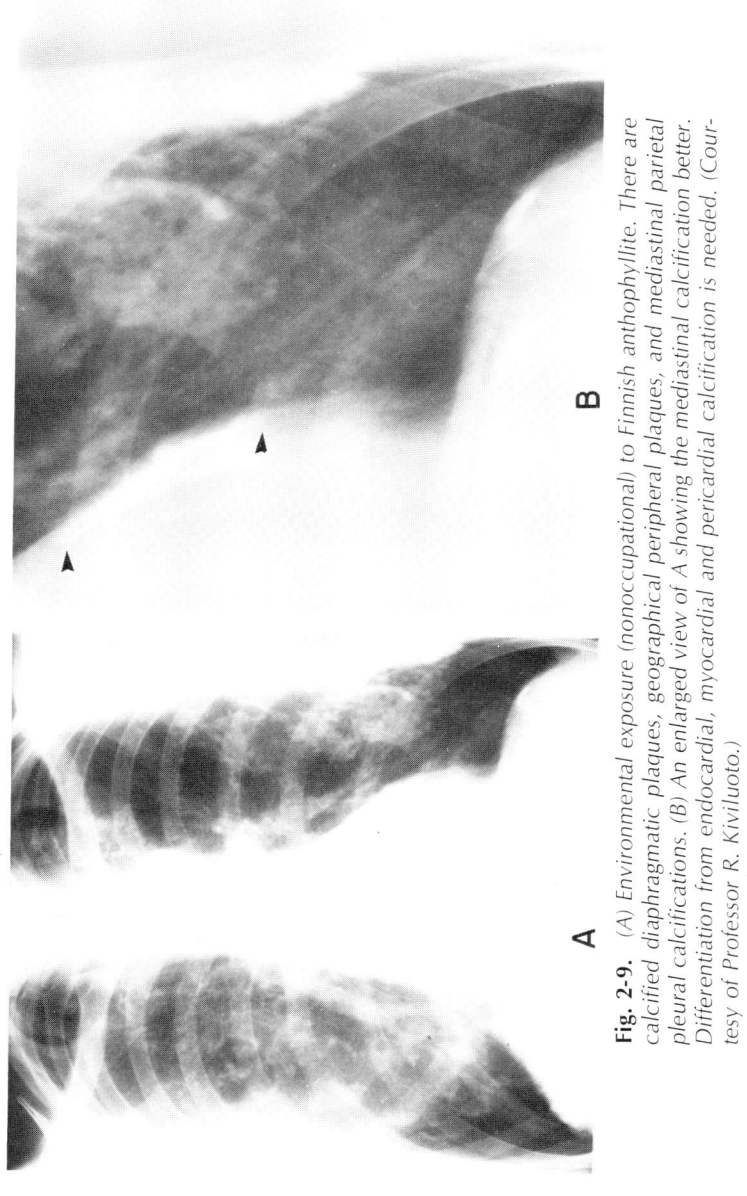

Fig. 2-9. (A) Environmental exposure (nonoccupational) to Finnish anthophyllite. There are calcified diaphragmatic plaques, geographical peripheral plaques, and mediastinal parietal pleural calcifications. (B) An enlarged view of A showing the mediastinal calcification better. Differentiation from endocardial, myocardial and pericardial calcification is needed. (Courtesy of Professor R. Kiviluoto.)

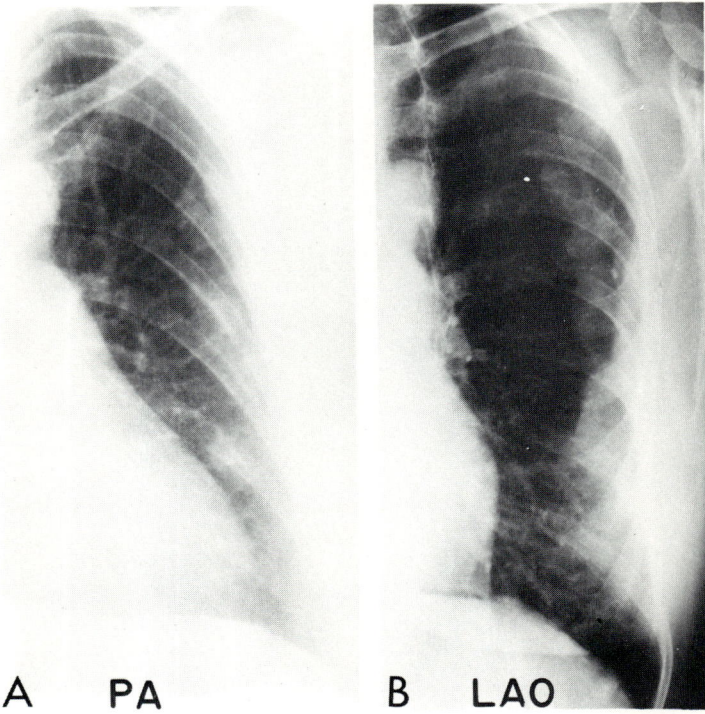

Fig. 2-10. *Conjugal asbestos plaques. A woman with plaques that are better seen in the LAO view (B) than in the PA (A).*

asbestos may develop plaques. In the past, asbestos workers might bring home fibers in their hair, clothes, and footwear. Families of these workers occasionally develop household contact (conjugal) asbestosis[17] (see Fig. 2-10). For centuries, villages in southeast Turkey around Cermik have used chrysotile asbestos for painting walls and floors. The nature of this material was not realized until recently. The villagers have a high incidence, up to 14 percent, of plaques, and the condition was known in Turkey as Cermik disease; only recently has it been realized that the raw material dug up by these villagers was chrysotile ore with some talc included.[18]

3. *Nonexposed groups.* In virtually every patient with large calcified bilateral plaques typical of asbestos exposure, an appropriate history of exposure is obtainable. In some urban patients with small noncalcified plaques, a definite history of exposure is not obtainable. Are these plaques due to unusual susceptibility to the low levels of exposure in ordinary urban life

or to some unelicited or forgotten exposure? A dentist the author has followed for some years may be in the latter group. His chest film showed small bilateral subaxillary plaques, and a history of asbestos exposure was not apparent until some years later, when he remembered that for some 35 years he had used asbestos string to line casting rings used in dental plate construction.[19]

CLINICAL MANIFESTATIONS

Hyaline or calcified pleural plaques may be present alone or in combination with visceral pleural fibrosis. They are most frequently found as an isolated finding and indicate asbestos exposure with all its significance to the clinician for the possible development of pulmonary fibrosis, intrathoracic (pleural and pulmonary malignancy) and extrathoracic (larynx, peritoneal, esophagus, colon, and possibly pancreas, kidney and breast) neoplasia, and splenic and hepatic capsular thickening. In the absence of other findings, the plaques do not produce symptoms. Lung function tests are not usually impaired if the worker does not smoke,[20,21] but some do show minor reductions in lung volumes.[22] Thus, although they themselves do not produce symptoms, the presence of plaques may be ominous; Fletcher,[23] in a survey of 408 shipyard workers with pleural plaques but with no pulmonary fibrosis, noted 3 workers with mesothelioma and 16 with bronchogenic carcinoma. Smoking history was not recorded. Edge[24] found a 2.5-fold increase in bronchial carcinoma in shipbuilders with plaques but no radiographic evidence of pulmonary fibrosis, as compared with controls from neighboring areas whose x-rays were strictly normal but who may have had some degree of asbestos exposure. The pleural plaques are not premalignant; however, Lewinsohn[25] reported a tubulopapillary mesothelioma with some undifferentiated cells arising by a narrow stalk from mesothelia cells covering a hyaline parietal pleural plaque. This case appears to be exceptional, if not unique.

When parietal pleural plaques are associated with diffuse visceral thickening (which may have resulted from a prior asbestos exudative effusion) and when there is lower lobe parenchymal fibrosis, the prognosis is different. About 20 percent of those with plaques have radiographically diagnosable pulmonary fibrosis. This condition has been termed "complicated hyalinosis," as opposed to simple hyalinosis, in which parietal pleural plaques are not accompanied by diffuse visceral pleural changes. Navratil studied a group of 50 present or former asbestos workers,[26] and his data are shown in Table 2-1. The difference between data for simple and complicated hyalinosis is statistically significant.

Table 2-1

	Simple Hyalinosis	Complicated Hyalinosis
Length of exposure	21.0 years	22.4 years
Elapsed time since onset of exposure	27.6 years	33.7 years
Mortality data	12%	40%

RADIOGRAPHIC APPEARANCE

Three problems confront the clinical radiologist:

1. Choice of optimal radiographic technique to demonstrate plaques;
2. The identification and differentiation of pleural plaques from other similar pleural shadows;
3. Pleural plaques may be associated with, and obscure, more serious asbestos-related thoracic disease.

Choice of Optimal Radiographic Techniques to Demonstrate Plaques

Film Size

Since pleural plaques have a peripheral location on a standard PA chest film, a 14 in. × 14 in. (355 mm × 355 mm) film, as used in the United Kingdom, or 14 in. × 17 in. (355 mm × 432 mm), as used in the United States, may not include the periphery of a large thorax. Although inconsequent, if films are inspected at the time of development prior to the patient leaving the department, the use of standard films in surveys or in rolls where film is examined when the patient is not available for exposure of a better centered or additional film may be a major disadvantage. Audsley[27] has therefore suggested a film size of 400 mm × 400 mm so that less than 2 percent of the population screened would not be fully covered by a single film. There is no published data on the efficacy of plaque detection by 100-mm films and photofluoroscopy compared with conventional size film.

Applied Kilovoltage

For many years, radiologists have used a high-kilovolt technique (110–140 kV) in preference to the older standard kilovolt technique (60–80 kV) for routine radiography (see Fig. 2-11). High-kilovolt techniques have a practical advantage in that there is a large latitude in exposure, so that variations in milliampere-seconds (mAs), which control film blackening or density, may be

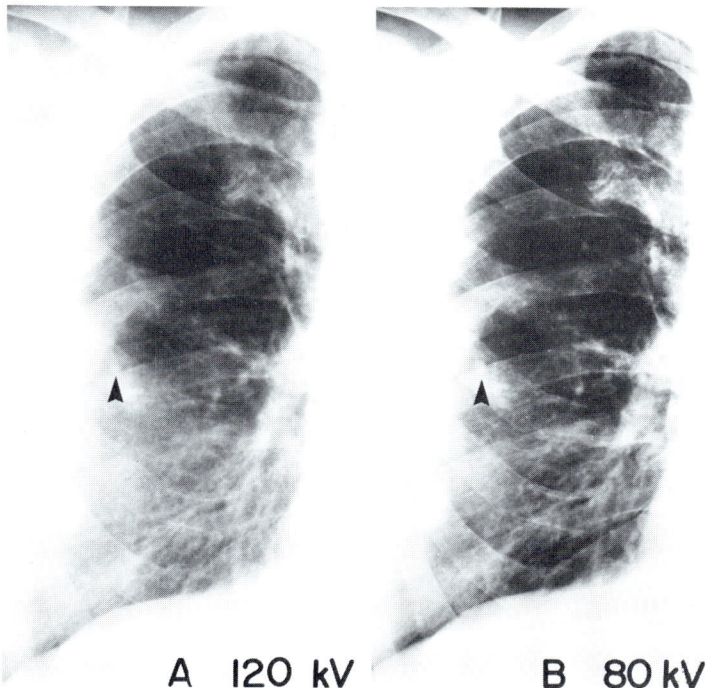

Fig. 2-11. *High- and low-kilovolt techniques. In A (120 kV), hyaline plaques are seen along the lateral chest wall, but the calcified plaque projected over the right fourth rib anteriorly is poorly visible (arrow); it is seen better in B (80 kV). The minimal fibrotic changes in the right lower lobe are seen better in A (120 kV). In C (120 kV), the calcified plaque overlying the left sixth rib anteriorly (see next page) is seen less well than in D.*

made over a relatively large range and an acceptable film still be obtained. This safety margin is at the expense of production of the film with less subject contrast (long-scale contrast), so that there is a long scale of shades of gray between the lightest and darkest parts of the film image. This is an advantage in separating adjacent and overlapping images, since the more radiographically dense image does not fully obscure the less dense. Noncalcified hyaline plaques adjacent to the ribs are therefore seen more easily with the high-kilovolt technique.

Conversely, low-kilovolt techniques produce an image with high subject contrast because there is large variation in the intensity of the transmitted x-ray beam through the various organs of the chest. This is based on the physical fact that low-kilovolt x-rays show more photoelectric type absorption in substances with high atomic numbers such as bone ($Z = 13.8$) as compared with muscle

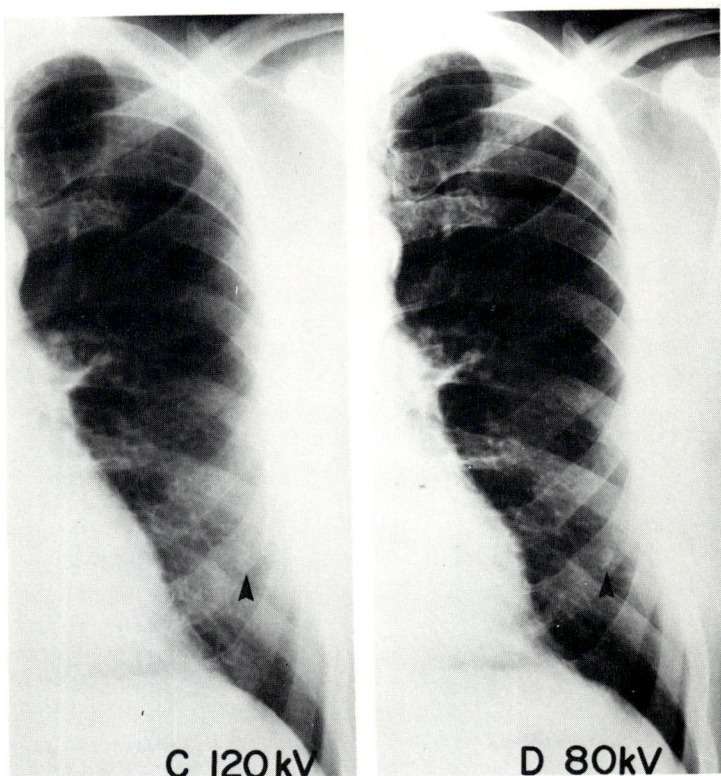

(Z = 7.4). Calcified pleural plaque will therefore be the more visible, since its Z number will approximate that of bone, whereas a noncalcified plaque will be less apparent, since its Z number will be similar to that of adjacent intercostal muscle. Many of the epidemiologic surveys have been made with mobile units carrying x-ray generators capable of generating a low kilovolt only, and although images so produced may show calcified plaques clearly, noncalcified plaques may be inapparent.

The information regarding the choice of technique may be tabulated as shown in Table 2-2 (altered from Bohlig and Gilson[28]).

General Radiographic Principles Affecting Image Quality

These principles are well known to all practicing radiologists and are succinctly described in modern texts on radiological physics.[29] Briefly, the important controlling factors are contrast and image quality. Contrast, as seen

Table 2-2

Lesion	High Kilovolt	Low Kilovolt
Pulmonary fibrosis	+	−
Hyaline plaque	+	−
Calcified plaque	−	+
Pleural effusion	+	−
Visceral pleural thickening	+	−
Mesothelioma and lung cancer	+	−

+ signifies preferred technique. Thus, because absorption of x-rays by calcium decreases with a rise in kilovolts, small areas of calcification may be inapparent on a high-kilovolt film, and two exposures, at high and low kilovolts, may need to be made for optimal detection of both types of plaques

on a film, depends on the contrast of the subject, film contrast (an inherent photographic property of the x-ray film used which may amplify subject contrast), fog, and scattered radiation. Image quality, the ability for point-for-point reproduction of parts of the subject x-rayed on the film, is governed by the degree of radiographic mottle, the ability of the apparatus (x-ray machine, grid, film, and screens) to define a sharp edge, and the resolving power, or the ability to record separate images of small objects near together.

Ultrasound Techniques

The use of ultrasound to identify pleural effusions, to select a suitable aspiration site,[30] and to monitor removal of fluid by use of special needle-transducer assemblies is now routine. Less utilized is ultrasonic detection of pleural plaques. Using A and B modes, plaques thicker than 2–3 mm are detectable whether calcified or not. Ease of detection increases with thickness and presence of calcification. Plaques thinner than 2 mm usually contain little or no calcium. The plaques appear as echo reflectant linear structures 2–5 cm from the skin surface. It is not possible to differentiate asbestos-related plaques from pleural thickening due to other causes. Plaques may be detected by ultrasound examination when not apparent on conventional radiographic examination. Viikeri[31] suggested that ultrasound be used for epidemiologic surveys, but despite the advantage of utilizing a nonionizing form of radiation, the technique is time-consuming.

Xerography

Xeroradiographic images have enhanced edges, and this technique permits greater latitude in the choice of exposure factors than does conventional filming. Edge enhancement should permit easier identification of plaques, but in practice, the increased radiation dose to the patient is a controlling factor,

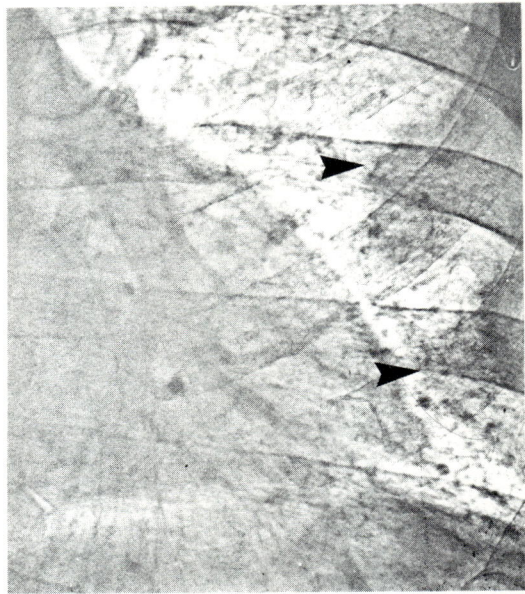

Fig. 2-12. *Xerogram of an insulating worker showing noncalcified pleural plaques.*

and conventional film oblique views are preferable. The plaques outlined in Figure 2-12 were easily apparent on conventional films; the xerograms were part of an examination to assess a malignancy in the opposite lung.*

Computed Tomography Techniques

Parietal and visceral pleural thickening, diffuse or plaquelike, calcified or not, causes an increase in soft tissue attenuation of x-ray beam and so is demonstrable by computed tomography (CT) techniques[32] (see Figs. 2-13 and 2-14). Diffuse and localized areas of thickening may be seen when inapparent in routine chest films and, if seen conventionally, may appear larger with CT. The inner (nearer lung) margins of plaques visualized by CT are denser than the

---

*It was reported recently that pleural plaques, thickening, and linear opacities of early parenchymal fibrosis are seen better on xeroradiographs (exposed at 10–30 *m*As 200 kilovolts at 1.35 *m* without grid or air gap and developed in positive mode) than silver halide films taken at 200 kilovolts. Xeroradiographic films are too small to cover the whole lung field and may be used as a supplement to conventional radiography. (Thomas RG and Sluis-Cremer GK: Two-hundred kilovolt xeroradiography in occupational exposure to silica and asbestos. Br J Ind Med 34:281–289, 1977)

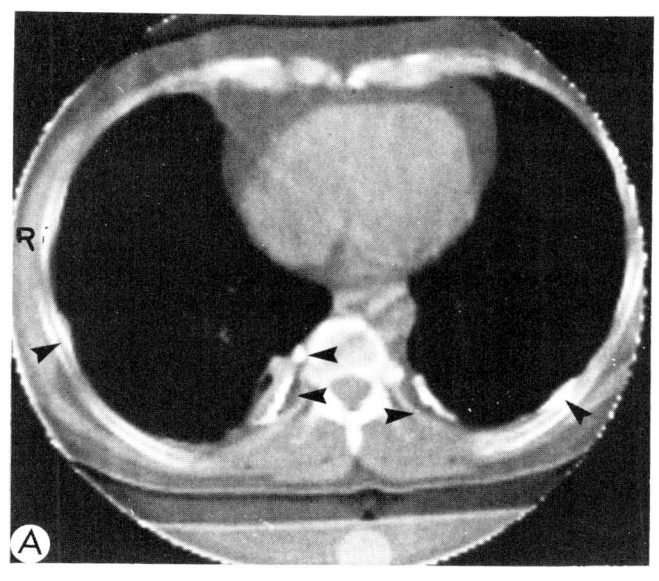

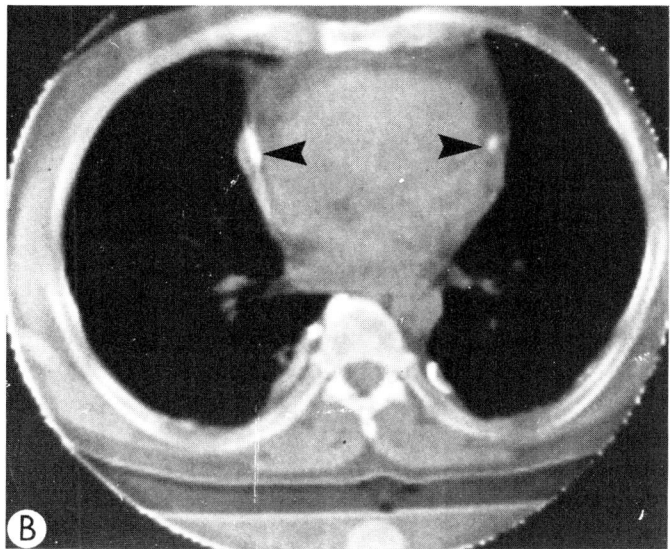

Fig. 2-13. CT demonstration of pleural plaques. (A) Calcified paravertebral (horizontal arrows) and peripheral plaques (oblique arrows). (B) Calcified mediastinal (horizontal arrows), paravertebral, and peripheral plaques. (C) Calcified diaphragmatic (horizontal arrows) and paravertebral plaques; also seen is wedge-shaped area of fibrous tissue in right lung (oblique arrows) (see next page).

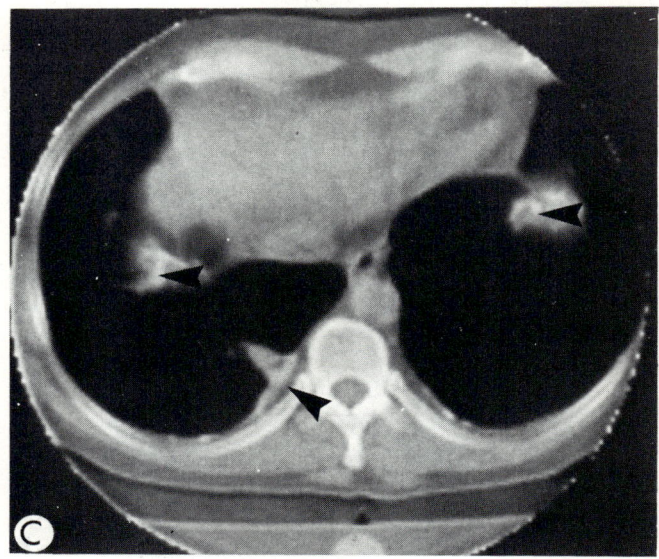

Fig. 2-13C

outer margins. Some changes are detectable only by this technique, e.g., extension of plaques along diaphragmatic crura below the level of the lungs, subpleural localized infiltrates that appear to be related to visceral pleural thickening as described by Solomon,[33] and bands, presumably fibrous, crossing the pleural cavity, especially at the cardiophrenic angle. This latter change is of extreme interest in that the absence of pleural adhesions at necropsy and thoracotomy had prompted the concept that parietal pleural plaques are noninflammatory in origin. Detection of these bands by CT should prompt a reassessment of the incidence of adhesions in asbestosis. Computed tomography is especially helpful in detection of plaques in the posterior mediastinum, adjacent to the heart, and those penetrating the diaphragm and lying adjacent to the liver and spleen (see Fig. 2-15). The latter may have been in part responsible for capsular fibrosis of liver and spleen described in asbestosis by pathologists in the past. The overall value of CT is shown by Kreel's[32] data: 11 of 13 patients, with exposures ranging from 1 to 40 years, have plaques demonstrable by CT, but only 8 of 13 were visible on chest films. Another value of CT lies in the detection of peripheral pulmonary malignancies that may be in part obscured by large plaques when using conventional techniques. Its value in the detection of pulmonary fibrosis, small nodular densities, and visceral pleural thickening is described in Chapter 2, Section 2.

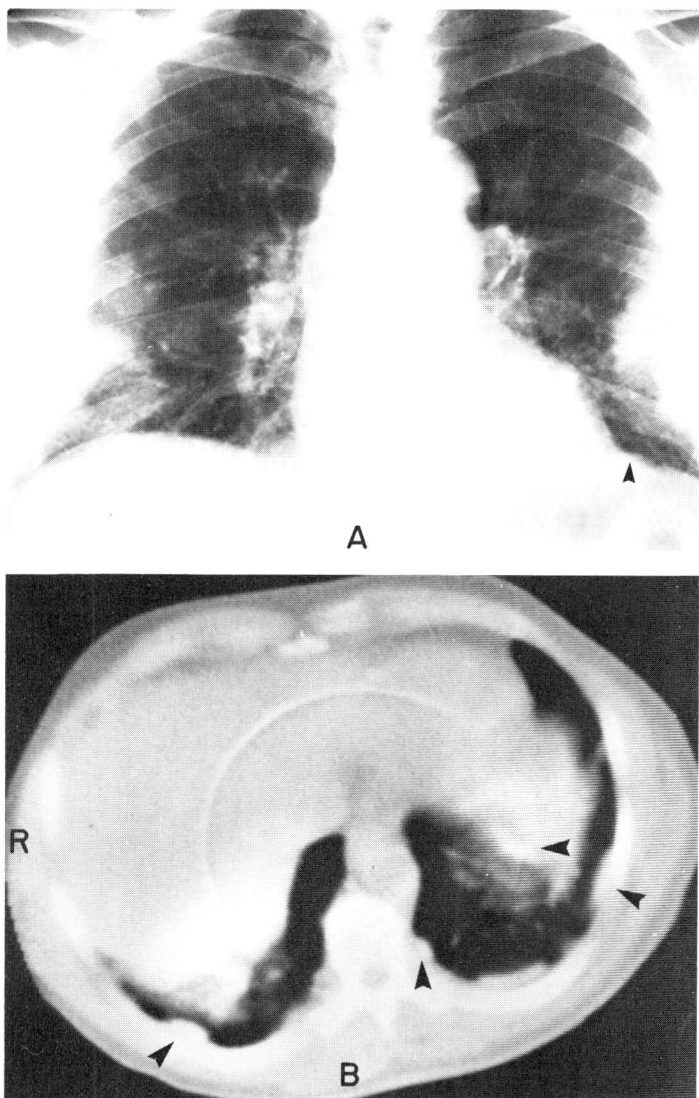

Fig. 2-14. (A) PA chest film of patient with an 18-month history of asbestos exposure while working in a shipyard in World War II. Large subaxillary plaques are seen, but plaque on left diaphragm is seen poorly (arrow). (B) CT section shows plaque on left diaphragm (horizontal arrow) as well as peripheral (oblique arrows) and paravertebral plaque (vertical arrow). (C and D) CT sections show that peripheral plaques may be present anteriorly (horizontal arrow) in addition to more typical posterolateral location (see next page).

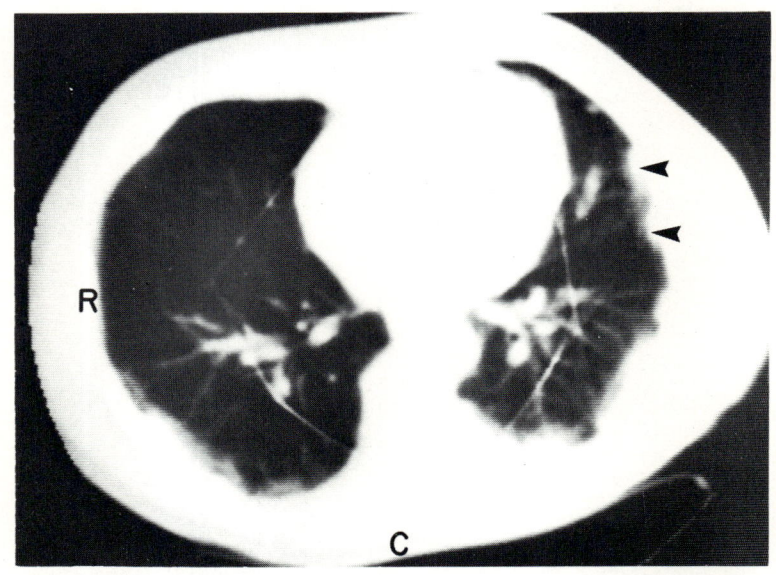
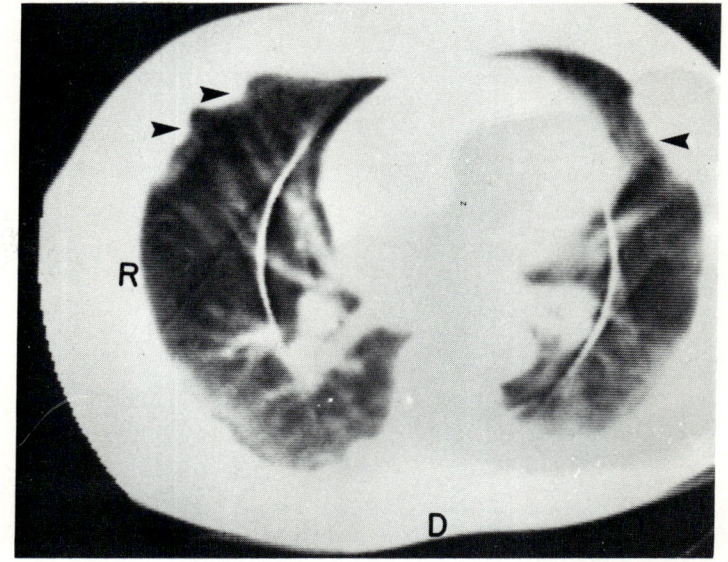

Fig. 2-14C,D

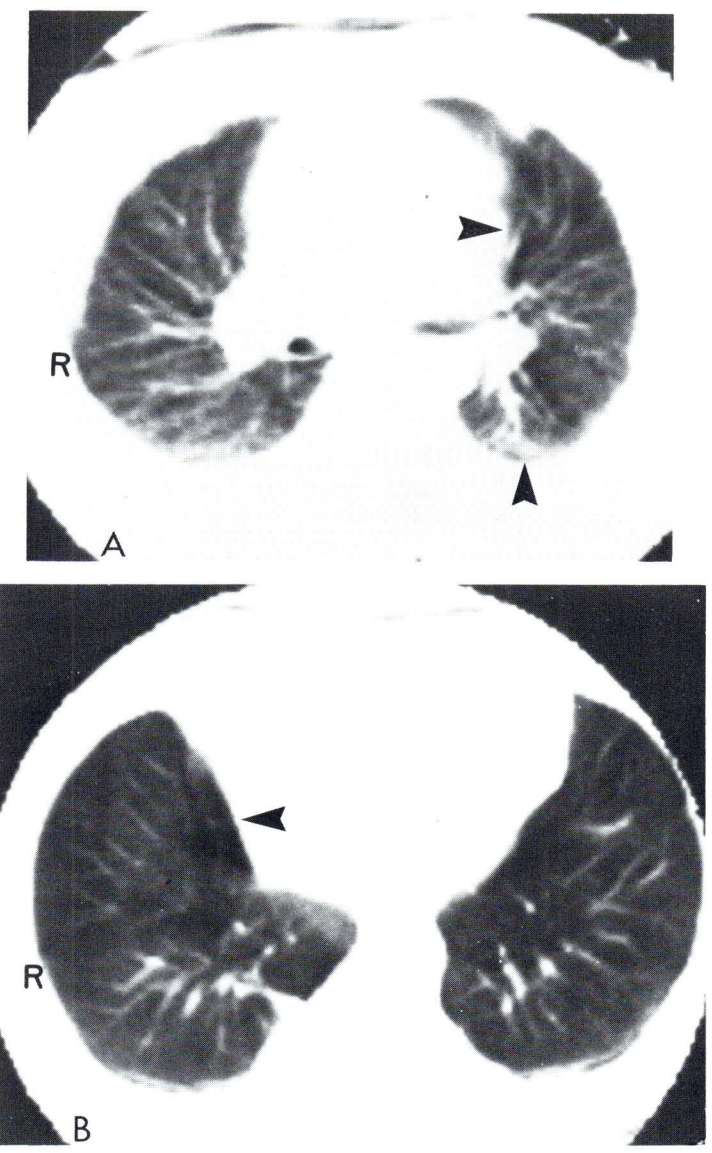

Fig. 2-15. Computed tomography (A) Irregular border of left side of the mediastinum due to plaques (horizontal arrow); there is also fibrosis in the posterior part of the left lung (vertical arrow). In (B) there is flattening of the right side of mediastinum due to mediastinal pleural plaques.

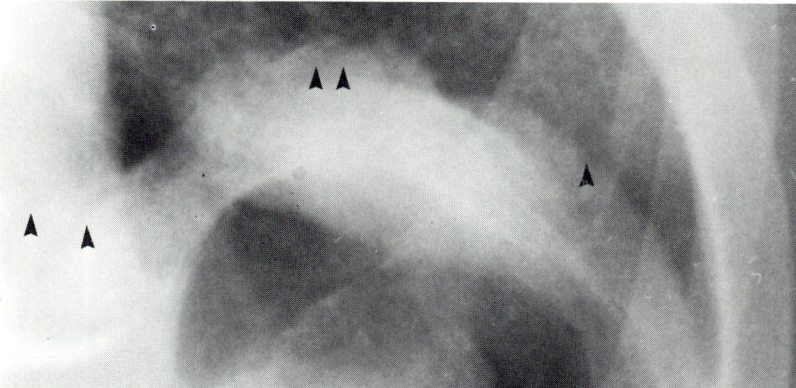

Fig. 2-16. *Diaphragmatic plaque in a lobulated diaphragm. Diaphragmatic plaques when noncalcified are best seen in full inspiration, which helps straighten out lobulated diaphragm. In this patient, the medial and lateral lobulations (arrows) do not have the plateau shape of the typical central diaphragmatic plaque (double arrows).*

Identification of Plaques and Their Differentiation from Similar Pleural and Chest Wall Shadows

Detection of Small Hyaline (Noncalcified) Plaques

Small, noncalcified hyaline plaques of mediastinal parietal pleura are not recognizable by conventional techniques. When adjacent to the diaphragm, parietal pleural plaques should be searched for assiduously in the middle one-third (the tendinous aponeurotic area); they are not found less than 2.5 cm from the costophrenic angles. A film exposed in full inspiration is needed, so that the raised plaque will stand out from the relatively flat, adjacent, uninvolved diaphragm (see Fig. 2-16). With poor inspiration and a domed diaphragm, the smaller plaques may be inapparent. The lobulations of diaphragmatic contour may obscure a plaque or be mistaken for one (see Fig. 2-17). Pleurodiaphragmatic adhesions at the lower end of the major fissure may obscure adjacent plaques (see Fig. 2-18). The shape of the plaque varies from slight elevations, difficult to separate out from the diaphragmatic contour, to localized buttonlike or plateaulike masses when larger. The small diaphragmatic plaques are usually not distinguishable on lateral projections. Since they are more common posterior to the midcoronal plane of the diaphragm, oblique views are helpful.

Small lateral hyaline noncalcified pleural plaques should be searched for

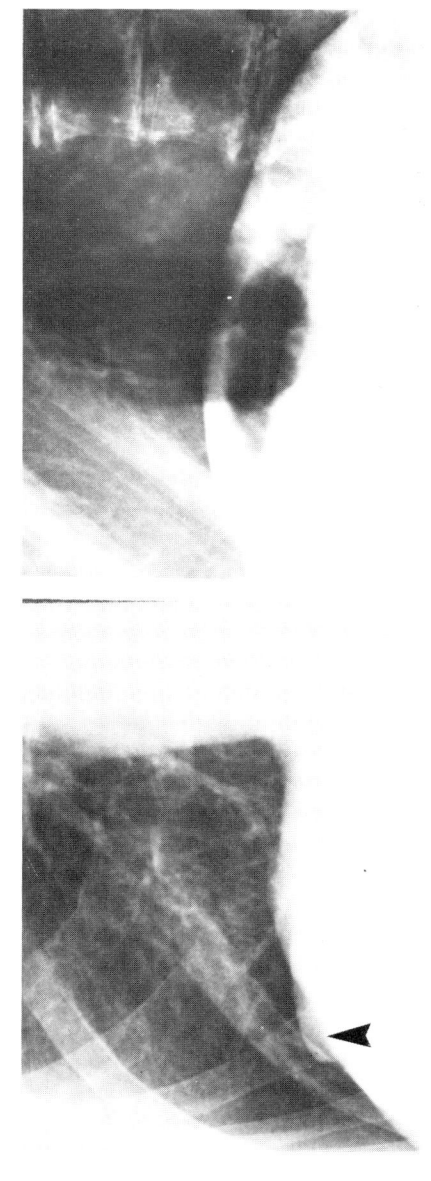

Fig. 2-17. PA view of right lung and lateral view. Muscle slips in frontal view may simulate diaphragmatic plaques; no plaques are evident in the lateral view.

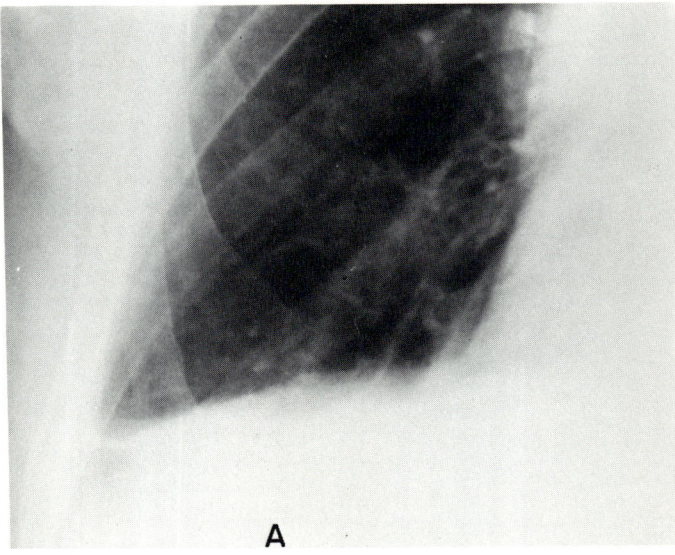

Fig. 2-18. *Diaphragmatic linear calcified plaques may be obscured by adjacent nonaerated lung or fluid. Linear atelectasis in A obscures the fine diaphragmatic calcification, which becomes apparent when this area is reinflated (B) (arrow) (see facing page).*

on the lateral chest wall between the sixth and ninth ribs and on the posterolateral chest wall between the fifth and tenth ribs (see Fig. 2-19). The apices and sulci are not involved. Small noncalcified plaques are usually not discernible on the lateral view because of the overlap of the left and right posterior rib ends and vertebrae. If the lateral projection is not true but slightly oblique, small plaques may occasionally be seen, but in general this is more helpful in detecting small calcified plaques. Any overlap of soft tissue of the arm may obscure lateral plaques. This is especially important if oblique views are made, since the arm nearest the cassette may be difficult to move out of the way and still maintain good contact of the patient with the cassette holder. Oblique projections are of great value in showing a tangential view of small plaques not visible on routine PA projections; several films taken at different obliquities are sometimes of value. Fluoroscopy helps in choice of appropriate degree of obliquity.

The line diagram in Figure 2-20 shows that the radiographic image of a plaque whose long axis is parallel to the x-ray beam may be enlarged by the use of appropriate oblique projections. In doubtful cases, both oblique (left and

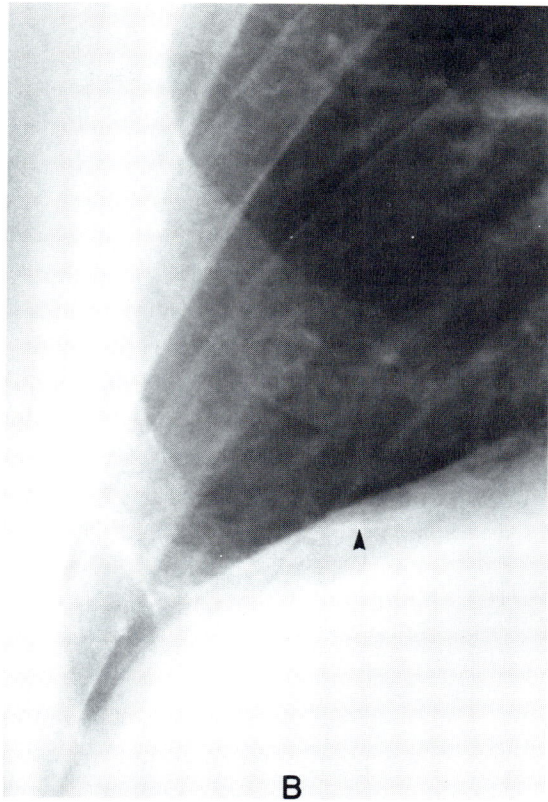

B

right) views should be used (Fig. 2-21). Views that are too steep an oblique will project the semispinalis and sacrospinalis muscles adjacent to the spine and will obscure the plaques, since they often are present adjacent to the spine.*

*The semispinalis muscle arises by a series of long muscle bundles from the backs of the tips of the first to tenth thoracic transverse processes and articular processes of third to seventh cervical vertebrae. It passes upwards to insert as three bundles. Semispinalis capitis inserts on the occipital bone between the superior and inferior nuchal lines close to the midline and immediately under the trapezius. Semispinalis cervicis inserts onto the spines of C2 to C5 vertebrae. Semispinalis thoracis inserts on the spines of C6 to C7 and T1 to T4 vertebrae. The sacrospinalis muscle arises from the sacral spines and lateral mass, the lumbar and lower thoracic spinous processes, and the posterior part of the crest of the ilium. It inserts as three columns—outer, intermediate, and medial—in a complicated manner from the mastoid process superiorly, all cervical vertebrae except C1, all thoracic and lumbar vertebrae, and all the ribs inferiorly.

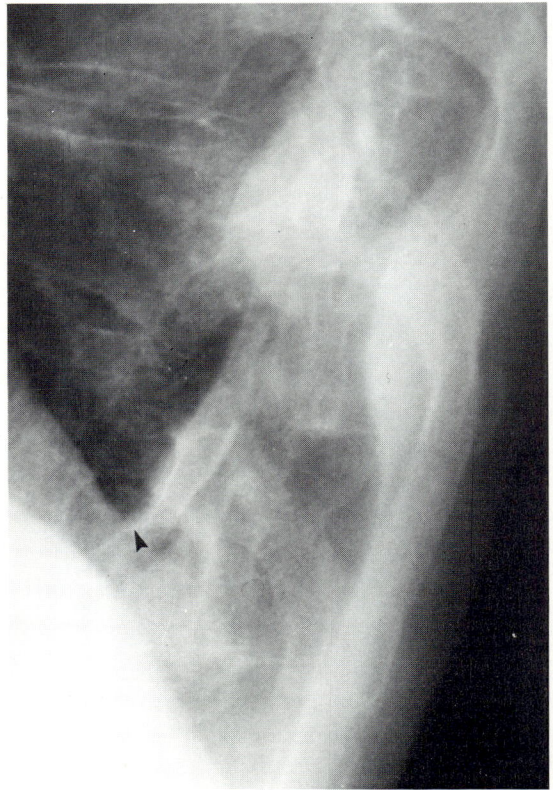

Fig. 2-19. A not-quite-true left lateral view of the chest shows large noncalcified plaques against left and right ribs adjacent to costovertebral angle. The left pleural gutter is obliterated (arrow); recurrent benign pleural effusions may follow asbestos exposure and, when remitted, leave a blunted costovertebral angle.

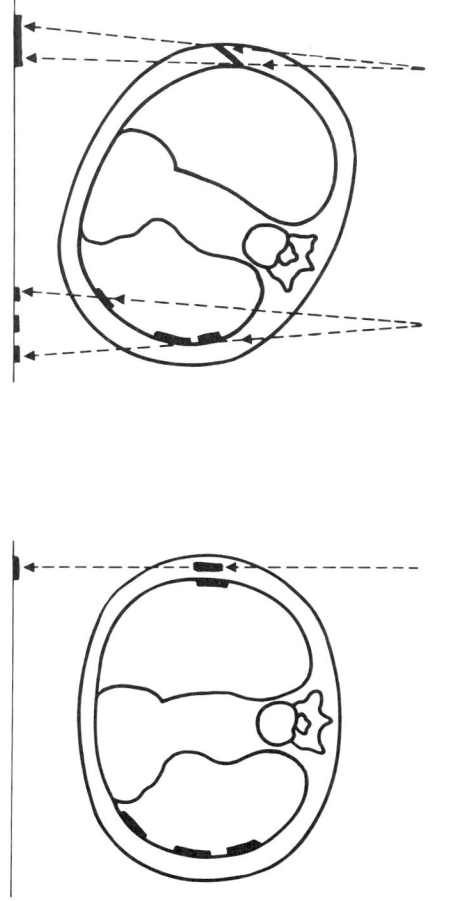

Fig. 2-20. Values of oblique projections. An oblique view will present more of a surface of a plaque "en face" to the incident beam. This is especially important in the detection of noncalcified plaques. (After H. Bohlig.)

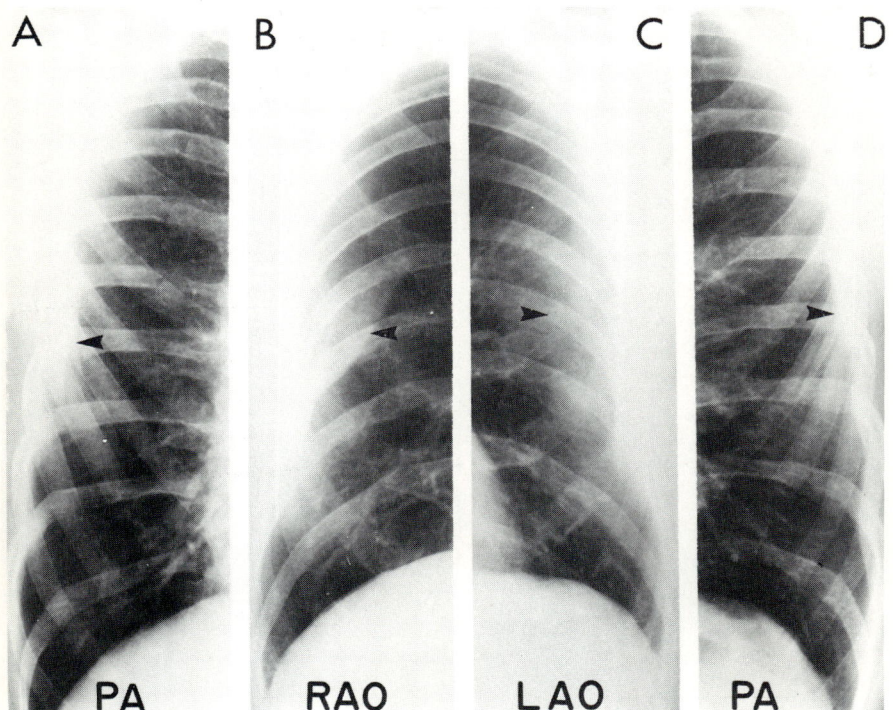

Fig. 2-21. *Value of oblique projections. Subaxillary plaques are largest in the posterolateral area between fifth and tenth ribs. Plaques are seen in A and D (PA views of right and left lung), those on left being barely visible. In the RAO (B) and LAO (C) views, the plaques become much more apparent.*

The plaques on oblique views may appear larger, and their shape will alter, usually from a flat or flangelike density to a more rounded one. Sometimes a coin lesion may be simulated; but plaques are usually less dense than a pulmonary coin lesion of similar size. Reference to Figure 2-21 will show that an oblique view may demonstrate several plaques, while a PA (or AP) view will show but one. In doubtful cases, instead of oblique PA films, oblique AP films may be helpful.

A major problem in the identification of small hyaline plaques is their differentiation from the normal companion shadows of the chest wall. In the subaxillary areas of the chest wall the shadows of interest are those due to serratus anterior and external oblique muscles, rib companion shadows, overlapping ribs and extrapleural fat (see Figs. 2-22 and 2-23). Overlapping rib shadows may be traced out satisfactorily with a high-kilovolt technique and have clearly definable borders, which is often not the case with a plaque that usually has a poorly definable medial border unless it is very thick. Extrapleural fat in obese patients is usually symmetrical over many intercostal spaces. The companion shadow on the under surface of ribs is usually more marked in the upper ribs, and pleural plaques are more common nearer the lower ribs. The interdigitations of serratus anterior and external oblique muscles as they arise from the ribs are a problem. A line diagram (Fig. 2-22A) shows that the serratus anterior slips have an isosceles triangle shape, while the external oblique slips may be triangular, V-shaped, or quadrilateral. Since the shadows from both sets of muscle slips are superimposed on a radiograph, the composite image may appear as a series of triangles, diamond shapes, or V or inverted V shapes. Differentiation from plaques may be difficult and is summarized in Table 2-3.

The line diagram of the anterior wall of the thorax shows the original of the external oblique muscles of the anterior abdominal wall from the outer surfaces of the lower eight ribs by slips, the upper of which interdigitate with the serratus anterior and the lower with the latissimus dorsi. The latissimus dorsi lies posteriorly and so is not shown in this diagram. The other muscle to be differentiated from pleural plaques is the serratus anterior, which originates by digitations from the outer surfaces of the upper eight ribs.*

Bilateral pleural thickening from prior inflammatory disease or hemothorax is usually not a problem in differential diagnosis because costophrenic sulci or costovertebral sulcus is usually obliterated. Pleuropericardial

---

*Another confusing shadow has been described as paralleling the medial surface of the upper 3 or 4 ribs along the lateral chest wall. It is more apparent on its oblique than PA view. It tapers inferiorly and may be up to 1 cm wide on the oblique view. It is caused by intercostal muscles, with subcostal muscles, endothoracic fascia, and fat contributing. (Sargent NE, Jacobson G, Gordonson JS: Pleural plaques: A signpost of asbestos dust inhalation. Semin Robentgenol 12(4):287–297, 1977)

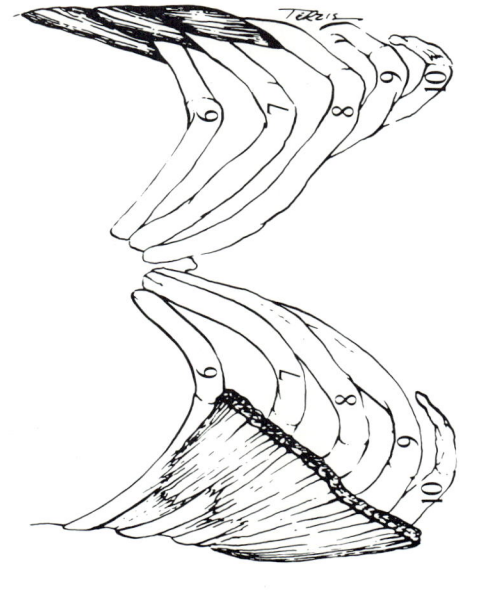

ORIGIN OF SERRATUS ANTERIOR FROM OUTER SURFACE OF UPPER 8 RIBS

ORIGIN OF EXTERNAL OBLIQUE FROM OUTER SURFACE OF LOWER 8 RIBS

A

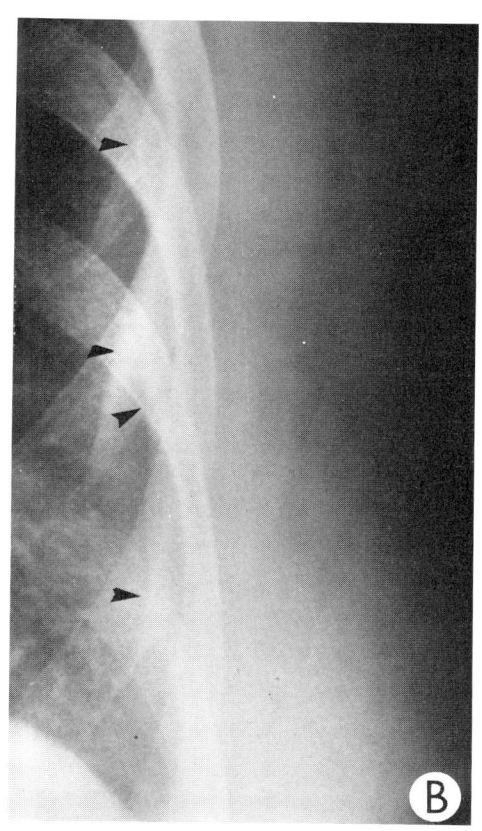

Fig. 2-22. Diaphragmatic representation of origin of muscle slips of external oblique and serratus anterior (A) (see facing page). The triangular shape of these slips is seen in B.

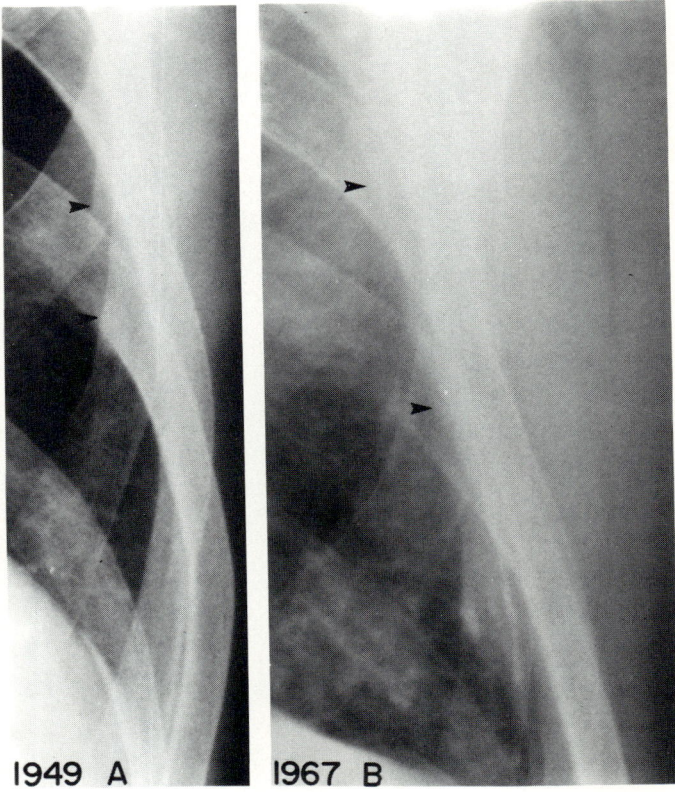

Fig. 2-23. Development of pleural plaques. In A (1949), the muscle slips of the serratus anterior are visible. In B (1967), noncalcified pleural plaques have obscured the muscle slips and more inferiorly calcified plaques are seen. The value of an overpenetrated oblique film to show calcified plaques is seen in C (1967). In D (1972), the noncalcified plaques are larger, and the calcification is more extensive (see facing page).

and pleurodiaphragmatic adhesions occasionally are problems. If a pleuropericardial adhesion is tentlike, differentiation is easy. If it is a localized area of thickening, as occurs as a sequel of transmural myocardial infarction, its differentiation from a plaque of the mediastial parietal pleura may be difficult. Fortunately, such plaques are usually not isolated, and others are apparent in the subaxillary or diaphragmatic area. Similarly, pleural diaphragmatic adhesions, if tentlike, are identifiable, and even if such an appearance is absent on frontal view, it may be seen in lateral view to lie adjacent to the major fissure, while most plaques usually lie more posteriorly, at least in the lower zones. In

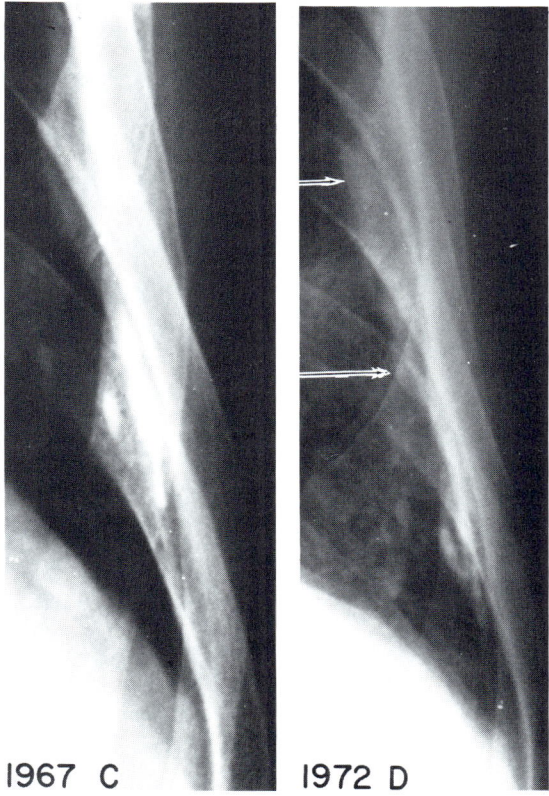

1967 C 1972 D

general, asbestos plaques are characterized by an absence of adhesions, and it is rare but not unknown to have an adhesion and a plaque coexist in the same area. The lack of distinctness of the medial part of the diaphragm seen in some patients with tiny pleural effusions or pectus excavatum is not a problem, since this area is not prone to plaque development. Plaques are most common in the approximate mid-third of the diaphragm in frontal view. Noncalcified callus seen soon after rib fractures, especially bilateral fractures, may be a radiographic problem in the absence of clinical information.

Assessment of Unilateral Plaques

Asbestos exposure produces bilateral plaques. Unilateral plaques are nearly always due to some other cause, e.g., pleural thickening subsequent to rib fractures or callus in a rib fracture simulating a plaque (see Fig. 2-24).

Table 2-3

Muscle Insertion	Pleural Plaques
Disappear on oblique view	More obvious on oblique view
Usually uniform in shape and size in any individual	Not uniform in shape and size
More apparent in muscular patients and those with much adjacent fatty tissue	Muscularity may obscure small plaques
Medial borders sharp	Medial border indistinct
Extends over ribs 4 to 12, but last two ribs may not be apparent on PA view	Typically occur adjacent to sixth to ninth ribs of lateral chest wall and seventh to tenth ribs posterolaterally, but usually only a few are involved in early cases; in advanced disease, differentiation from muscle slips is easier

Modified from Fletcher and Edge.[6]

Unilateral asbestos-related plaques may occur, however, if there has been a pleural synthesis on one side preventing plaque development. Potential causes include hemothorax, empyema, tuberculous pleurisy, and thoracotomy. Pre-existing unilateral chronic pulmonary parenchymal disease may prevent airway passage of asbestos fibers to initiate plaque development.

Detection of Small Calcified Plaques

Calcified pleural plaques occur in the same location as fibrohyaline plaques, i.e., parietal pleura adjacent to the lateral, posterolateral chest walls and, to a lesser extent, anteriorly, the mediastinal pleura, and the diaphragmatic area (see Fig. 2-25). The same projections as mentioned for detection of noncalcified plaques will therefore be useful. Because of the reduction of x-ray absorption with increasing kilovolts, a low-kilovolt technique is preferred. For mediastinal and diaphragmatic calcifications, an overpenetrated film frequently shows calcifications more clearly. While conventional tomography has a limited use in the detection of noncalcified plaques, it is helpful in the detection of small calcifications. The conventional lateral view is especially useful in identifying diaphragmatic calcifications. Although in North America and the United Kingdom posterolateral calcifications are more common, in the Finnish anthophyllite group, anterolateral calcifications predominate.

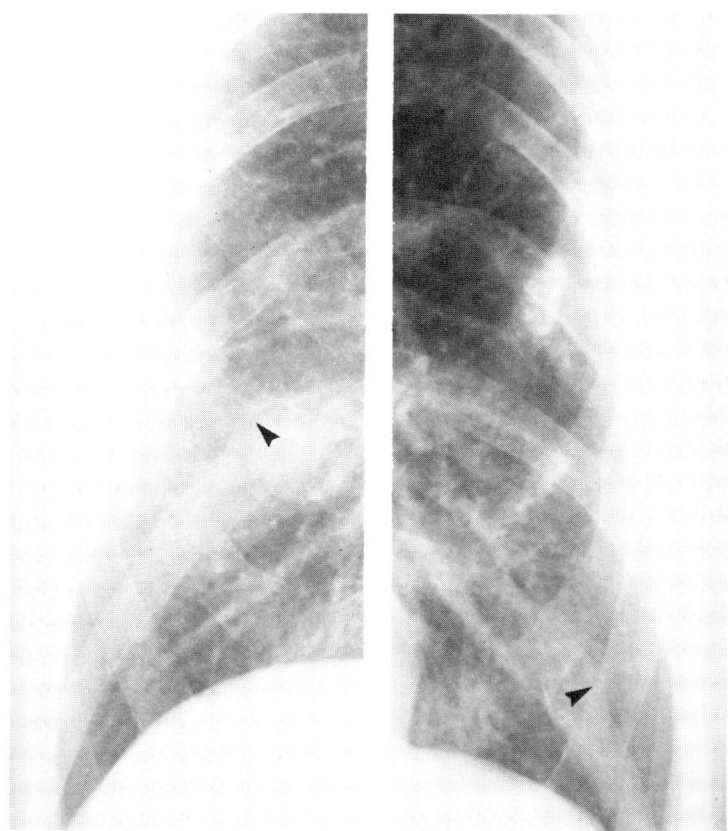

Fig. 2-24. Unilateral pleural plaques are frequently due to old rib fractures, and their calcification is linear. This ex-asbestos worker has old fractures of the right tenth and left eleventh ribs (arrows). Plaques, both noncalcified and calcified, are present only on the left, are superior to the rib deformity, and are typically the shape of asbestos plaques. Unilateral plaques due to asbestos are an extreme rarity and usually an alternative cause should be considered.

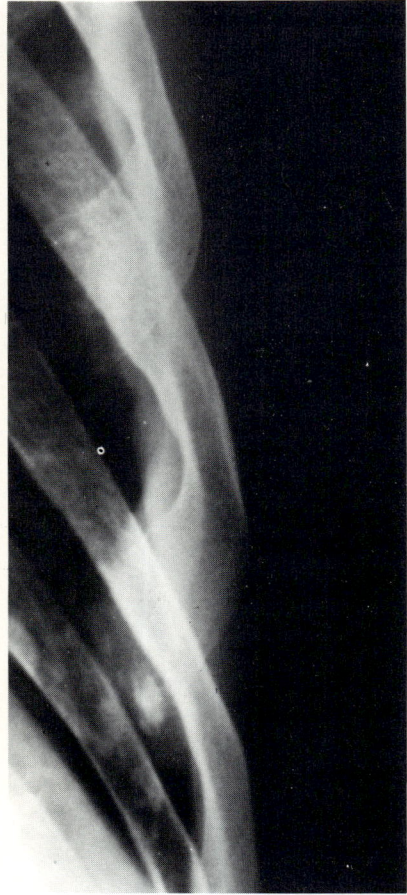

Fig. 2-25. *Oblique projection; rib detail techniques to show calcified and noncalcified plaques.*

The shape of the calcifications differs according to location. Peripheral plaques (as opposed to mediastinal and diaphragmatic plaques) may exhibit the forms shown in Figure 2-4A. Usually in the geographic, rectangular, and circular forms the periphery is more dense on the x-rays. The steplike and lobulated forms that usually lie closely adjacent to the lateral chest wall on frontal views may appear homogeneously dense on the x-ray. The areas appearing most dense will alter with varying projections as thicker parts of the plaque become tangential to the beam.

Mediastinal plaques do not show such a varied radiographic appearance.

They are almost always linear shadows, continuous or interrupted, of varying thicknesses and length. They present in frontal radiographs as long plaques of calcification, 0.5–2 cm on either or both sides of the vertebral column. If both the anterior and posterior mediastinal pleural reflections are calcified, there will be a double or tramline shadow, about 1 cm apart. On the left side, differentiation from calcification of the descending aorta is needed. The mediastinal pleura may also be calcified where it lies against the heart. It is indistinguishable from localized periocardial calcifications or myocardial calcifications. In some asbestos surveys, in fact, it was considered as being pericardial in location. Like paravertebral mediastinal pleural plaques, it is linear. It parallels the heart border, being more common on the left side. It may lie adjacent to the left atrial appendage, near the area of opposite pulsations, i.e., just below the outflow tract of the right ventricle or in the area of the left ventricular wall. In the latter position, differentiation from pericardial calcification, calcification in a transmural myocardial infarct, or intracavitary myxoma may be difficult. The rare calcifications along the right heart border are adjacent to the right atrium. The preponderance along the left heart border compared with the right has been stated to result from the increased mechanical irritation of the asbestos fibers when adjacent to the pumping heart. Since more of the plaques have been reported adjacent to the left atrium than adjacent to the left ventricle, this concept may be incorrect.

Calcifications along the diaphragm are restricted to the more rigid central aponeurotic area, as are the hyaline plaques. On lateral view, they are seen beginning at the posterior border of the heart and extending backwards. Since the deeper parts of the plaques calcify, and the outline of the diaphragm on the frontal view may be anterior or posterior to the plane of calcification, the calcifications may or may not parallel the diaphragm. In the lateral view, however, such parallelism usually exists. Low-kilovolt techniques in full inspiration are needed. The shapes are less varied than the subaxillary shadows, with the linear form predominating. Lower rib costal cartilage calcifications projected along or below the diaphragm on the frontal view may simulate a calcified plaque. Some examples are seen in Figure 2-26.

"Talc plaques" described in x-rays of talc workers appear as linear calcifications similar to the above. These calcified plaques were described in the early reports on talcosis. Talc is a hydrated magnesium silicate closely related chemically to several types of asbestos (chrysotile, tremolite, and anthophyllite), and talc deposits usually contain one or more of these minerals.[34,35] Plaques occurring after talc exposure are probably due to an associated asbestos content rather than to talc fibers, but current evidence is not

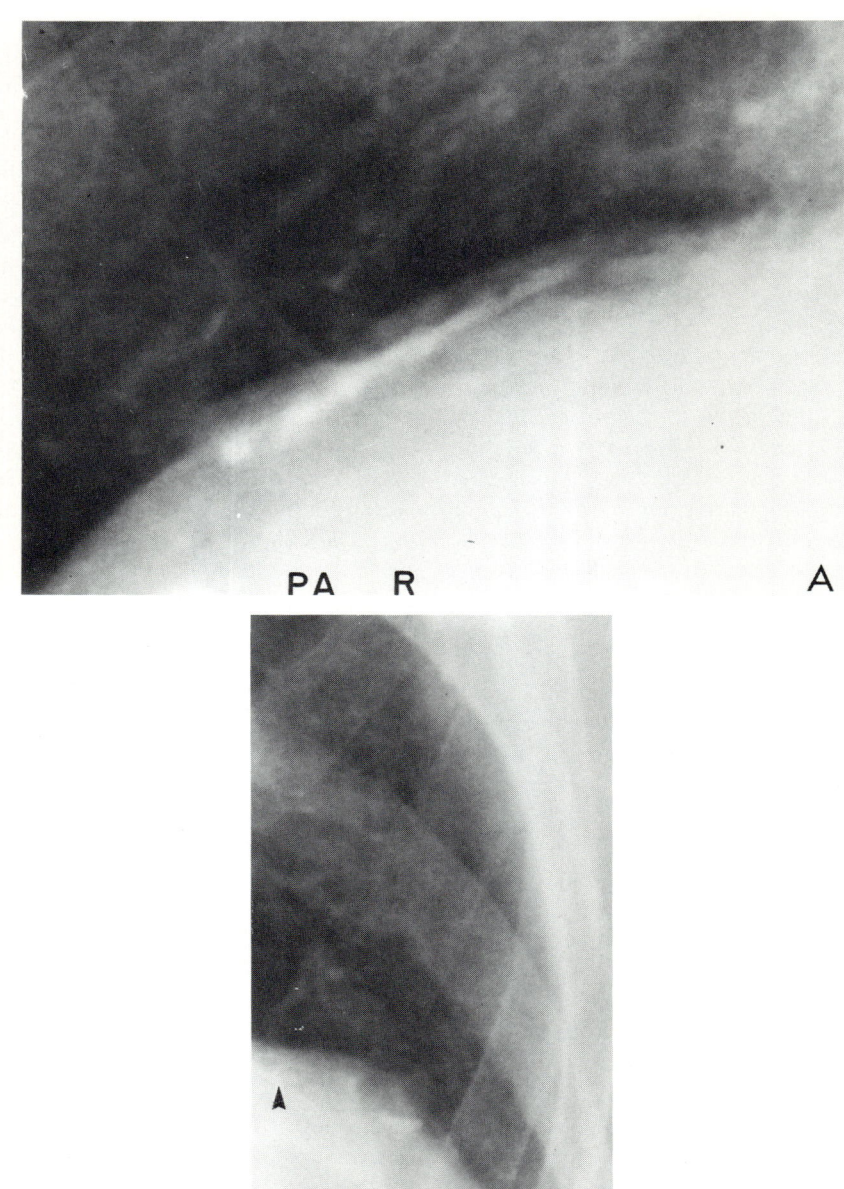

PA R A

B PA L

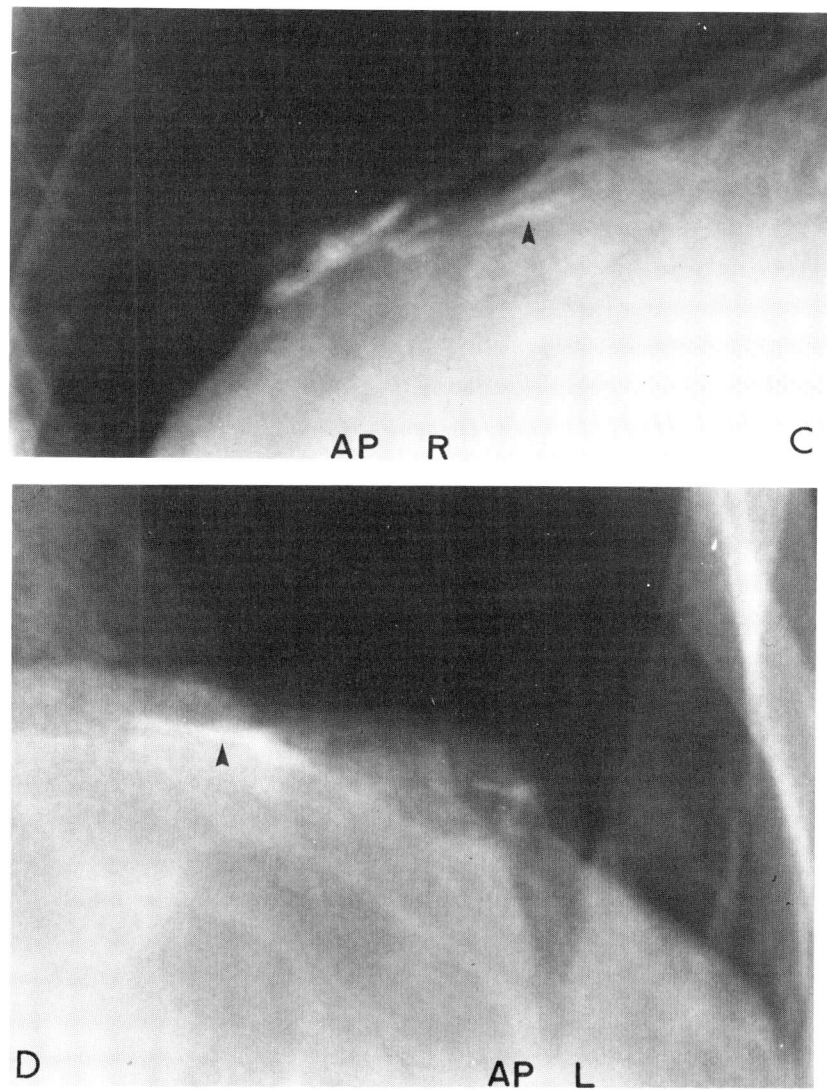

Fig. 2-26. *Value of AP and PA projections. A and B are PA views of the right and left hemidiaphragm. In C and D which are the AP views, the calcification in medial parts of the hemidiaphragms (arrows) become more apparent. For geometric reasons, better definition of posterior located diaphragmatic calcification will be obtained by AP views. An overpenetrated view (D) is an additional aid.*

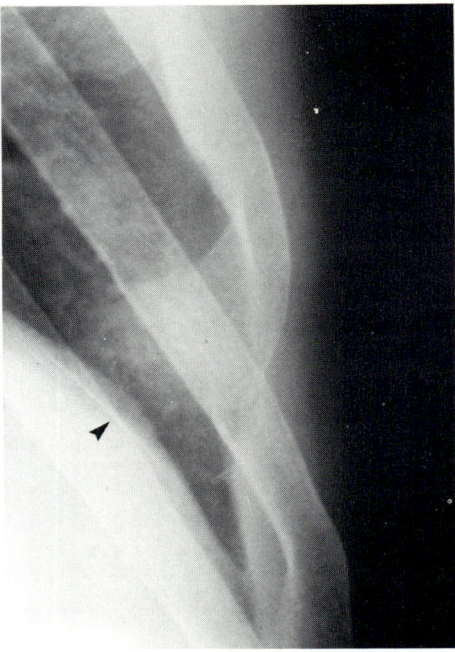

Fig. 2-27. *Anterior pleural plaques. Oblique view shows pleural plaques in unusually anterior locations. There is also linear diaphragmatic calcification (arrow).*

conclusive. Occasional case reports have described calcified pleural plaques in chronic mineral oil aspiration, sceroderma, and after irradiation.

Significance of Visceral Pleural Thickening After Asbestos Exposure

Radiography cannot distinguish between diffuse thickening of visceral and parietal pleura (interlobar fissures excepted) (see Fig. 2-27). Diffuse thickening of the visceral pleura is seen after asbestos exposure as a "dry" pleurisy[33] or as residual from a resolved asbestos effusion. Diffuse lateral chest wall shadowing and thickening of the interlobar fissures may result from many types of pleural exudates and transudates, and in an asbestos worker the contribution from asbestos exposure is always conjectural.

Pleural Plaques Associated with and Obscuring More Serious Asbestos-related Lung Disease

Masking of Small Peripheral Pulmonary Carcinoma by Large Parietal Pleural Plaques

There is a predominance of asbestos-related lung cancer in the lower lobes, the areas that usually contain the greatest proportion of ferruginous bodies and the greatest degree of pulmonary fibrosis. The difficulty in the early detection of bronchogenic carcinoma in severely fibrotic regions is discussed in Chapter 2, Section 2. Since parietal pleural plaques predominate adjacent to the sixth to tenth ribs and the diaphragm, and since many asbestos-related lung cancers are peripheral in location, especially the adenocarcinoma, the early radiographic detection of these tumors may be difficult. Stereoscopic and oblique projections should be used, but their value is limited if a large plaque and a small peripheral carcinoma are adjacent. Tomographic sections at close intervals should be made (Fig. 2-86). Oat cell and squamous cell carcinomas are also common in patients with asbestos exposure, but these tumors are usually more central and less likely to be masked by plaques. CT may prove very helpful. The axial images should be valuable in separating the adjacent shadows due to a plaque and those due to a peripheral carcinoma.

Asbestos Pleural Effusion Masking Parietal Pleural Plaques

A pleural effusion is a rare stigma of asbestos exposure (Chapter 2, Section 3) (see Fig. 2-28). In may be unilateral or bilateral and may resolve completely or be recurrent over many years. The fluid is an exudate that does not contain asbestos fibers. For this reason and also because such effusions are rarely associated with recognizable plaques, the cause is often difficult to ascertain. The easiest technique for identification of any accompanying plaques is a steep Trendelenburg* decubitus view which permits the exudate to move toward the lung apex and so uncover the pleura adjacent the lower ribs. Unlike the usual decubitus view for pleural effusion, the exposure should be made in both the inspiratory and expiratory phases. An elevated diaphragm in the expiratory phase may obscure some of the lower plaques, although the effusion is seen more easily in this phase.

*Friederich Trendelenburg (1844–1924) is alleged to have performed the first unsuccessful pulmonary embolectomy! (Brauerei Schwechat A.G, Hopfen-Archiv.)

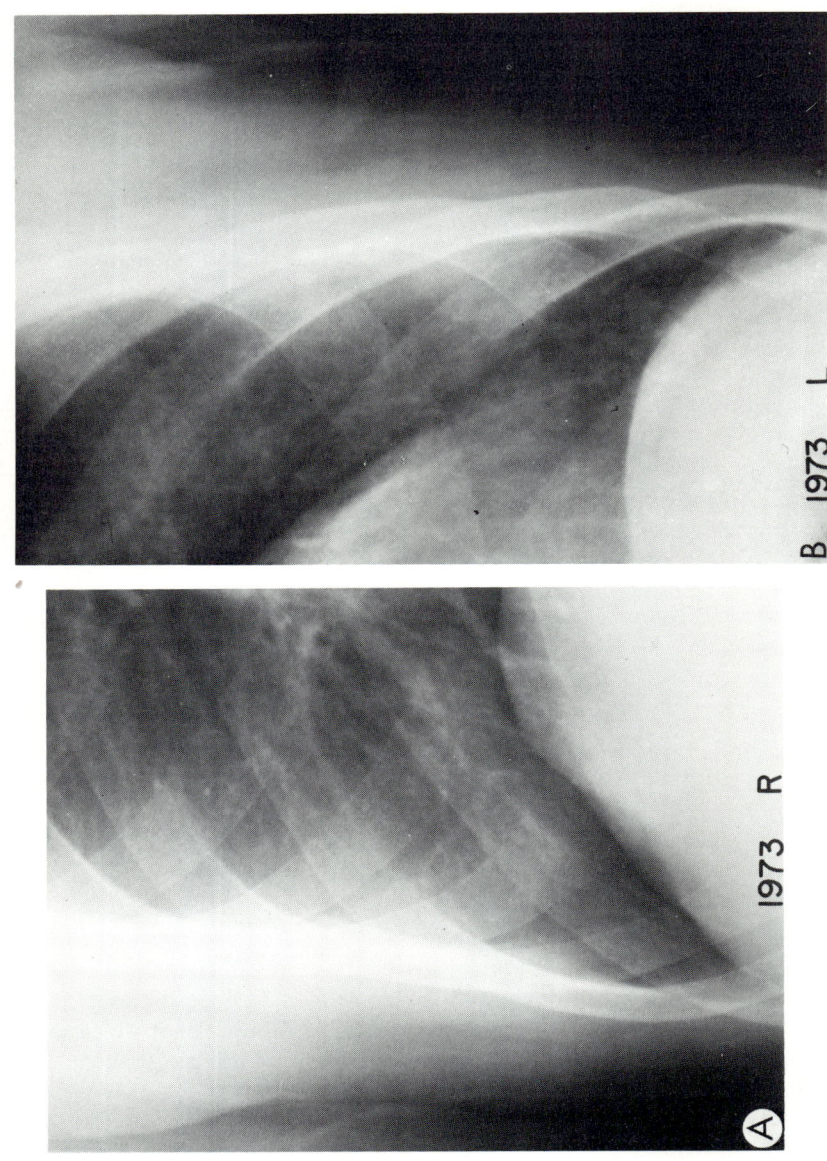

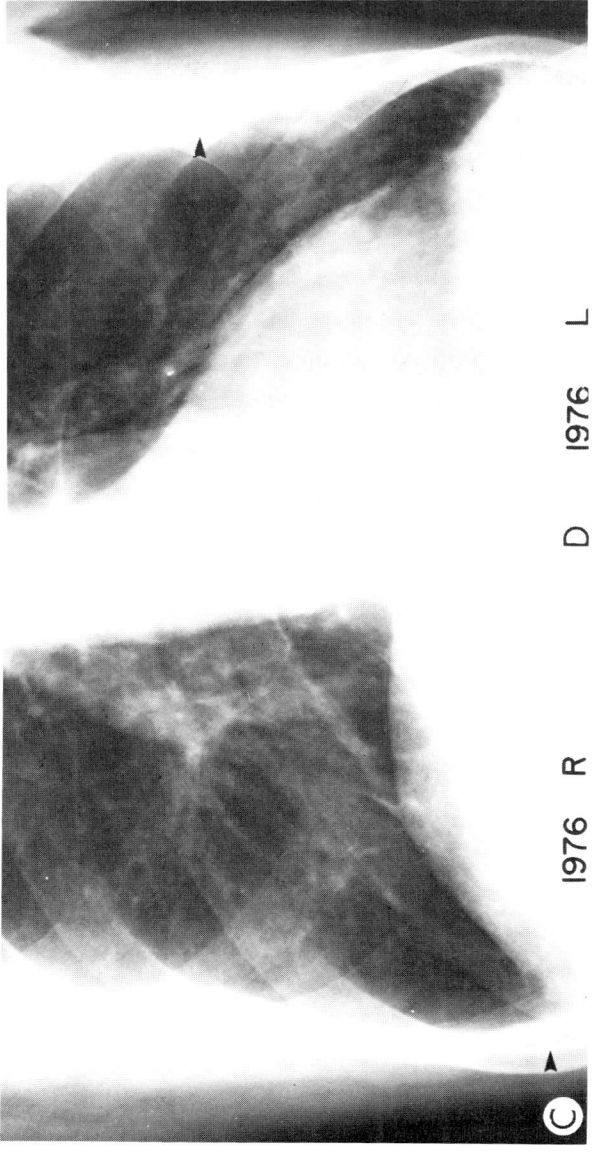

Fig. 2-28. Pleural plaques and pleural effusion. In 1973 (A and B), both lungs appear normal. In 1976 (C) an asbestos effusion had developed on the right (arrow), and on the left (D) noncalcified pleural plaques (arrow) and a tiny effusion are present.

Association of Plaques in Asbestos-related Mesothelioma

The presence of pleural plaques is a potentially useful "marker" in the radiographic diagnosis of mesothelioma. Unfortunately, very few x-rays of patients with pleural mesothelioma show identifiable plaques. Pleural plaques are more evident in association with peritoneal mesotheliomata. These patients have usually had a heavy crocidolite exposure, and it is conjectured[36] that the type of fiber is of importance. It is acceptable that a mesothelioma of any size would envelop and obscure parietal pleural plaques. But why are they so rarely visible beyond the radiographic shadow of a mesothelioma or on the contralateral side? Postulating that some fibers predispose to plaque formation and others to mesothelioma induction would appear reasonable because anthophyllite asbestos production in Finland is associated with a high incidence of parietal pleural plaque formation but not mesothelioma.[37-39] Furthermore, anthophyllite gives rise to plaque production at an early stage of exposure, and these should have attained a large size and be reasonably recognizable should mesothelioma have developed in exposed workers. Chrysotile mining is known to be related to a low incidence of mesothelioma. Yet in two Quebec chrysotile mines, the one with the higher dust exposure had a high incidence of both mesothelioma and pleural plaque formation, quite unlike the situation in Finland, where plaque formation is common and mesotheliomata rare. South African N.W. Cape crocidolite exposure entails a high risk of mesothelioma induction and of pleural plaque formation, but the incidence of mesothelioma combination varies with the manganese content of the asbestos.[40] Furthermore, crocidolite and amosite ore often intermingle in the same rock formation, although pure amosite is a lesser cause of mesothelioma induction.[16a,16b] Excluding anthophyllite, which causes pleural plaques only (only one anthophyllite worker is known to have developed mesothelioma), the other three major fibers all cause both pleural plaques and mesotheliomata to varying degrees. It ensues that some unknown factor is responsible for the relatively few pleural plaques seen in asbestos workers who develop mesotheliomata.

REFERENCES

1. Jones JSP, Sheers G: Pleural plaques, in Bogovski P, Gilson JC, Timbrell V, et al (eds): Biological effects of Asbestos. Lyon, IARC Scientific Publications, 1973, pp 243-248
2. Thomson JG: The pathogenesis of pleural plaques, 1969, in Shapiro HA

(ed): Pneumoconiosis. Proceedings of the International Conference, Johannesburg, 1969, Capetown OUP, pp 138–141
3. LeBouffant L, Martin JC, Durif S, et al: Structure and composition of pleural plaques, in Bogovski P, Gilson JC, Timbrell V, et al (eds): Biological Effects of Asbestos. Lyon, IARC Scientific Publications, 1973, pp 249–257
4. Kiviluoto R: Asbestosis: Aspects of its radiological features, in Shapiro HA (ed): Pneumoconiosis. Proceedings of the International Conference, Johannesburg, 1969, Capetown OUP, pp 253–255
5. Rom WM, Palmer PES: The spectrum of asbestos related diseases. West J Med 121:10–21, 1974
6. Fletcher DE, Edge JR: The early radiological changes in pulmonary and pleural asbestosis. Clin Radiol 21:355–365, 1970
7. Hourihane DOB, Lessof L, Richardson PC: Hyaline and calcific pleural plaques as an index of exposure to asbestos. A study of radiological and pathological features of 100 cases with a consideration of epidemiology. Br Med J 1:1069–1074, 1966
8. Meurman L: Asbestos bodies and pleural plaques in a Finnish series of autopsy cases. Acta Pathol Microbiol Scand Suppl 181:8, 1976
9. Roberts GH: The pathology of parietal pleural plaques. J Clin Pathol 24:348, 1971
10. Enticknap JB, Smithers WJ: Peritoneal tumors in asbestosis. Br J Ind Med 21:20–31, 1964
11. Black LF: The pleural space and pleural fluid. Mayo Clinic Proc 47:493–506, 1972
12. Roe FJC, Carter RL, Walters MA, et al: The pathological effects of subcutaneous injections of asbestos fibers in mice: Migration of fibers to submesothelial tissues and induction of mesothelioma. Int J Cancer 2:628–638, 1976
13. Navratil M: Pleural calcification due to asbestos exposure compared with relevant findings in the non-exposed population. Inhaled particles and vapors, III. Walton WH (ed): Proceedings of the British Occupational Hygiene Society Symposium, London, 1970. Old Woking, 1970, pp 695–701
14. Stanfield D, Edge JR: Circulating rheumatoid factors and antinuclear antibodies in shipyard asbestos workers with pleural plaques. Br J Dis Chest, 1974, pp 68–166
15. Rossiter CE, Bristol LJ, Cartier PA, et al: Radiographic changes in chrysotile asbestos mines and mill workers of Quebec. Arch Environ Health, Chicago, 1972, pp 388–400

16a. Selikoff IJ: The occurrence of pleural calcifications among asbestos insulation workers. Ann NY Acad Sci 132:351–367, 1965
16b. Selikoff IJ: Mortality of factory workmen exposed to amosite asbestos. Proceedings of the IV International Conference on Pneumoconiosis, Bucharest, 1971. Apimonch
17. Anderson HA, Lilis R, Daum S, et al: Household-contact asbestos neoplastic risk. Ann NY Acad Sci 271:311–323, 1976
18. Yazicioglu S: Pleural calcifications associated with exposure to chrysotile asbestos in southeast Turkey. Chest 70:43–47, 1976
19. Hazards of asbestos in dentistry. Council on dental therapeutics. Council on dental material and devices. J Am Dent Assoc 92:777–778, 1976
20. Leathart GL: Pulmonary function tests in asbestos workers. Trans Soc Occup Med 18:49–55, 1968
21. Rom W, Thornton J, Miller A, et al: Abnormal spirometry in shipyard workers with pleural disease. Am Rev Respir Dis 115(4)part 2:239, 1977
22. Becklake MR, Fournier-Massey GG, McDonald JC, et al: Lung function in relation to chest radiographic changes in Quebec asbestos workers. Bull Physiopathol Respir (Nancy) 6:637, 1970
23. Fletcher DE: Mortality study of shipyard workers with pleural plaques. Br J Ind Med 29:142–145, 1972
24. Edge J: Asbestos related lung disease in a British shipbuilding population with particular regard to the incidence of bronchial carcinoma in men with pleural plaques. A mortality study. Am Rev Respir Dis 115(4)part 2:211, 1977
25. Lewinsohn HC: Early malignant changes in pleural plaques due to asbestos exposure: A case report. Br J Ind Chest 68:121–127, 1974
26. Navratil M, Dobias J: Development of pleural hyalinosis in long term studies of persons exposed to asbestos dust. Environ Res 6:455–472, 1973
27. Audsley WP, Latham SM, Rossiter CE: Film sizes for radiography of the chest. Radiography 36:70–72, 1970
28. Bohlig H, Gibson JC: Radiology, in Bogovski P, Gilson JC, Timbrell V, et al (eds): Biological Effects of Asbestos. Lyon, IARC Scientific Publications, 1973, pp 25–30
29. Christensen EE, Curry TS, Nunnally J: An introduction to the physics of diagnostic radiology. Philadelphia, Lee and Febiger, 1973
30. Goldberg BB, Kotler MN, Ziskin MC, et al: Diagnostic uses of ultrasound. New York, Grune & Stratton, 1975, pp 137–142
31. Viikeri M: Ultrasound examination of pleural plaques. Acta Radiol (Suppl), 1970, p 301

32. Kreel L: Computer tomography in the evaluation of pulmonary asbestos. Acta Radiol (Diag) 17(4):4-5-412, 1976
33. Solomon A, Webster I: The visceral pleura in asbestosis. Environ Res 11:218-234, 1976
34. Smith AR: Pleural calcification resulting from exposure to certain dusts. Am J Roentgenol 67:375, 1952
35. Fehre W: Ueber doppelseitige Pleura-Verkalkungen infolge beruflicher Stubeinwirkungen. Fortschr Roentgenst 85:16, 1956
36. Parkes RW: Personal communication
37. Kiviluoto R: Pleural calcifications as a roentgenological sign of non-occupational endemic anthophyllite asbestosis. Acta Radiol (Suppl), 1960, p 194
38. Meurman L: Pleural fibrocalcific plaques and asbestos exposure. West J Med 121:10-21, 1974
39. Kiviluoto R, Meurman L: In Shapir HA (ed): Pneumoconiosis. Proceedings of the International Conference, Johannesburg, 1969, Capetown OUP, 1969, pp 190-191
40. Webster I: Malignancy in relation to crocidolite and amosite, in Bogovski P, Gilson JC, Timbrell V, et al (eds): Biological Effects of Asbestos. Lyon IARC Scientific Publications, 1973, pp 195-198

SECTION 2
PULMONARY FIBROSIS

Inorganic dusts may be fibrogenic, such as asbestos and free silica, or nonfibrogenic, such as iron and tin. Diffuse pulmonary fibrosis represents an end-stage lung response to many other causes, much as ulceration is common to many colonic diseases and nephrosclerosis to many renal insults. Thus, other conditions must be borne in mind when assessing the radiographs of those with asbestos exposure, since not only are there similarities but also two conditions may coexist, e.g. sarcoidosis and asbestos-related pleural plaques or changes due to silica and asbestos as in cement-asbestosis, and in addition, asbestos workers may be free of asbestos-induced lung disease but have pulmonary changes resulting from some other disease or drug causing fibrosis.

A brief classification of the causes of widespread pulmonary fibrosis is given based on pathophysiological etiology[1] and contains three main groups:

1. Fibrosis secondary to granuloma formation
2. Fibrosis secondary to alveolar exudate
3. Fibrosis secondary to inorganic dust

FIBROSIS SECONDARY TO GRANULOMA FORMATION

In the acute stages of sarcoidosis, berylliosis, and extrinsic allergic alveolitis due to inhalation of organic dusts, granulomas are formed in all zones of the lungs. However, in the healing stages, fibrosis is predominantly in the upper zones.

FIBROSIS SECONDARY TO ALVEOLAR EXUDATE

Inflammatory and noninflammatory exudates may progress to diffuse alveolar wall fibrosis. Cytotoxic agents such as O_2, busulphan, hexamethomium, bleomycin, beryllium, and vanadium may be responsible. Exudates resulting from hypersensitivity to nitrofurantoin and salazopyrine may lead to fibrosis. Aspiration and viral pneumonias and the changes due to disseminated intravascular coagulation may lead to diffuse fibrosis. All of the above may have definable radiographic changes. The fibrosis that may follow continuous elevation of left atrial pressure rarely is demonstrable radiographically. A final group, where immunologic factors are possibly important, include acute cryptogenic fibrosing alveolitis, systemic lupus erythematosus, and idiopathic hemosiderosis. In this broad group of diseases, pulmonary fibrosis is a sequel of tissue necrosis and occurs predominantly in the lower lobes (the necrosis may persist, so that healing is by scarring and not by resolution).

FIBROSIS SECONDARY TO INORGANIC DUST

It has been noted that fibrosis secondary to granuloma occurs predominantly in the upper lobes, while that following alveolar exudates occurs mainly in the lower lobes.[1] The fibrosis that follows inhalation of silica and coal dust is usually found in the upper zones, but that related to asbestosis is usually more apparent in the lower zones. There has been no acceptable explanation for this difference. Since there is preferential ventilation of the lower lobes, the corollary that there is impaired clearance from the upper lobes could be used to explain the upper lobe predominance of silicosis. It is apparent that no single theory can explain satisfactorily the upper lobe fibrotic changes in silicosis and the lower lobe changes in asbestosis, especially when recent reports state there is a more or less uniform distribution of inhaled ferruginous bodies[2] and asbestos fibers[3] throughout the lungs. Earlier reports stated a more basal distribution of these bodies.

MICROSCOPIC APPEARANCE

The basic lesion of asbestos-related pulmonary fibrosis is widespread peribronchiolar fibrosis. This is the end stage. Initially there is an intraluminal reaction within the alveoli to entrapped asbestos dust. Within the alveolar lumina the asbestos fibers, macrophages, and desquamated cell debris become organized by strands of reticulin and later collagen. The type I lining cells of the alveolar walls become replaced by type II granular pneumocytes. Some of the alveoli become walled off.[4] Initially, only the alveoli arising from scattered individual respiratory bronchioles are affected. With increasing asbestos dust exposure or with the advent of immunologic factors, an interstitial reaction spreads to involve other adjacent respiratory bronchioles and then spreads from these peripherally to their alveoli. It is customary to describe the fibrosis as interstitial despite the alveolar wall involvement.

The development of fibrosis has been studied in rats exposed to asbestos dust of varying intensity and for varying periods.[5] Transposing data obtained from experimental animals to humans may be misleading in that, for rats, the order of increasing fibrogenesis is anthophyllite and Canadian crysotile, crocidolite and Rhodesian crysotile, and finally amosite, which does not parallel clinical experience. Of value, however, is the similarity of histological appearances in animals and humans. In both experimental animals and patients, macrophages collect in the alveoli in which the fibers become deposited, and the alveolar walls react by replacing their type I lining cells by type II granular pneumocytes. This is reminiscent of the findings in desquamative interstitial pneumonia[6] in which type II granular pneumocytes line distal air sacs, and radiographs show a predominantly basilar change; desquamative interstitial pneumonia is probably an early stage in the development of diffuse fibrosis from many causes. As the experimental lesions progress, the reaction spreads to involve the adjacent respiratory bronchioles, alveolar ducts, atria, and alveoli, and coalescence of nearby involved areas occurs. Much of the lung parenchyma is eventually replaced by collagen, which distorts airways to leave air spaces that contribute to the honeycomb appearance seen on radiographs.

GROSS APPEARANCE

The lower lobe preponderance has been commented on. Involvement of the upper or middle lobes may be seen in severe cases or when the patient has been exposed to quartz (silica) or talc[7] in addition to asbestos. The fibrosis is usually plentiful in subpleural areas, giving the lung surface a whitish, puckered appearance up to 1 cm thick. The parenchyma when cut is brown-red and feels indurated. The lung volumes are reduced in severe cases; if there is much accompanying panlobar emphysema and only mild fibrosis, lung volume may be increased. Hilar node involvement does not occur unless there is a mixture of asbestos and silicosis. If bronchiole thickening and distortion are severe, the cut surface of the lung may exhibit a "honeycomb" appearance, the walls of the honeycomb "cells" being the interweaving fibrotic airway walls.

PATHOGENESIS

The laying down of collagen by fibroblast is termed fibrogenesis. In asbestosis, the fibrosis is diffuse, while in silicosis, it is more nodular. The pathogenesis of asbestos-related fibrosis may be considered under three aspects:

1. The role of macrophages
2. Influence of fiber size and shape
3. Immunologic factors

Role of Macrophages

The mechanism of fibrogenesis is probably the same for all asbestos fibers, even though amosite and crocidolite are more fibrogenic than chrysotile and anthophyllite. The wandering macrophages that are attracted to inhaled asbestos fibers play a key role. It is thought that the strongly fibrogenic fibers (amosite and crocidolite) stimulate macrophages to release substances that induce fibroblasts to lay down collagen and so produce fibrosis. The less fibrogenic fibers, chrysotile and anthophyllite, are more cytotoxic and may injure the macrophages to such an extent that these fibrogenic substances are not released[8] or are released in smaller amounts.

The degree of macrophage cytotoxicity of asbestos is related to magnesium content. Adherence of fibers to surface membranes of macrophages is in part dependent on the presence of magnesium hydroxide, the removal of magnesium, or its inactivation by chelation, which will reduce the surface cytotoxic effect of chrysotile.[9] Sialoglycoproteins in cell membranes interact with asbestos fibers to produce protein clusters that alter cell membrane permeability and may allow early release of fibrogenic substances from the macrophages. A defense mechanism is present in that the surface macrophage cytotoxic effect is inhibited by the presence of human protein or bronchial secretions.[10]

Following the attachment of asbestos fibers to macrophage surface membrane and initiation of the early cytotoxic effects described above, some of the fibers of small size are ingested and interact with membranes around secondary lysosomes. There is then a secondary release of enzymes, such as β glucoronidase, β galoctosidose and lactic dehydrogenase, lipids, and lipoproteins that cause adjacent fibroblasts to lay down collagen. Ferritin is synthesized in the secondary lysosomes containing asbestos fibers and contributes to asbestos body formation.[8]

Thus, asbestos probably does not have a direct effect on fibroblasts in producing pulmonary fibrosis. Instead, asbestos fibers are absorbed onto the surface of macrophages, the smaller particles ingested, and fibrogenic substances released in two phases as described above.

A purely mechanical effect of asbestosis fibers in the production of fibrosis is not generally accepted. However, evidence for a mechanical effect is quoted by Harrington.[11] There is, however, some conflicting evidence in regard to pleural fibrosis being produced by mechanical effect after inoculation of pleural space in experimental animals.[12]

The role of chemical factors, including trace elements associated with asbestos fibers in fibrogenesis, has been considered. Asbestos fibers are soluble to varying degrees, with chrysotile more soluble than the amphiboles (amosite, anthophyllite, and crocidolite), and silicic acid and metals in or on the surface of asbestos fibers are potential causes of fibrosis. The various biologically active metallic cations probably play a part via an effect on macrophages as indicated above.

Role of Fiber Size and Shape

Fiber size and shape govern penetration of and retention in airways, and particle size is a factor in ingestion of fibers fragmented by macrophages. The characteristic size and shape of asbestos fibers are shown in Figure 2-6; the amphiboles are rectilinear but of varying diameters, the largest being anthophyllite, then amosite, and finally crocidolite, while chrysotile is curly or serpentiform in shape. The diamteter of chrysotile bundles varies with aggregation of fibers, but the fibers fragment, and ultimate chrysotile fibers may have a diameter as small as 0.03 μm.

Asbestos fibers larger than 200 μm are unlikely to penetrate nasal passages but may reach the lower airways in mouth breathers. Once past the nose, even long thin fibers may pass through the trachea and major airways and reach respiratory bronchioles where they tend to be deposited at bifurcation sites. In addition to length, fiber diameter is important, the aerodynamic diameter of the asbestos fibers and particles controlling their falling speed. Asbestos fibers of diameters greater than about 3 μm are unlikely to reach alveoli. Most of inhaled fibers do not reach the lower airways because the ciliary escalator mechanism is so efficient that 99 percent is removed from the airways, although some of this will be subsequently passed over the epiglottis and swallowed, with implications in induction of gastrointestinal malignancy.[13]

The needlelike amphiboles penetrate the lung more effectively than do curly chrysotile fibers, but since chrysotile has a tendency to physically disintegrate into fibers of short arcs, these fragments may behave as the rectilinear amphiboles.[14] Further penetration of fibers and particles to the pleura occurs via interstitial lymph and macrophages. Experimental studies show fibers in subvisceral pleural location in the following order of descending concentration: crocidolite, amosite, anthophyllite, and chrysotile.[15] Relating penetrability to fiber type requires qualification in that fiber size varies with the stage of processing, being greatest in mining and least, and therefore of more penetrating power, in the asbestos textile industry. Size and shape may vary within mineralogic type, Australian crocidolite being of a smaller diameter than South African N.W. Cape crocidolite, which is, in turn, of finer diameter than Transvaal crocidolite.

Fiber particle size limits ingestion by macrophages. Short fibers (less than 5 μm) are completely ingested by macrophages, intermediate size particles (5–25 μm) may or may not be completely ingested, and long fibers (more than 25 μm) are never completely taken up. With the long fibers, several macrophages may be needed to completely engulf a single fiber.[8] Longer fibers are more fibrogenic than short ones. Long ones are less well phagocytosed and transported away.[11] Lauweryms and Baert provide a recent excellent and detailed account of alveolar clearance of particles and the role of the pulmonary lymphatics.[16]

Immunologic Factors

There is experimental work suggesting that antinuclear antibodies may accelerate disease started by a different agent, and antinuclear antibodies are found in 25 percent of asbestos patients,[1] those with severe fibrosis usually being ANA positive. Initial reports suggested that the presence of HLA-B27 antigens makes an asbestos worker more susceptible to the development of severe as opposed to mild pulmonary fibrosis. More recently, this has been disputed. In a group mainly exposed to chrysotile, there was no correlation between HLA-B27 antigen prevalence and the presence or absence of pulmonary fibrosis.[20] But HLA-B12 was more prevalent in those with pulmonary fibrosis and HLA-BW5 was more prevalent in those without pulmonary fibrosis, raising the possibility that these two antigens provide susceptibility to or protection from the development of fibrosis. The matter is discussed more fully in Chapter 1.

Relation Between Asbestos Dust Burden and Severity of Fibrosis

The retained asbestos load in the lung may be estimated by many techniques. If light microscopy is used, only fibers of 0.4 μm or greater in diameter will be seen; since most asbestos dust particles are less than 0.3 μm diameter, electron microscopy is needed for an accurate estimate. Fortunately, the percentage of optically visible fibers is reasonably constant between 12 and 30 percent of total, so that light microscopy data may be extrapolated to give an estimate of total asbestos load.[17]

Using these techniques, the dust load–fibrosis relationship for asbestos differs from that found with silicosis. In the latter the severity of pulmonary fibrosis is proportional to the silicic content of the lungs. With mild and moderate asbestos loads in the lungs, there is an increasing severity of pulmonary fibrosis, but in severe pulmonary fibrosis, there is no correlation with a further increase in fiber concentration.[18] Additionally, no relationship was found between severity of pulmonary fibrosis, duration of exposure, time from first exposure, or time from last exposure to death. The suggestion is made, at least for the amphiboles that were the predominant fiber, that mild and moderate degrees of pulmonary fibrosis are proportionately related to dust burden but that further transition to severe pulmonary fibrosis depends on the interaction of some additional factors. Infection is one possible factor,[19] and prompt treatment would thus be needed even in apparently minor respiratory infections in asbestos workers to halt progression of fibrosis. A second possibility is that the asbestos fibers may initiate fibrosis that may progress to a moderate severity but that an immune mechanism may intervene to produce severe fibrosis.

VARIANTS OF ASBESTOSIS

Asbestos-related pulmonary fibrosis may be atypical, and there are some variants of clinical and radiological interest:

1. Cryptogenic fibrosing alveolitis
2. Household contact asbestosis
3. Massive fibrosis
4. Caplan's syndrome
5. Cement asbestosis

Cryptogenic Fibrosing Alveolitis

A proportion of patients thought to have nonspecific interstitial pulmonary fibrosis (cryptogenic fibrosing alveolitis) may have an undetected history of asbestos exposure or a biopsy specimen may have been examined with light microscopy only and a false underestimate of asbestos burden obtained. This may apply especially to chrysotile, which fragments into tiny particles. In one patient, light microscopy revealed fibrosis and inflammatory changes but no ferruginous bodies.[21] Electron microscopy showed large numbers of small (less than 5 μm) chrysotile fibers. The inference was made that some patients diagnosed as having fibrosing alveolitis or desquamative interstitial pneumonia may, in fact, have asbestosis.

This inference produced some engagingly sarcastic correspondence in the *New England Journal of Medicine,* with Miller et al.[22] restating their belief that particles of less than 5 μm are fibrogenic, while Gross et al.[23] found this statement questionable.

Household Contact Asbestosis

Within the group of cryptogenic alveolitis patients, there are some who had household contacts with former asbestos workers who carried asbestos in their clothes, shoes, or hair. Anderson et al., in a study of 326 individuals who have had household contact with amosite asbestos workers, found 36 percent with pleural or parenchymal changes typical of asbestos exposure; children had a greater proportion of involvement than wives or siblings.[24] Pleural changes without pulmonary fibrosis were seen more frequently than pulmonary fibrosis alone. There were 4 patients in this group with pleural mesothelioma.

Massive Fibrosis

A third group includes those with massive upper lobe fibrosis.[7] The reason is unknown, but two-thirds of this group had positive PPD skin tests even though there was no clinical evidence for active tuberculosis. If one accepts the relationship between immunologic status and severity of pulmonary fibrosis in severely asbestotic patients, an analogy *may* be the upper lobe fibrosis seen in ankylosing spondylitis in which there is a strong association with HLA-B27 antigen. Discrete areas of massive fibrosis extending over areas of more than 1 cm may occasionally be seen in both upper and lower lobes. These have been reported in miners, and it may be that the high quartz content (16 percent of South African asbestos) is responsible.[25]

Caplan's Syndrome

An unusual group comprised those with asbestos-related pulmonary fibrosis who have or develop rheumatoid arthritis. Multiple rounded nodules appear on the chest radiographs, sometimes in crops and mainly in the lower lobes, but any area may be involved. Occasionally, the nodules are unilateral. The nodules vary in size from a few millimeters to a few centimeters; some may cavitate and, if so, may have thick or thin walls. The cavities may fill in later.

They are necrobiotic nodules, similar to those seen in the lungs of some patients with rheumatoid arthritis, but they differ in that they contain asbestos fibers and ferruginous bodies and are not accompanied by subcutaneous nodules. The nodules may proceed, accompany, or follow the onset of rheumatoid arthritis.

In deference to Anthony Caplan, who first described the nodules accompanying coal workers' pneumoconiosis,[26] this entity has been termed Caplan's syndrome in asbestosis.[27-30] This syndrome has also been noted in those

those exposed to silica and pottery manufacture, sand blasting, and brass and iron foundries.[31]

Cement Asbestosis

A large group of patients includes those with cement-asbestos pneumoconiosis. About two-thirds of world production of asbestos is used in cement production. The fiber type will vary with need; crocidolite is preferred when tensile strength and resistance to acid is important, and chrysotile is used if flexibility is needed. The asbestos is mixed in the proportion of 15 to 20 percent with artificial Portland cement that consists of calcium silicate, tricalcium aluminate, and tricalcium ferrite. Portland cement also contains 1 to 5 percent free silicate (SiO_2) and smaller amounts of other oxides (Al, Fe, Mg). Exposed workers may develop a combined pneumoconiosis due to asbestos and silica. Asbestos produces mainly lower lobe fibrosis with irregular and linear opacities, while silica causes rounded parenchymal densities, progressive massive fibrosis, and hilar enlargement with egg shell type calcification.

CLINICAL FEATURES

The symptoms of pulmonary fibrosis may be summarized as dyspnea, frequently with dry cough, and occasionally chest pain. Physical signs may include restricted chest movement, end inspiratory crepitations, and digital clubbing. A broader account is given in Chapter 1.

RADIOGRAPHIC CHANGES

General

Parenchymal radiographic changes resulting from asbestos exposure are not specific (see Figs. 2-29 and 2-30). Excluding the characteristic pleural plaques, the parenthymal changes are those of interstitial fibrosis, which is more severe in the lower lobes, and this finding is common to many disease entities, e.g., scleroderma, desquamative interstitial pneumonia, recurrent aspiration pneumonia, and bronchiectasis. It is therefore important to examine radiographs showing pulmonary fibrosis for the presence of calcified and noncalcified plaques, since these may act as biological markers to suggest the

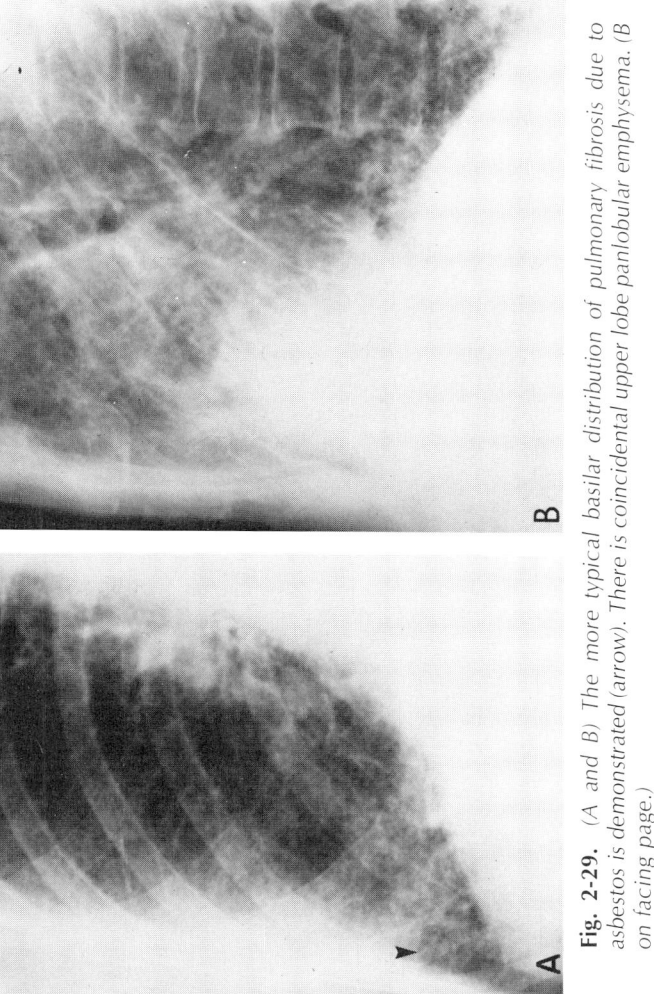

Fig. 2-29. (A and B) The more typical basilar distribution of pulmonary fibrosis due to asbestos is demonstrated (arrow). There is coincidental upper lobe panlobular emphysema. (B on facing page.)

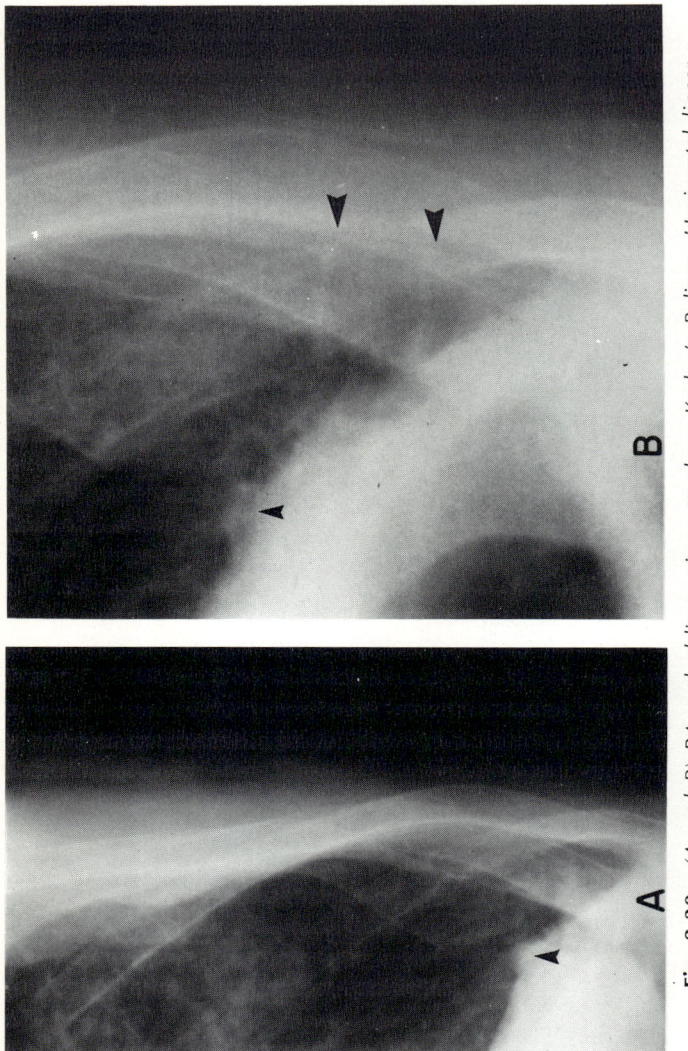

Fig. 2-30. (A and B) PA and oblique views to show Kerley's B lines. Horizontal linear stranding (horizontal arrows in B) as a result of thickening of interlobular septa is common in asbestosis. The interlobular septa may be widened into broad fibrous bands, frequently wider than usually seen with B lines of cardiogenic or oncogenic origins. The interlobular septa may be more apparent in oblique view (B) (see facing page). There are subaxillary and diaphragmatic plaques, (vertical arrows). The incidence of plaques in pulmonary fibrosis has been underestimated with conventional techniques. CT shows many plaques not seen conventionally.

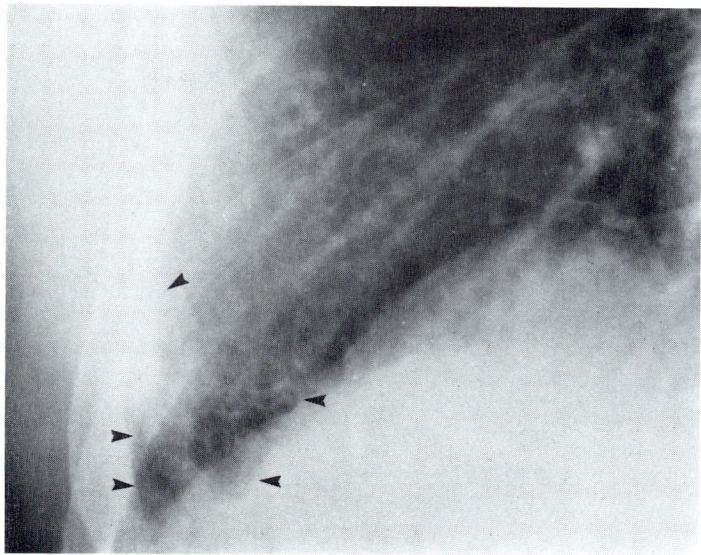

Fig. 2-31. *Lower lobe fibrosis and bullae adjacent to diaphragm (arrows). Contraction of fibrous areas frequently leads to bullae development. A subaxillary plaque is present (oblique arrow).*

cause of the fibrosis (see Fig. 2-31). A proportion of patients with asbestos-related pulmonary fibrosis do not show plaques. In Solomon's series, 25 percent of the South African miners with pulmonary fibrosis did not have pleural plaques in chest x-rays.[32] A similar percentage is stated by Soutar et al. in a study of 84 patients with industrial (nonmining) exposure to asbestos.[33] The absence of plaques has been attributed to differing etiologic mechanisms in the development of plaques and fibrosis or the entrapment of fibers in fibrotic areas so that the pleura is not reached. The latter seems improbable, since the number of plaques increases with the severity of the fibrosis.[34]

The parenchymal fibrotic changes may be classified according to the ILO U/C classification (see Chapter 3) into opacities that may be small or large, rounded due to silica or irregular due to asbestos. Both rounded and irregular opacities coexist if there has been exposure to both of these substances, such as in asbestos cement workers. Rounded and irregular opacities may be present in those who have had asbestos exposure only. There is evidence (discussed later in this section) showing that true summation of overlying shadows will produce a more rounded density of the p, q, r type, while imperfect superimposition tends to produce an s, t, and u type pattern. Profusion of densities is thus of more significance than is the type of density when ILO Classification is used for epidemiological or compensation purposes. The notation is thus purely descriptive and noninterpretative. This has value in epidemiologic surveys and compensation work. It avoids the dangers met with in clinical radiology, where descriptive terms have acquired an interpretative significance. Thus, "honeycombing" (Fig. 2-32) was first used to describe the late phase of histiocytosis-X but is currently commonly applied to the pattern resulting from a variety of interstitial changes, whether from fibrosis as in pulmonary fibrosis, hamartomatous change as in tuberous sclerosis, or inflammation as in bronchiectasis.

In routine radiological assessment of pulmonary fibrosis, one may retain the use of descriptive terms such as round or irregular opacities, but search should also be made for septal lines, ring shadows (honeycombing), and longer hair line shadows.

Most septal lines seen radiographically, are of two types, A and B (see Fig. 2-33). B lines are usually 1–2 cm long and are seen in the lower lung zones touching the pleura at the outer ends. A lines are less easily identified in pulmonary fibrosis because although they are longer than the B lines (2–4 cm), their position radiating from the hilus toward the pleura is often obscured by the fibrotic changes. A lines are therefore best seen in asbestosis in the upper zones, where pulmonary fibrosis is less severe. The B lines are best seen in the anterior and lateral parts of the lower zones in both frontal and oblique x-rays, because in the lingula and middle lobe the connective tissue septa are well developed and the lobules are arranged vertically, resulting in short horizontal septa. The septal lines become thickened, and when extreme, part of the thickness is due to merging with alveolar interstitium that has fibrosed. The thickening extends to the visceral pleura. Retraction of these thickened septa may result in localized areas of panlobular emphysema. Thickened septal C lines producing a reticular pattern result from the visualization of connective tissue septa between peripheral lobules seen en face and superimposed on deeper septa randomly distributed in deeper parts of lung.[35] Confident radiographic identification is greatest with the B lines, less for the A lines, and least for the C lines. B-line identification is complicated by the similar appearance of fine fibrotic lines that occur in early pulmonary fibrosis as a result of thickening of the alveolar interstitium. When they extend to the pleura, differentiation from B lines is impossible. In Solomon's series,[32] 5 of 32 patients had such fine fibrotic lines, which Solomon characterized as fine fibrosis not due to Kerley's B lines, while in Soutars series,[33] 36 percent had septal lines.

Long hairline shadows on radiographs in areas of otherwise normal-appearing lung are an occasional finding; if they do not result from an accessory fissure or linear alveolar atelectasis, they may be due to a prior granulomatous or nongranulomatous inflammatory focus that has healed and

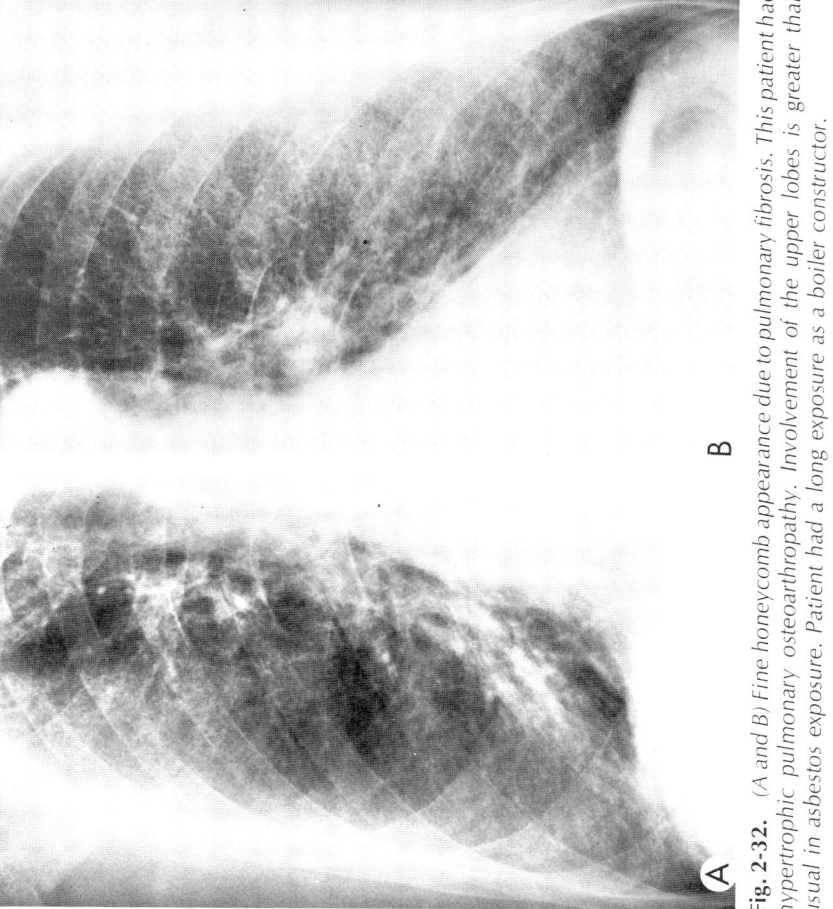

Fig. 2-32. (A and B) Fine honeycomb appearance due to pulmonary fibrosis. This patient had hypertrophic pulmonary osteoarthropathy. Involvement of the upper lobes is greater than usual in asbestos exposure. Patient had a long exposure as a boiler constructor.

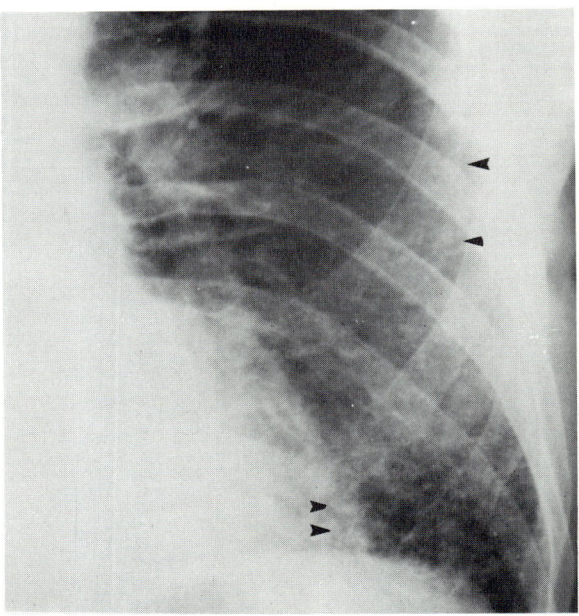

Fig. 2-33. *Pulmonary fibrosis in an asbestos worker. There are thickened interlobular septa (some are indicated by arrows). The increased translucency due to a bulla at the left base allows better visualization of multiple irregularly shaped opacities typical of asbestos exposure. Note the ill-defined cardiac border due to adjacent fibrosis and mediastinal pleural thickening.*

disappeared. The length of these lines may be out of proportion to the preceding focus.

Honeycombing is a radiographic finding in interstitial lung disease, the term being borrowed from the gross pathological finding. Since examination of x-ray films for most twentieth-century physicians has replaced the autopsy room organ recital of prior years, it seems a good term to retain. It indicates replacement of normal lung by small cystlike spaces amidst extensive pulmonary fibrosis.[36] The spaces result from confluence of distal air spaces, and they are lined by atypical cells that have spread distally from the more proximal airways.[37] The pattern is easily assessed with the naked eye on cut surfaces of fibrotic lung. On a chest radiograph, the appearance is recognizable without too much difficulty, but the radiolucent spaces among the fibrotic areas may represent not only the confluent air spaces lined by atypical epithelium but also areas of normal and uninvolved lung and foci of panlobular emphysema. It has been suggested that the diagnosis of honeycombing should be made only when the radiolucencies are round or oval and when the margins are traceable for about 360 degrees.[35] This system is analogous to that used in the diagnosis of other lung cavities. By convention, these radiographic spaces are not greater than 4–10 mm wide and the thickness of their walls vary from hairline to 2 mm.[38] Honeycombing was found in 36 percent of the Brompton Hospital series of industrial asbestos users.[38]

Honeycombing is one type of ring shadow. A second type seen in pulmonary fibrosis results from thickening of connective tissue around the more proximal airways. If seen end on, the airway will present a ring shadow, and if seen along its length, the airway will exhibit a more linear shadow. Because of distortion, the linear appearance is generally more difficult to see in asbestos-related pulmonary fibrosis, although it is a classical sign of fibrosis associated with bronchiectasis. The ring shadow may be of hairline thickness or wider if the fibrotic process has extended deeper into the previously aerated alveoli. The central lucency is due to intraluminal gas.

A shaggy outline of the cardiac silhouette is a nonspecific sign. It has been described in mediastinitis, chronic adhesive pericarditis, and pertussis. It may be due to disease of the pericardium, mediastinal pleura, or lung parenchyma adjacent to the heart. In asbestosis, it may be due to thickening by plaques of the mediastinal parietal, pleural residua of benign pleural effusion affecting the mediastinal visceral pleura, or interstitial fibrosis in those parts of lingula and middle lobe adjacent to the heart. It was seen in 8 percent of William's series.[39]

Small opacities, usually irregular and occasionally rounded in shape with margins that may be sharply or poorly defined, are seen as a result of asbestos exposure. They become obscured if a severe degree of fibrosis develops. Their size varies from a pinpoint to up to 4 mm in diameter for irregular opacities. Large opacities are rarely seen except in variants such as cement asbestosis and as part of Caplan's syndrome with asbestosis. Based on histological studies,[40] these small irregular opacities may originate in terminal air spaces in early stages or in peribronchial interstitium in more advanced phases. The former, which are air space shadows, may spread by extension through airways and pores of Kohn, coalesce, and be characterized by indistinct margins. The latter, being interstitial in location, are surrounded by aerated air spaces and theoretically should have distinct margins. From a practical point of view, this distinction cannot be made on radiographs, since the densities seen, even though some may be rounded and some may be irregularly marginated are composite shadows resulting from summation of overlying densities.[41] Superimposition of opacities not in direct contact will result in poor marginal definition,[35] while perfect superimposition will produce shadows of greater density that may

Table 2-4
Parenchymal Changes in Asbestosis

Findings	Frequency
Pinpoint	29% (many 18%, few 11%)[a]
Irregular opacities 2–4 mm diameter	75% (many 29%, few 46%)
More than 4 mm diameter	20%
Diffuse haze (ground glass appearance, not obviously due to pleural changes)	18%
Septal lines	36%
Honeycombing	36%

[a]The designation "few" is equivalent to the ILO classification of profusion 1/1, and "many" to a profusion of 2/2 or more (see Chapter 3).

falsely suggest sharper margins. With widespread imperfect superimposition, a diffuse gray haze, sometimes referred to as having a "ground glass" appearance, will ensue.

In the group of 84 industrial asbestos workers seen by Soutar et al.,[33] the incidence of the above changes is given in Table 2-4.

Suboptimal radiography may result in an erroneous diagnosis of interstitial fibrosis. A radiograph that is underexposed may produce too dense a shadow of the pectoral muscles, simulating fibrosis. In such an instance the normal lung inferior to the muscle mass will have a greater transradiancy while asbestos related fibrosis in this area would show reduced translucency. A radiograph exposed during an incomplete inspiration, especially in a heavy patient, will show reduced translucency in the basal areas. The use of too low a kilovoltage may make identification of fibrosis difficult. In general there is a tendency to diagnose fibrosis too frequently when interpreting films of those known to have had exposure to asbestos. In particular, the presence of large confluent plaques seen en face produces a hazy appearance that may simulate fibrosis and it is especially in this situation that high kilovoltage techniques are helpful.*

VARIANTS OF X-RAY APPEARANCE

Massive Fibrosis

Massive upper lobe fibrosis is usually symmetrical, but one side may be more involved, producing a tracheal shift. The upper lobes are diffusely involved with hilar retraction, fissural elevation, and rib crowding. Large

*Felson, B. Radiology of the pneumoconioses. Symposium sponsored by American College of Radiology. Jan 13–15, 1978, Washington D.C. (unpublished).

fibrotic masses are occasionally present in the lower lobes, either alone or in combination with upper lobe fibrosis. The role of prior tuberculous infection or the quartz content of asbestos has been noted. The appearance has, however, been seen in some U.S. asbestos workers where quartz content is not a factor.

Caplan's Syndrome

The multiple nodular densities may be unilateral or bilateral, they can vary in size from a few millimeters to a few centimeters, they can necrose to produce thick or thin wall cavities, and they are occasionally accompanied by pleural effusion. The radiological differential diagnosis includes metastatic disease, Hodgkin's disease, septic infarcts, infectious granulomatous disease, Wegener's granulomatosis, staphylococcal pneumatoceles, fungal infections, especially in those with altered immunity, and rheumatoid nodules unrelated to any pneumoconiosis.

Cement Asbestosis

Silico-asbestosis is seen in cement workers who are exposed while mixing asbestos fibers with synthetic Portland cement, which contains calcium silicate. The mixture is then ground, which entails exposure to silica. Those workers exposed develop a mixed pneumoconiosis. Asbestos inhalation is responsible for the characteristic mid and lower zone fibrosis described earlier. Silicosis is responsible for occasional densities of progressive massive fibrosis (Fig. 2-34). In addition, there may be enlarged hilar nodes with eggshell calcification. The large fibrotic areas migrate medially, unlike the very rare localized areas of pulmonary fibrosis in pure asbestosis, which remain in unchanged location, usually in upper lobe. In addition, numerous small opacities are present. These are rounded or irregular in shape. The rounded shadows are due to the effect of silica and the irregular ones, to asbestos. A comparison of the opacities seen in asbestos workers[42] is outlined in Table 2-5. These data differ somewhat from the Bromptom analysis,[33] which although agreeing that irregular opacities are characteristic of asbestos, did include some tiny rounded densities (29 percent of those examined), but the radiographic findings were not related to the type of asbestos exposure. The profusion of rounded opacities correlates better with total mixed dust exposure than does the profusion of irregular opacities.[43] The fact that asbestos exposure alone, as opposed to mixed dust, produces mainly irregular small opacities is further suggested by data from workers in a Finnish anthophyllite mine.[44] Forty percent had small

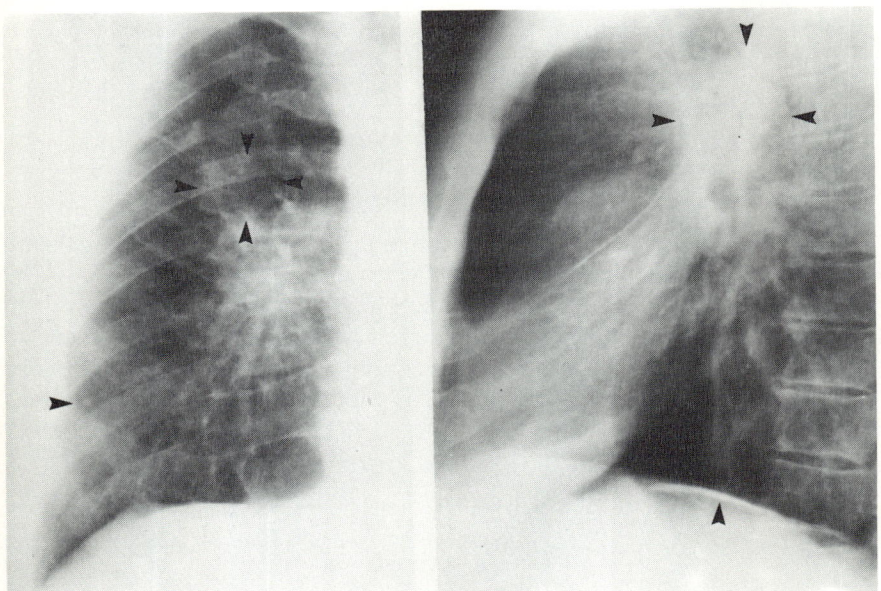

Fig. 2-34. Cement asbestosis. The cement component of cement asbestosis is responsible for the large fibrotic mass in the upper lung fields and the smoothly rounded opacities which are more randomly distributed, both being attributed to the calcium silicate and free silica present in cement. The large fibrotic mass in the upper zone is outlined with arrows. If the frontal view is examined with a hand lens, multiple rounded opacities will be seen; a prominent one is indicated by an arrow in the frontal view. Lateral view shows diaphragmatic calcification due to asbestos.

Table 2-5
Cement Asbestosis

		Exposure	to:
Density Type	Cement Only	Cement-Asbestos	Asbestos Only
Irregular	33%	66%	75%
Rounded	18%	10%	0–2% (none had rounded shadows alone, 2% had both)
Pleural plaques			
Noncalcified	25%	25%	16%
Calcified	2%	7%	9%

parenchymal opacities that were classified as irregular small opacities (86 percent), rounded small opacities (7 percent), and both types (7 percent).

The type of asbestos end product is of importance. Asbestos cement used for production of shingles contains chrysotile but no crocidolite, and those engaged in their manufacture have an immense excess burden of pulmonary fibrosis, while workers manufacturing asbestos cement pipe, which currently contains 3 percent crocidolite and higher percentages in the past, have a 5 to 6 percent burden of lung cancer.

RELATION BETWEEN RADIOGRAPHIC APPEARANCE, EXPOSURE DOSE, AND PULMONARY FIBROSIS

In cement asbestos workers with mainly mild to moderately severe pulmonary fibrosis, the profusion of irregular and rounded opacities is related to total dust exposure.[45] Lung volumes and maximal exploratory flow rates decreased in relation to increasing cumulative asbestos dust exposure. Pulmonary diffusing capacity was not related. Crocidolite exposure produced lower expiratory flow rates and reduced diffusion capacity when compared with chrysotile exposure.[45] Weill et al. concluded for their patients, who generally did not exhibit severe radiographic changes, that both radiological monitoring and pulmonary function testing were necessary to detect the earliest abnormalities in the largest number of exposed workers, since in individual patients, abnormalities may first be identified by radiograph, with pulmonary function tests being normal, or vice versa.

More recently, Roberts et al.[46] in reviewing a large number of patients with pulmonary fibrosis but without an asbestos occupation exposure, thought that a rough estimation of the disease activity may be obtained from the radiographs in the early phases when changes in the alveolar walls and lumen are predominant. This produces a hazy pattern. Since the distribution is focal and scattered, an air bronchogram appearance is not seen, as opposed to the air bronchogram effect that may be seen in the early stages of more diffusely spread air space diseases, e.g., lobar pneumonia. In the intermediate stages, disease severity is more accurately assessed by physiological tests. It is at this phase that the smaller irregular densities of asbestosis become apparent. Radiographs again become of value in the later stages of the disease for detecting honeycombing due to severe fibrosis.

RADIOGRAPHIC DETECTION OF CANCER IN FIBROTIC LUNGS

A primary carcinoma is difficult to detect in a fibrotic lung (see Fig. 2-35). All types—adenocarcinoma, alveolar cell carcinoma, oat cell and squamous carcinomas—have been described,[47] although adenocarcinoma and alveolar carcinoma are common distally and oat cell is common in the proximal airways. Some central bronchial carcinomas may be metastatic from a small undiscovered primary carcinoma lying peripherally in fibrotic lung. Conventional techniques including tomography and bronchography may not reveal a primary malignancy in an area of severe distortion until the mass is huge (see Chapter 2, Section 5). Hemoptysis is not a symptom of uncomplicated pulmonary fibrosis and should indicate the need for an intensive investigation to exclude a neoplasm. A similar problem is seen in scar carcinoma developing in areas of pulmonary fibrosis as a result of systemic sclerosis, sarcoidosis, rheumatoid arthritis, and idiopathic interstitial pulmonary fibrosis. Pleural mesotheliomata may rarely present as localized peripheral masses and may be similar in appearance to a carcinoma. Pulmonary fibrosis sufficient to be radiographically evident occurs in about 20 percent of pleural mesotheliomata. The incidence of pulmonary fibrosis with peritoneal mesothelioma is greater, since the latter is more often associated with a more intense exposure, especially to crocidolite.[48]

COMPUTED TOMOGRAPHY IN ASBESTOS-RELATED PULMONARY FIBROSIS

Peripheral malignancies are more accurately identified with computed tomography* (CT) than conventional radiography.[49] The author has not read any report of the accuracy of CT in detecting scar carcinoma in fibrotic lungs. A

---

*A description of the physics of computed tomography is beyond the scope of this section. For those unfamiliar with CT, two good "starting off" references are G. N. Hounsfield, Computerized transverse axial scanning (Tomography): Part 1. Description of system, Br J Radio 46: 1016–1022, 1973, and J. Ambrose, Computerized transverse axial scanning (Tomography): Part 2. Ibid. pp. 1023–1047. The technique allows for radiographic differentiation of tissues of different absorptive capacity to x-rays. It is more than 100 times more sensitive than conventional x-ray systems. The absorptive capacity of a substance may be expressed in different ways, e.g., new or old Hounsfield units, so that on this scale, water is equivalent to 0, fat to −50, and calcified tissue and bone to 40–500 old Hounsfield units. Varying the window width allows for the visual demonstration of only those tissues with a chosen range of absorptive value. Varying the window level enables the center

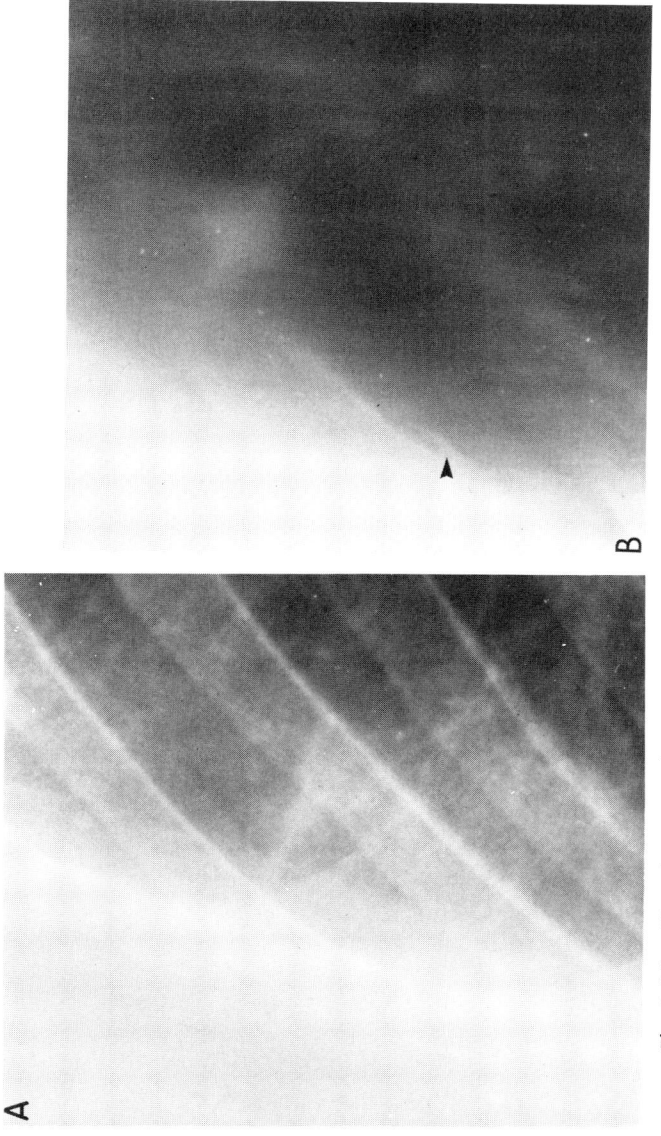

Fig. 2-35. (A and B) Frontal view and tomogram of patient with alveolar cell carcinoma. A prominent linear fibrotic scar is seen in right upper lobe; the associated cancer is barely seen (A). Tomographic section demonstrates not only the tumor but also a linear plaque adjacent to a rib (arrow). The presence of the plaque acts as a biological marker of prior asbestos exposure.

density that appears homogenous on a conventional radiograph may have a honeycomb appearance on CT examination. At first thought, this might lead one away from the diagnosis of malignancy, but this could be erroneous; some carcinomas are multifocal in origin or extend irregularly along preexisting tissue planes. The use of measure mode in the assessment of pulmonary masses is currently being explored. In this technique, the window width is narrowed to 001, the lowest possible, and the window height is manipulated so that the tissue of interest has an equal number of black and white dots. The corresponding window height is termed the tissue density and expressed in new or old Hounsfield units (CT No.). CT tissue density is determined by tissue compactness (among other factors, e.g., Z number and effective kilovoltage). The value of this technique in the detection of scar carcinoma is uncertain. A malignant mass, which is a solid compact homogenous entity, should have greater tissue density than a similar x-ray shadow as a result of superimposition of many areas of pulmonary fibrosis. It seems improbable, however, that this technique could differentiate between a multifocal carcinoma arising over a small area and a malignancy spreading along preexisting tissue planes. CT does have a part in radiotherapy planning, both in estimation of tissue depth and dose and in tumor regression during radiotherapy.

Kreel[50] has described CT findings in asbestosis. Large triangular homogenous dense masses inapparent on conventional radiographs may be seen on CT sections (see Figs. 2-36 and 2-37). These have been described with their base against the mediastinal surface of the lung in both the lower and middle lobes. Their nature is uncertain but probably represents composite shadows due to parenchymal fibrosis and thickening of the visceral pleura.

Transpulmonary bands are bands of soft tissue with parallel borders (unlike the triangular shadows described above) that are present in the costophrenic and cardiophrenic angles as well as near the diaphragm; they are not apparent on routine radiography and again are presumed to be due to fibrosis merging with the thickened visceral pleura (see Figs. 2-38 and 2-39).

Aggregates of honeycomb areas in subpleural locations are frequently seen on CT sections more clearly than on radiographs (see Figs. 2-40 and 2-41). The ease of identification of subpleural fibrotic areas confirms the impression from conventional radiography that pulmonary fibrosis begins in subpleural locations.

In addition to the major changes, nodules of varying sizes comparable

---

of the selected window width range to be set at any desired point to suit the tissue of interest; thus, for examination of mediastinal fat the window level would be optimal at −50 old Hounsfield units. Measure mode gives an assessment of the absorptive value of the tissue being examined, and it is hoped that it may be of value in the more precise identification of different types of normal and abnormal tissue.

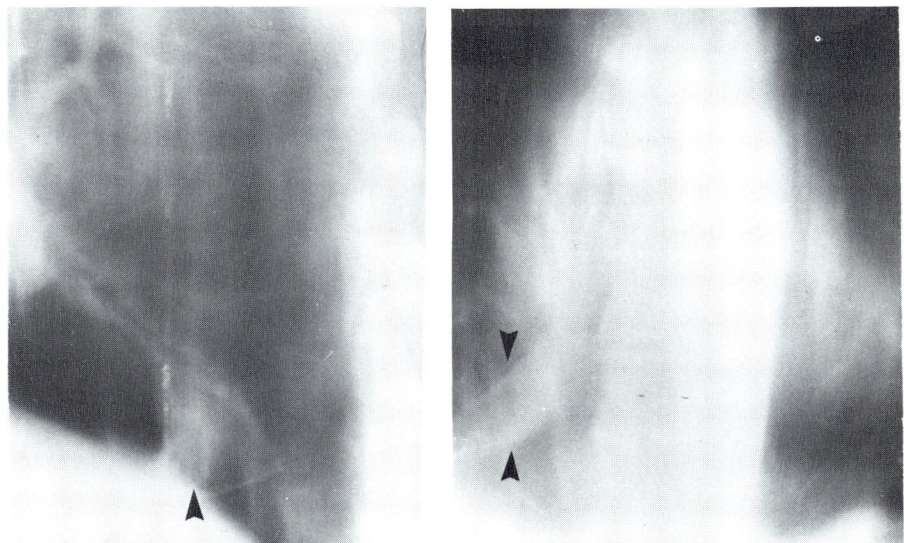

Fig. 2-36. Frontal and lateral tomograms show wedge-shaped areas of pulmonary fibrosis that were inapparent on conventional films of a 48-year-old male with long exposure to asbestos in boiler factory. These tomograms were made because of findings on CT examination (Fig. 2-37)

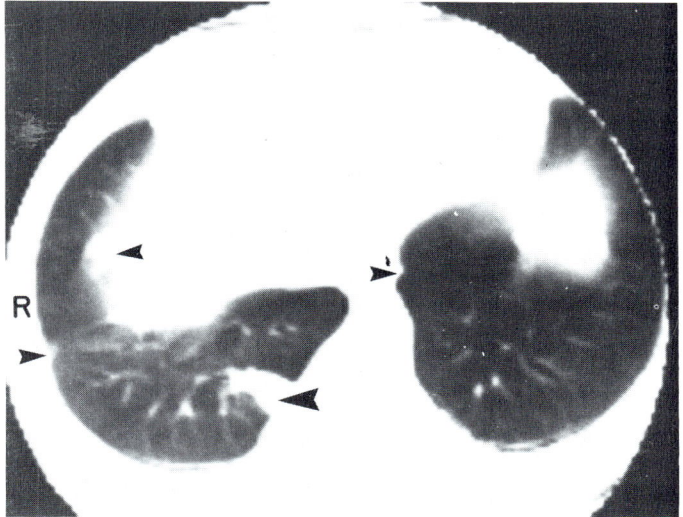

Fig. 2-37. CT examination. Wedge-shaped area of pulmonary fibrosis is in right lower lobe (large arrow), which was not apparent on conventional frontal and lateral chest films. Small arrows indicate mediastinal and pleural plaques.

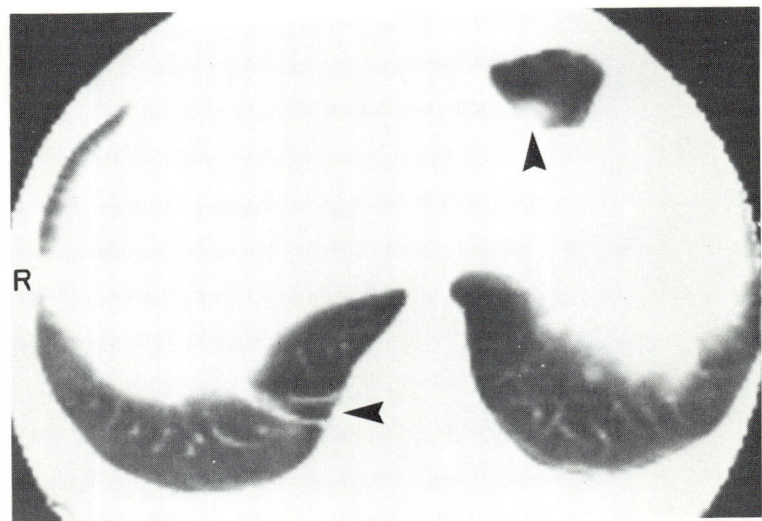

Fig. 2-38. CT examination. Transpulmonary bands of fibrous tissue are seen in the right lung near the diaphragm (horizontal arrow); diaphragmatic plaques on the left are indicated by vertical arrow.

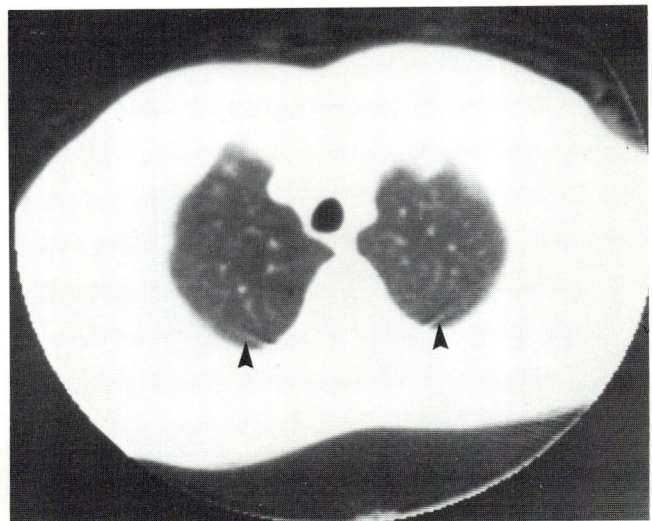

Fig. 2-39. CT examination. Section through the upper lobes. Artifacts simulate transpulmonary fibrous bands (arrows).

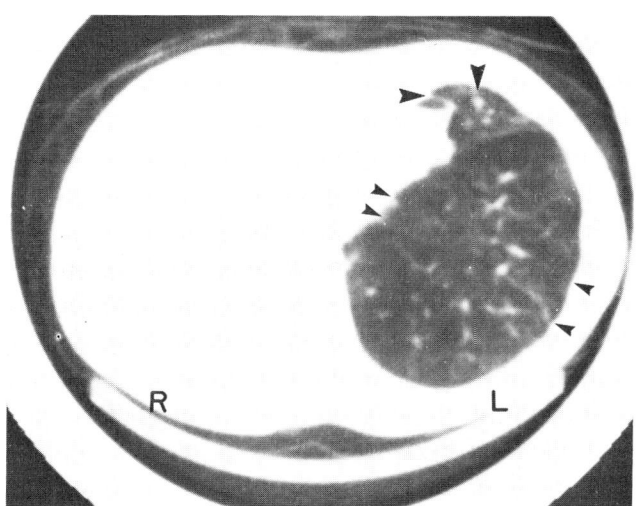

Fig. 2-40. CT examination. In the anterior portion of the left lung is a small transpulmonary band of fibrous tissue (horizontal arrow); slightly lateral are small areas of nodular densities that were interpreted as fibrosis (vertical arrow); mediastinal and peripheral plaques are indicated by small oblique arrows. The appearance of the right lung is due to radical irradiation for a prior adenocarcinoma. Patient is an ex-asbestos worker, who is free from recurrence three years after irradiation.

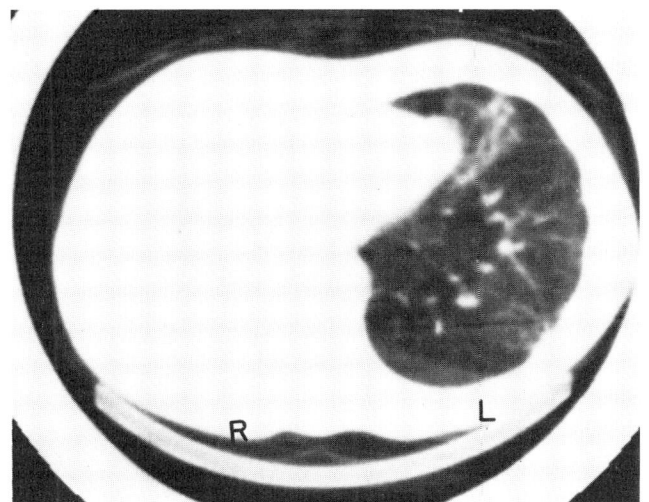

Fig. 2-41. CT examination. Slightly more inferior than the view in Fig. 2-40, the fibrotic area is more diffuse. On the conventional chest films the differential diagnosis between a new primary malignancy, metastases, or focal area of fibrosis was difficult. An absolute differentiation between pulmonary fibrosis and a malignancy infiltrating lung tissue planes is still not possible with CT.

with the ILO U/C classification of rounded opacities (p less than 1.5 mm; q, 1.5–3.0 mm; and r, 3–10 mm diameter) and irregular opacities of varying thickness (s linear, t medium, and u coarse thickness) may be identified. Even when conventional radiography suggest a linear type of fibrosis, CT may demonstrate a honeycomb appearance and thus a greater degree of involvement.

Parietal pleural plaque appearance with CT is described in Chapter 2, Section 1, but it may be noted that subpleural areas of fibrosis may be seen adjacent to noncalcified plaques that are inapparent on conventional radiography. Similarly, the predilection of the visceral pleura of the lesser fissure to show thickening has a counterpart in that homogenous areas of high attenuation with irregular areas may be seen adjacent to the minor fissure. On occasion, CT has demonstrated a diffuse symmetrical and bilateral pleural thickening.[51] The cause is unknown, but it may represent the diffuse thickening in the visceral pleura that has been noted at autopsy in some patients.

CT is also helpful in detecting changes in the vascular bed of fibrotic areas. The vessels may show abrupt tapering and be abnormally straight and thin or tortuous toward the periphery. This may also occur in areas without apparent fibrosis. Where parenchymal fibrosis is apparent, increased perfusion in the more dependent parts as a gravity-related response may be abolished. This is demonstrated if CT is performed with the patient supine and prone. Cardiovascular motion at slow scan speeds make this difficult to detect. Contrast enhancement using intravenous injection is unlikely to yield useful information in this area because of dilution in the pulmonary vascular bed.

CT may show bullae that are inapparent on plain films. Their presence in an otherwise healthy asbestos worker may suggest the need for alternative employment, since such patients would have an additional burden should asbestos-related pulmonary fibrosis develop subsequently.

NONOCCUPATIONALLY RELATED PULMONARY FIBROSIS IN ASBESTOS WORKERS

The syndrome of "a dog with lice and fleas" may be mentioned. Asbestos workers may develop pulmonary fibrosis as a result of other causes. Figure 2-42 is a radiograph of a man with an occupational exposure to asbestos whose pulmonary fibrosis was due to histologically proven sarcoidosis. The pulmonary fibrosis spares the upper zones, which is unusual in sarcoidosis and more typical of asbestosis. The subaxillary noncalcified plaques are partly obscured by the fibrotic areas. There is thickening of the visceral pleura of the major

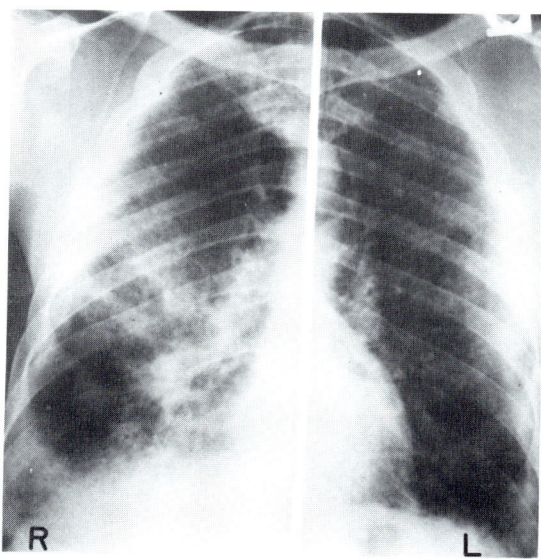

Fig. 2-42. *Sarcoidosis and pleural plaques. There are bilateral thick noncalcified parietal pleural plaques related to prior occupational exposure to asbestos. Because of systemic symptoms (fever and loss of weight) and rapid onset of lung parenchymal changes, an open biopsy, which revealed sarcoidosis, was performed.*

fissure. Pleural involvement is rare in sarcoidosis, but visceral pleural thickening is occasionally seen in asbestos workers. It is never seen in absence of parietal pleural changes and may be the residual of a benign asbestos pleural effusion. The tissue diagnosis of sarcoidosis may be difficult in such an instance because the presence of "sarcoidlike" granuloma in fibrotic lungs with a heavy asbestos test load has been reported.[52]

NUCLEAR SCANNING

Nuclear scanning methods are used in the assessment of pulmonary fibrosis. The author has not read of its use in asbestos-related pulmonary fibrosis. The use of isotopic methods in idiopathic pulmonary fibrosis is described in detail by Roberts et al.[46] Three isotopic techniques are used: macroaggregated albumin labeled with technetium 99m (^{99m}Tc MAA) to evaluate lung perfusion; xenon 133 (^{135}Xe) or xenon 127 (^{127}Xe) to evaluate ventilatory functions; and gallium 67 citrate (^{67}Ga) to quantitate lung inflammation, or alveolitis.

REFERENCES

1. Turner-Warwick M: A perspective view on widespread pulmonary fibrosis. Br Med J 2:371–376, 1974
2. Oldham PD: A trial of techniques for counting asbestos bodies in tissues, in Bogovski P, Gilson JC, Timbrell V, et al. (eds): Biological Effects of Asbestos. Lyon, IARC Scientific Publications, 1973, pp 45–49
3. Beattie J, Knox JF: In Davies CN (ed): Inhaled Particles and Vapors. London, Pergamon Press, 1961, p 419
4. Seals RME, Wagner JC: Pathological reactions of the lung to dust, in Morgan WKC, Seaton A (eds): Occupational Lung Diseases. Philadelphia, WB Saunders, 1975
5. Wagner JC, Berry G, Skidmore JW, et al: The effects of the inhalation of asbestos in rats. Br J Cancer 29:252–269, 1974
6. Liebow AA, Steer A, Billingsley JG: Desquamative interstitial pneumonia. Am J Med 39:369–404, 1965
7. Gree RA, Dimcheff DG: Massive bilateral upper lobe fibrosis secondary to asbestos exposure. Chest 65:52055, 1974
8. Allison AC: Experimental methods—cell and tissue culture: Effects of asbestos particles on macrophages, mesothelial cells and fibroblasts, in Bogovski P, Gilson JC, Timbrell V, et al. (eds): Biological Effects of Asbestos. Lyon, IARC Scientific Publications, 1973, pp 89–93
9. Harrington JS, Miller K, Macnals G: Hemolysis by asbestos. Environ Res 4:95–117, 1971
10. Allison AC: Lysosomes and the toxicity of particulate pollutants. Arch Intern Med 128:131–139, 1971
11. Harrington JS: Fibrogenesis. Environ Health Perspect 9:271–279, 1974
12. Stanton MF: Some etiological considerations of fiber carcinogenesis in Bogovski P, Gilson JC, Timbrell V, et al. (eds): Biological Effects of Asbestos. Lyon IARC Scientific Publications, 1973, pp 289–294
13. Timbreel V: Physical factors as etiological mechanisms, in Bogovski P, Gilson JC, Timbrell V, et al. (eds): Biological Effects of Asbestos. Lyon, IARC Scientific Publications, 1973, pp 295–303
14. Pooley FD: Electron microscope characteristics of inhaled chrysotile fibers. Br J Ind Med 29:146–153, 1972
15. Timbrell V, Pooley F, Wagner JL: Characteristics of respirable asbestos fibers, in Shapiro HA (ed): Pneumoconiosis. Proceedings of the International Conference, Johannesburg, 1969. London, OUP, 1970, pp 120–125
16. Lauweryns JM, Baert JH: Alveolar clearance and the role of the pulmonary lymphatics. State of the art. Am Rev Respir Dis 115:625–683, 1977

17. Ashcroft T, Heppleston AG: Asbestos fiber concentration in relation to pulmonary reaction, in eds. Bogovski P, Gilson JC, Timbrell, et al. (eds): Biological Effects of Asbestos. Lyon, IARC Scientific Publications, 1973, pp 236–237
18. Ashcroft T, Heppleston AG: The optical and electron microscope determination of pulmonary asbestos fiber concentration in its relation to the human pathological reaction. J Clin Pathol 26:224–234, 1973
19. Elder JL: Asbestos in western Australia. Med J Aust 2:579–583, 1967
20. Evans CC, Lewinsohn HC, Evans JM: Frequency of HLA antigen in asbestos workers with and without pulmonary fibrosis. Br Med J 1 (6061):603–605, 1977
21. Miller A, Langer AM, Teirstein AS, et al: "Nonspecific" interstitial pulmonary fibrosis in association with asbestos fibers detected by electron microscopy. N Engl J Med 292:91, 1975
22. Miller A, Teirstein AV, Langer AM, et al: Submicroscopic asbestos particles and disease. Letter to Ed. N Engl J Med 292:1195, 1975
23. Gross P, Hairky RA, Carrington CB: Submicroscopic asbestos particles and disease. Letter to Ed. N Engl J Med 292:1195, 1975
24. Anderson HA, Lilis R, Daum S, et al: Household contact asbestos neoplastic risk. Ann NY Acad Sci 271:311–323, 1976
25. Solomon A, Goldstein B, Webster I, et al: Massive fibrosis in asbestosis. Environ Res 4:430–439, 1971
26. Caplan A: Certain unusual radiological appearance in the chest of the coal miner suffering from rheumatoid arthritis. Thorax 8:29–37, 1953
27. Mattson S-B: Caplan's syndrome in association with asbestosis. Report of a case. Scand J Respir Dis 53(3):153–161, 1971
28. Rickards AG, Barrett GM: Rheumatoid lung changes associated with asbestosis. Thorax 13:185–193, 1958
29. Tellison WG: Rheumatoid pneumoconiosis (Caplan's syndrome) in an asbestos worker. Thorax 16:372–377, 1961
30. Morgan WKC: Rheumatoid pneumoconiosis in association with asbestosis. Thorax 19:433–437, 1964
31. Caplan A, Cowen EDH, Gough J: Rheumatoid pneumoconiosis in a foundry worker. Thorax 13:181–184, 1958
32. Solomon A: Radiology of asbestos, in Shapiro HA (ed): Pneumoconiosis. Proceedings of the International Conference, Johannesburg, 1969. London, OUP, 1970
33. Soutar, CA, Simon G, Turner-Warwick M: The radiology of asbestos induced diseases of the lungs. Br J Dis Chest 68:235–252, 1974
34. Weill H, Waggenspack C, Bailey W, et al: Radiographic and physiologic

patterns among asbestos workers engaged in manufacture of asbestos-cement products. J Occup Med 15:248–252, 1973
35. Heitzman ER: The Lung: Radiological-Pathological Correlation. St Louis, CV Mosby, 1973, p 49
36. Oswald N, Parkinson T: Honeycombed lungs. Q J Med 18:1–20, 1949
37. Meyer EP, Leibow AA: The relationships of interstitial pneumonia, honeycombing and atypical epithelial proliferation to cancer of the lung. Cancer 18:322–351, 1965
38. Simon G: Principles of Chest X-ray Diagnosis. London, Butterworth, 1962
39. Williams R, Hugh-Joines P: The radiological diagnosis of asbestos. Thorax 15:103–108, 1960
40. Webster I: The pathogenesis of asbestos, in Shapiro HA (ed): Pneumoconiosis. Proceedings of the International Conference, Johannesburg, 1969. London, OUP, 1970
41. Resink JEJ: Is a roentgenogram of fine structures a summation image or a real picture. Acta Radiol 32:391–403, 1949
42. Scansetti G, Coscia GC, Piscani W, et al: Cement, asbestos and cement-asbestos pneumoconiosis. Arch Environ Health 30:272–275, 1975
43. Enterline E, Weill H: Asbestos in asbestos cement workers, in Bogovski P, Gilson JC, Timbrell V, et al. (eds): Biological Effects of Asbestos. Lyon, IARC, Scientific Publications, 1973, pp 179–183
44. Kiviluoto R: Asbestosis: Aspects of its radiological features, in Shapiro HA (ed): Pneumoconiosis. Proceedings of the International Conference, Johannesburg, 1969. London, OUP, 1970, pp 253–255
45. Weill H, Ziskind MM, Waggenspack C, et al: Lung function consequences of dust exposure in asbestos-cement manufacturing plants. Arch Environ Health 30:88–97, 1975
46. Roberts WC, Moss ML, Line BR, et al: Idiopathic pulmonary fibrosis, clinical, histologic, radiographic, physiologic, scintiographic, cutologic and biochemical aspects. Ann Intern Med 85:760–788, 1976
47. Fox B, Risdon RA: Carcinoma of the lung and diffuse interstitial fibrosis. J Clin Pathol 21:486–491, 1968
48. Parkes RW: Personal communication
49. Muhm JR, Brown LR, Crowe JK: Use of computed tomography in the detection of pulmonary nodules. Mayo Clin Proc 52:345–348, 1977
50. Kreel L: Computed tomography in the evaluation of pulmonary asbestosis. Acta Radiol (Diag) 17:405–412, 1976
51. Kreel L: Personal communication
52. Tayot J, Henin-Landes D, Fondimara A, et al: Asbestos with sarcoid-like pulmonary lesions. A propos of one anatomical clinical case report. Ann Anat Pathol (Paris) 21(2):269–276, 1976

SECTION 3
PLEURAL EFFUSIONS

Exudative pleural effusions etiologically related to prior asbestos exposure have been described in recent years. Assessment for an effusion is now part of the ILO U/C radiographic work chart (Chapter 3). Pleural effusions related to asbestos exposure may be secondary to bronchogenic carcinoma, mesothelioma, cor pulmonale due to pulmonary fibrosis, or so-called benign asbestos effusion.

This additional entity, "benign asbestos effusion," has been described by many authors.[1-3] The criteria for diagnosis are prior history of asbestos exposure, absence of any other predisposing cause for the effusion, and spontaneous remission of the effusion. Excluded are those patients with an asbestos exposure history and carcinoma, mesothelioma, or cor pulmonale due to severe pulmonary fibrosis or in whom some other identifiable cause such as lymphoma is detectable. Acceptance of the entity of benign asbestos effusion is widespread, thus Becklake[4] writes, "The justification for this diagnosis increases, and asbestos exposure can reasonably be added to the long list of causes of benign *recurrent* pleural effusion." Fletcher and Edge[5] state, "The only occasion when benign asbestos pleurisy with effusion can be diagnosed with confidence is when a chronic effusion is persistently negative for tuberculosis on culture, when no other cause can be found, and where the condition spontaneously improves."

In the author's opinion, the diagnosis of benign asbestos effusion is fraught with hazard. It cannot be made without a long-term follow-up to ensure that spontaneous complete resolution of a single or multiple episode of pleurisy has occurred. Even in such cases, an occult cause such as thromboembolic disease may be responsible. More worrisome is that an effusion may be present for months or years, culminating in a diagnosis of mesothelioma. In addition, the pleural cavity in health contains a small amount of pleural fluid, with a protein content similar to that of interstitial fluid. The amount is sufficiently great that it may be demonstrated by lateral decubiti radiographs in 4 percent of healthy persons; this technique will detect amounts of fluid greater than 3–5 ml.[6]

CLINICAL FEATURES

Bearing in mind the author's skepticism expressed above, the following reflects current published descriptions mentioned in the references.

The effusion may be unilateral, bilateral, or recurrent. Regression of an

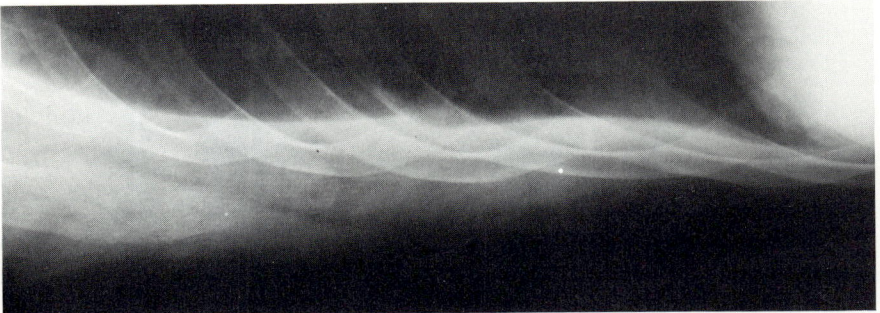

Fig. 2-43. *Shipyard worker who complained of dull chest pain. Right decubitus view showing pleural effusion; no plaques are visible.*

effusion on one side may be followed by a contralateral occurrence. Up to four separate episodes in 1 patient are recorded. The effusion may recur over many years without evidence of mesothelioma development. In others, a mesothelioma may be accompanied by a pleural effusion on the contralateral side, apparently benign in that the radiographic appearance on that side may be normal. If the effusion is prolonged, the prognosis with regard to eventual development of mesothelioma must be guarded. The onset is usually insidious but occasionally acute. By definition the effusion must resolve without specific treatment. The effusions are small and usually need lateral decubiti radiographs for adequate visualization (see Figs. 2-43 and 2-44). Pleuritic chest pain is present in patients with acute onset, whereas only a dull ache may be present in insidious effusions, and some patients are asymptomatic. Physical signs will vary with the amount of fluid, and in acute cases there may be fever, usually low grade. Digital clubbing may be present in prolonged effusions, especially if there is much accompanying parenchymal fibrosis. Dry crepitations due to associated interstitial fibrosis may be heard.

Over 50 benign asbestos effusions have been recorded as of 1977. Thus, Gaensler and Kaplan[1] report 21 percent of their asbestos patients to have had a pleural effusion, and in their series of 91 pleural effusions of various etiologies, 13 percent were believed related to asbestos exposure as compared with the following:

Congestive failure	22%
Malignancy	24%
Infection	14%
Collagen disease	9%
Pulmonary infarct	3%
Chronic interstitial pneumonia	3%

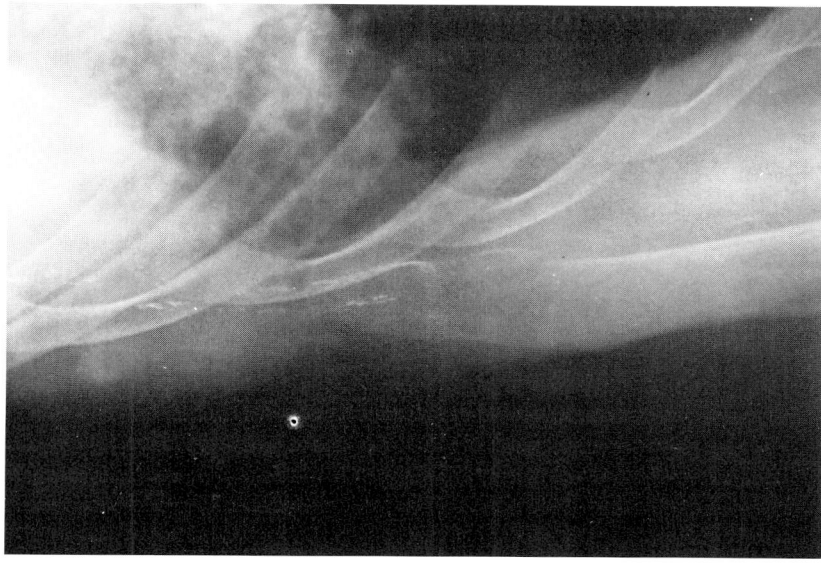

Fig. 2-44. Left decubitus view in steep Trendelenburg and expiration shows mobile pleural effusion, fibrotic changes, and panlobular emphysema in left lower lobe of ex-shipyard worker. Again, no plaques are seen. The white streaks are artifacts.

    Laennec's cirrhosis   2%
    Undetermined   9%

In their series, a single episode of effusion was seen in 6 patients, two to four episodes in 5 patients, and a persistent effusion in 1 patient. Unlike Gaensler and Kaplan, the author subscribes to the opinions of Fletcher, Edge, and Becklake that a definition of benign asbestos pleural effusion must include complete resolution. In Gaensler and Kaplan's series the effusion was unilateral in 3 patients and bilateral (simultaneously or in sequence) in 9. The interval between the last asbestos exposure and the development of pleurisy has varied from a few months to 31 years,[2] while duration of exposure has been from 3 to 38 years.[1]

    When the effusion has an acute onset, it may be accompanied by fever, leukocytosis, fast sedimentation rate, and general systemic symptoms. A few may show a positive latex agglutination test for rheumatoid factor; circulating antinuclear antibodies are usually absent. Many other diseases may thus be simulated. Analysis of the exudate is of limited value (see below); if the effusion is prolonged a limited thoracotomy should be performed to examine pleural and parenchymal biopsy material for asbestos fibers and fragments using specialized techniques and, more important, to exclude other causes by appropriate histological and microbiological examinations.

PLEURAL FLUID ANALYSIS

Asbestos related pleural fluid is an exudate with a protein content varying from 3.4 to 7.5 gm/100 ml.[1] Red blood cells may be absent, but counts in the range of 5,000 to 50,000 cells per cubic millimeter are usually present.[4] The inflammatory cell content, polymorphonuclear leukocytes, monocytes, lymphocytes, and eosinophils are variable; eosinophils in some patients and lymphocytes in others are disporportionately frequent. Asbestos fibers or fragments have not been reported in the exudate.

Pleural exudates will usually have a pleural fluid-to-serum protein ratio of greater than 0.5, a pleural fluid LDH (lactic dehydrogenase) of greater than 200, and a pleural fluid-to-serum LDH ratio of greater than 0.6. Simultaneous use of both pleural fluid protein and LDH levels better differentiates exudates from transudates than do the previously used pleural protein level of 3.0 gm/100 ml.[7] Exfoliative cytology of the exudate is necessary to exclude an underlying malignancy, especially mesothelioma and bronchogenic carcinoma, in those with a history of asbestos exposure. The cytological identification of benign and malignant mesothelial cells and their differentiation from cells shed from a carcinoma or from a mesothelial reaction are difficult. It is especially important to note that atypical macrophagelike cells, similar to cells found in proven mesothelioma, may be found. In 2 of 6 patients who initially were thought to have benign pleural effusions and in whom such cells were found, the eventual clinical course was that of mesothelioma.[8] A progression over many years of apparently benign asbestos effusion to mesothelioma has been noted by others.[9-11] To repeat, an effusion in a person with prior asbestos exposure that does not remit cannot be considered as a benign asbestos effusion, and even then, some other cause may be responsible (see Fig. 2-45).

PATHOLOGY

The underlying lung usually shows some degree of fibrosis, the visceral pleura is thickened, (see Fig. 2-46) the parietal pleural usually has some degree of lamellar thickening, but localized plaque formation large enough to be apparent radiographically is usually absent.

The visceral pleura may be as thick as 15 mm and is white in appearance. There is gross hyaline connective tissue proliferation, with well-formed collagen fibers arranged in bundles and an occasional cleft lined by flattened cells. If papillary formation is present, the possibility of a developing mesothelioma cannot be discounted. Cellular infiltration is usually slight, and if great, other etiologies need careful consideration.[13] Blood vessels are usually scanty but

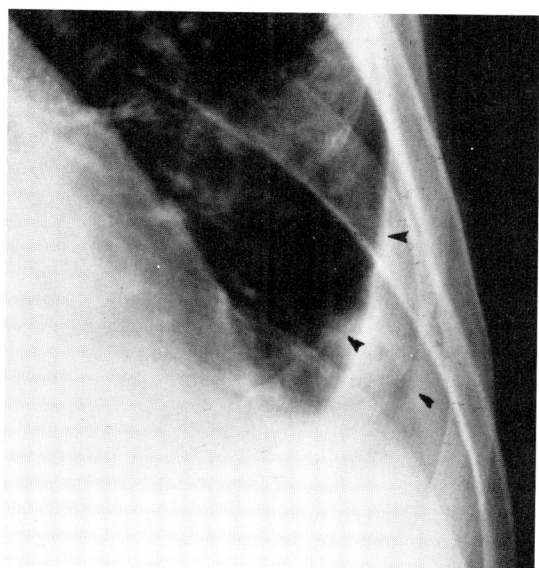

Fig. 2-45. Left pleural effusion and plaques in an ex-shipyard worker. A small mesothelioma was present on the right. Because of the small size of the mesothelioma, it was thought unlikely to have produced mediastinal lymphatic obstruction, and the etiology of the left effusion was therefore in doubt. The left pleural aspirate did not contain any cells.

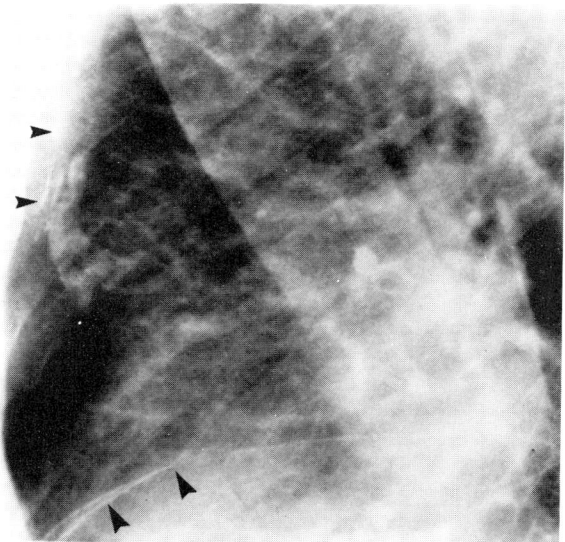

Fig. 2-46. Lateral view of chest of an ex-shipyard worker. Oblique arrows indicate thickening of visceral interlobar fissure; horizontal arrows point to anterior mediastinal parietal pleural calcification.

occasionally are frequent and help explain the sanguineous nature of some effusions.

The parietal pleura may show a diffuse thickening, but localized plaque formation on the side of the effusion occurs in a minority of cases, and calcification of plaques is rare. Parietal pleural plaques, calcified or noncalcified, may be present on the uninvolved side.

The underlying lung is invariably abnormal. There are varying degrees of pulmonary fibrosis. Minimal involvement may entail pleural thickening and edema of interlobular septa and extension of pleural fibrosis into the septa; more severe involvement is characterized by increased collagen formation in the interstitium of the lung and obliteration of alveoli and bronchioli by fibrosis. A fuller account is given in Chapter 2, Section 2 on pulmonary fibrosis.

Although asbestos fibers and particles are not apparent in the exudate, they may be detected in the affected pleura and lung. Specialized techniques may be needed.

All the main types of asbestos fibers have been associated with benign asbestos effusion.[10,12–16] The author has not read of pleural effusion developing in experimental animals subjected to asbestos inhalation.

RADIOLOGY

In the identification of an asbestos-related exudate, decubiti views in expiration, with a Trendelenburg tilt, are frequently essential, since volumes of fluid are usually small. As mentioned previously, small amounts of pleural fluid may be demonstrated in normal persons with this technique.[6] When the exudate is recurrent, a prior episode may have resulted in obliteration of costophrenic angle and subsequent effusions may not be clearly apparent initially. Lamellar diffuse thickening of the parietal or visceral pleura may simulate an effusion, but in these instances the costophrenic angles are usually not obliterated. Thickening of interlobar fissures may be a sequel of a prior effusion or may be due to asbestos exposure without an effusion. Interlobar visceral pleural thickening due to "dry" asbestos pleurisy without a current effusion is most common in the minor fissures and is always associated with parietal pleural changes.[17]

The "biological markers" of calcified and noncalcified parietal pleural plaques should be sought. For unknown reasons, calcification is extremely rare on the side of an asbestos exudate. Noncalcified plaques may be seen, although their frequency is stated as less than 50 percent in most radiological series of asbestos exudates; this is probably an understatement related to assiduity of search, lack of employment of oblique projections, tomography, and CT. The differentiation of lamellar diffuse parietal pleural thickening from visceral pleural thickening (interlobar fissures excluded) is not possible radiographically. Parenchymal pulmonary fibrosis should be sought; it may not be evident on a chest radiograph except in the more severe forms or by using oblique views. Ultrasound techniques may be helpful in locating optimal sites for diagnostic thoracentesis, since exudate volumes are usually small.[18] Thoracentesis under fluoroscopic control has been recommended when small volumes of fluid are aspirated.[19]

In addition to excluding causes of effusion unrelated to asbestos exposure, a search must be made for bronchogenic carcinoma and mesothelioma. In bronchogenic carcinoma, mediastinal node involvement is statistically much more important than pleural involvement in the formation of an effusion.[20] Fifty-five degree oblique tomography of the hila is useful for this assessment[21] and is, in the author's opinion, often superior to frontal or lateral tomography, although assessment of the left hilus and adjacent mediastinum is more difficult than that of the right.

Mesothelioma may simulate, be accompanied by, or be preceded by a pleural effusion for many months. In addition, mesothelioma may produce bilateral effusions by involvement of the superior vena cava, mediastinal nodes, thoracic duct, and pericardium. If the azygous vein is involved, superior caval involvement will raise parietal pleural capillary pressure and so increase filtration from parietal pleura, but there is usually an accompanying element of lymphatic obstruction which, by reducing fluid and protein absorption, is of greater significance.[22] Pericardial involvement and subsequent tamponade or restrictive pericardial disease will have a similar hemodynamic effect in addition to the effect of lymphatic obstruction.

At the risk of being repetitious, the author believes that whenever the diagnosis of a "benign asbestos pleural effusion" is made, arrangements for repeated later clinical and radiographic assessment must be made to ensure that patients with mesothelioma are not missed.

REFERENCES

1. Gaensler EA, Kaplan AJ: Asbestos pleural effusion. Ann Intern Med 74:1 178–191, 1971
2. Chahinian P, Hirsch A, Bignon J et al: Les pleuresies asbestosiques non tumurale. Rev Fr Mal Respir 1:5–39, 1973
3. Eisenstadt HB: Pleural effusions in asbestosis. N Engl J Med 290:1025, 1974
4. Becklake MR: Asbestos related disease of the lung and other organs:

Their epidemiology and implications for clinical practice. Am Rev Respir Dis 114:187–227, 1976
5. Fletcher DE, Edge JR: The early radiological changes in pulmonary and pleural asbestosis. Clin Radiol 21:355–385, 1970
6. Black LF: The pleural space and pleural fluid. Mayo Clin Proc 47:493–506, 1972
7. Light RW, MacGregor I, Luchsinger PC et al: Pleural effusions: The diagnostic separation of transudate and exudate. Ann Intern Med 77:507–513, 1972
8. Butler EB, Berry, AV: Diffuse mesotheliomas, diagnostic criteria using exfoliative cytology, in Bogovski P, Gilson JD, Tembrill V, et al. (eds): Biological Effects of Asbestos. Lyon, IARC Scientific Publications, 1973
9. Kiviluoto R, Meurman L, Shapiro HA (eds): Pneumoconiosis. Proceedings of the International Conference, Johannesburg, 1969. Capetown, OUP, 1970, pp 190–191
10. Collins TFB: Pleural reactions with asbestos exposure. Br J Radiol 41:655–661, 1968
11. Eisenstadt HB: Asbestos pleurisy. Disease of chest. Chest 46:78–81, 1964
12. Sluis-Cremer GK, Webster I: Acute pleurisy in asbestos exposed persons. Environ Res 5:380–392, 1972
13. Mattson SB: Monosymptomatic exudative pleurisy in persons exposed to asbestos dust. Scand J Resp Dis 56:263–272, 1975
14. Mattson SB, Ringquist T: Pleural plaque and exposure to asbestos. Scand J Resp Dis Suppl, 1970, p 75
15. McNulty JC: Asbestos mining, Wittenoom, Western Australia, in Proceedings of the First Australian Pneumoconiosis Conference, Sydney, pp 447–466
16. Navratil M, Dobias J: Development of pleural hyalinosis in long term studies of persons exposed to asbestos dust. Environ Res 6:455–472, 1973
17. Solomon A, Webster I: The visceral pleura in asbestosis. Environ Res 11:218–234, 1976
18. Goldberg BB, Pollack HM: Ultrasonically guided renal cyst aspiration. J Urol 109:5–7, 1973
19. Collins JD, Byrd SE, Bassett LW: Thoracentesis under fluoroscopic control. JAMA 237:2751–2, 1977
20. Brinkman GL: The significance of pleural effusion complicating otherwise operable bronchogenic carcinoma. Chest 36:152–154, 1959
21. McLeod RA, Brown LR, Miller, WE et al: Evaluation of the pulmonary hila by tomography. Radiol Clin North Am 14:1 51–84, 1976
22. Carlson HA: Obstruction of the superior vena cava: An experimental study. Arch Surg 29:609–677, 1934

SECTION 4
PLEURAL AND PERITONEAL MESOTHELIOMATA

Mesothelial tissue, which lines the pleural, pericardial, and peritoneal spaces, may be the site of mesothelioma formation. These tumors may be benign or malignant. Benign pleural tumors include lipoma, hemangioma, benign mesothelioma, and simple cyst. Malignant primary tumors of mesothelium include malignant mesothelioma and sarcoma.

EPIDEMIOLOGY

Wagner et al.[1] in 1960 suggested that mesotheliomata were related to asbestos exposure. This initial observation has been subsequently confirmed by many sources, including surveys of workers with known occupational exposure in mining, milling, shipbuilding and repairing, insulation, cement, and textile industries, as well as those living near these industries who are not occupationally exposed but who are environmentally at risk.

The incidence of mesothelioma in the general population, using evidence from autopsy series,[2] is about 2 to 3 per million per year. An appreciation of the incidence of mesothelioma in asbestos workers is difficult to obtain, since the population at risk is undefined. Some 3.5 to 4.0 million men and women worked at one time or another in the U.S. shipyards during World War II,[3] and it is impossible, even in a developed country, to investigate such numbers. The problem in less developed areas is greater. The South African Asbestos Reference Panel totals 375 cases of mesothelioma; there is an annual work force of about 20,000 persons in the asbestos mines of South Africa, but many of these are migrant workers in the tribal tribute system, and so the total population at risk cannot be determined.[4]

The recorded incidence based on mortality studies of those known to have been engaged in asbestos industries varies. In Finnish anthophyllite mines and adjacent areas, only one death from mesothelioma has been recorded. In the chrysotile mills of northern Italy, no deaths from mesothelioma are known, while in Quebec similar workers have a 0.2 percent mesothelioma-related death rate. The Soviet Union, which produces over 2 million tons of chrysotile per year, has not released data on mortality due to mesothelioma. Selikoff et al. have surveyed the mesothelioma risk in 17,800 asbestos insulation workers in the United States and Canada over the period 1967–1971.[5,44] They noted 213 pleural and 26 peritoneal mesotheliomas. This reflects approximately five times the expected incidence when compared with age-matched controls. These people have been exposed to chrysotile and amosite but not to crocidolite. In the same survey, a group of 337 amosite insulation workers had 16 peritoneal and 4 pleural mesotheliomas. Most of the above employees were men. In a study of a factory with a large female work force employed in spinning (crocidolite), weaving and mattress making (chrysotile and amosite), gas mask filter assembly (crocidolite and amosite), brake lining (chrysotile), and rubber jointing manufacture (chrysotile and crocidolite), of those workers followed for more than 20 years, 1.5 percent of females and 1 percent of the males died of mesothelioma.[6]

The majority of mesotheliomata are asbestos-related; in a few, no asbestos exposure can be discovered. A familial incidence has been described. In Australia, it is estimated that only 16 percent of mesothelioma patients have had no occupational exposure.[7] The end occupation can be misleading, however; two-thirds of the Australian mesothelioma patients developed mesothelioma while they were in an unrelated occupation, although they did have prior occupational exposure to asbestos, usually in the form of crocidolite. Australian crocidolite has very fine fibers that can penetrate pleura the more easily and so induce mesothelioma. Matching the Australian experience, 15 percent of U.K. mesothelioma patients,[8] 16 percent of the South African patients,[9] and 11 percent of the Mayo Clinic series patients[10] have had no known asbestos exposure. Higher proportions of mesothelioma patients with no detectable history of asbestos exposure are recorded by Elmes, 33 percent,[11] and Oels, 62 percent,[12] but occupational histories were incomplete. At the other end of the spectrum, only 6 percent of the males and none of the females in a U.S. series developed mesotheliomata that were apparently unrelated to asbestos exposure.[13]

An unusual group of mesothelioma patients are those who have had household contact with asbestos workers. In a group of 326 persons who lived in the same house as amosite asbestos workers, 4 have died from mesothelioma.[14]

The incidence of mesothelioma is rising rapidly, having increased about sevenfold in the last decade in the United Kingdom. More detailed mortality reporting, the setting up of mesothelioma registers, and a greater awareness on the part of internists, radiologists, and pathologists, especially in urban and shipbuilding areas, play a part in this increase, but much must be blamed on inadequate dust control in the years leading up to and including World War II and shortly after and the belated recognition in the 1960s of the association between mesothelioma induction and asbestos. Because of the long latent period between first exposure and development of mesothelioma, averaging 30 to 40 years in most series, and the fact that adequate dust control has only been achieved in the late 1960s and 1970s, the incidence of mesothelioma is expected to be high until the turn of the century. The mesothelioma disease wrought by naval shipbuilding in World War II is being observed by the current generation of physicians, much as the disease related to World War I battleship construction was seen by previous generations, although the situation went unappreciated. The next generation of physicians will undoubtedly see mesothelioma related to naval construction during the "cold war" period, although synthetic substitutes for asbestos are being used increasingly.

FACTORS AFFECTING THE PATHOGENESIS OF MESOTHELIOMA

The pattern of response to most toxic agents varies in large population samples and in general follows an S-shaped curve, but very low doses of a toxic substance may preferentially affect susceptible persons.[15] Caplan's syndrome, the association of pulmonary nodules and raised titers of circulating rheumatoid factor in coal miners, and drug toxicities associated with the lack of the enzyme glucose-6-phosphate dehydrogenase are two well-known examples. Although there are conflicting accounts of the association between raised titers of circulating antibodies (see Chapter 1) and pleural plaques, there are no published data on the relationship between pleural plaques, circulating antibodies, and the later development of mesothelioma.

Effect of Dose

In a study of U.K. asbestos textile workers, Newhouse has shown a dose–response relationship to length of exposure and degree of exposure to dust for mortality due to mesothelioma (and lung cancer).[16] The incidence of mesothelioma more than doubles if exposure is greater than 2 years; for short exposures of less than 2 years, the ratio is about three times greater for heavy as compared to light exposure. Pipe laggers in the textile factory studied had much higher rates than did asbestos textile production workers.

A dose–response relationship between amphibole asbestos exposure and induction of mesothelioma is suggested[17a,17b] by an electron microscopy study of lung parenchyma from mesothelioma specimens compared with random autopsy controls. Of the mesothelioma specimens, over 50 percent had a sufficient amount of asbestos fibers to indicate an intermediate, short-, or long-term exposure, while only 10 percent of the controls had such an intensity of fibers. A dose–response relationship for chrysotile fibers is harder to elicit, since these fibers fragment into smaller particles, and their detection in tissues is more difficult.

Cocarcinogens are not known to be relevant in the induction of mesothelioma. Although asbestos is highly adsorbent, there is no evidence that by-products of combustion from smoking are additive to the risk of mesothelioma formation, unlike the increased risk of bronchogenic carcinoma. Similarly, trace metals in the fibers, organic substances in asbestos (paraffinlike fraction, polycyclic hydrocarbons) and antioxidants incorporated in polyethylene bags currently used, or oils in jute bags previously used for asbestos packing and transport are not cocarcinogenic for mesothelioma induction.[18]

Effect of Fiber Type

Fiber type is associated with a potential for mesothelioma induction. The danger is greatest with crocidolite, minimal with amosite but risk is slightly greater for amosite than chrysotile, and virtually zero for anthophyllite. The main variable is fiber diameter. Of the amphiboles, this diameter is smallest with crocidolite, intermediate with amosite, and greatest for anthophyllite. The greater incidence of mesothelioma with fine-diameter fibers such as crocidolite is related to less deposition in the proximal airways and easier penetrability of the pleura and peritoneum. The fiber shape is important; although the long curly chrysotile fiber would not be expected to reach the pleura easily, once fragmented, the short chrysotile fibers have a short arc and behave aerodynamically like the straight amphiboles. Current belief is that asbestos fibers up to 10 μm in length and less than about 1 μm in diameter may cause mesothelioma. A fuller account of the subject relating the problem to clinical practice is given in Chapters 1 and 2, Section 2.

PATHOLOGY AND NATURAL HISTORY

Site

Mesothelioma may arise from any mesothelial surface. Origin from pericardium is extremely rare and denied by some. Determining the point of origin when both the pericardium and the pleura are involved is difficult. Most thoracic mesotheliomata arise from the pleura. Figure 2-47 illustrates a tumor that probably first arose in the pericardium or adjacent pleura. No cases are reported of simultaneous origin in both pleural and peritoneal cavities. In later phases of their natural history, a mesothelioma arising in one cavity, either pleural or peritoneal, may invade the diaphragm to involve the other cavity

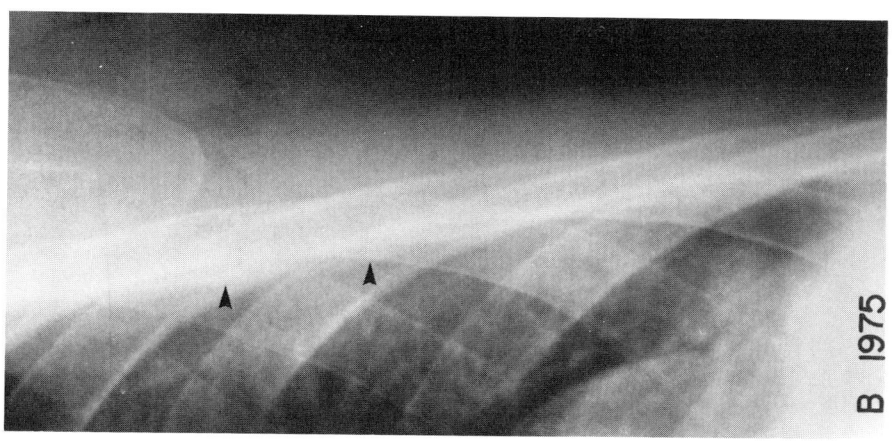

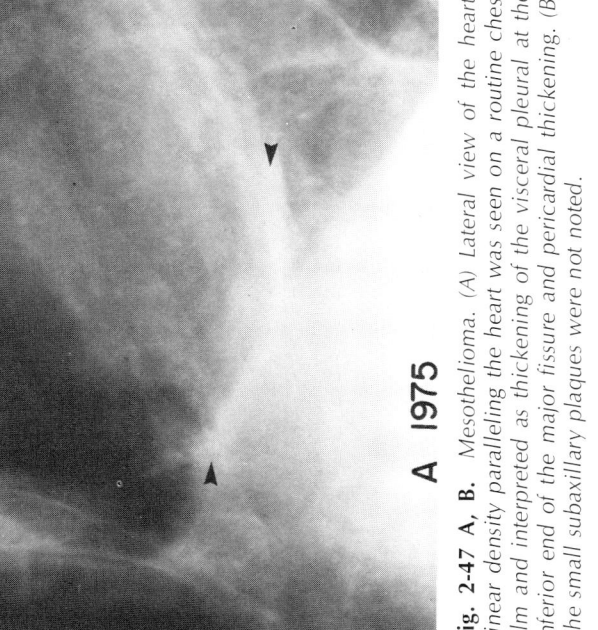

Fig. 2-47 A, B. Mesothelioma. (A) Lateral view of the heart. Linear density paralleling the heart was seen on a routine chest film and interpreted as thickening of the visceral pleural at the inferior end of the major fissure and pericardial thickening. (B) The small subaxillary plaques were not noted.

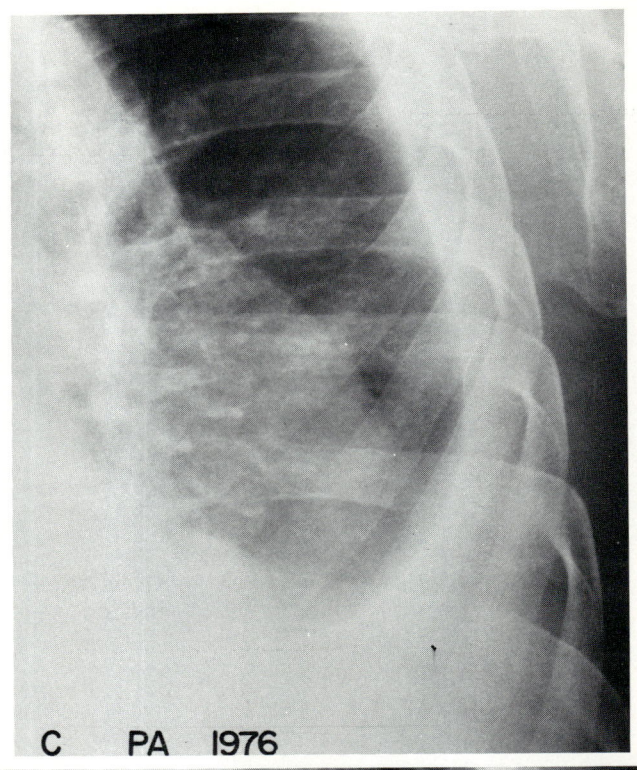

C   PA   1976

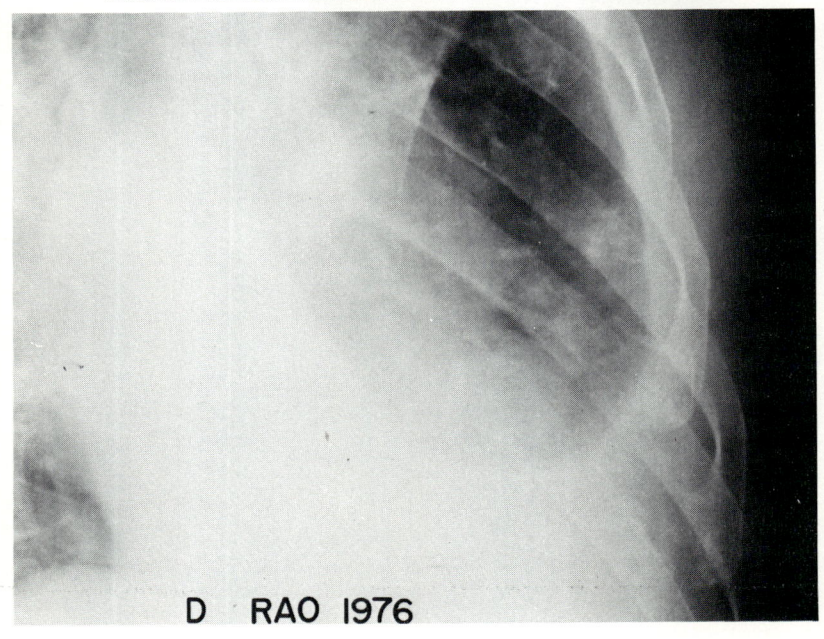

D   RAO   1976

Table 2-6
Ratio of Pleural to Peritoneal
Mesotheliomata

Author	Patient Sex	Ratio
Borow[10]	M and F	2:1
Greenberg[8]	M and F	26:1
Edge[19]	M	28:1
Harris[20]	M	54:1
Milne[7]	M	10:1
Elmes[40]	M and F	7:1

(Fig. 2-48). The difficulty in distinguishing a mesothelioma arising in the female pelvis from papillary adenocarcinoma of the ovary is described on page 217. The ratio of pleural to peritoneal mesothelioma is shown in Table 2-6. In other earlier series which included women workers, in whom there is always a problem of separating pelvic mesothelioma from ovarian cancer, a higher proportion of peritoneal mesothelioma is recorded.[6,10,16] Borow reported on a group of patients, 11 percent of whom were females, and found a ratio of pleural to peritoneal mesothelioma of 2:1.[10] Most mesothelioma patients are males, which is not surprising because the type of work utilizing asbestos is usually physically arduous. When this is not a limiting factor, as in gas mask filter assembly using crocidolite, female mortality is high.

Pleural Mesothelioma

The tumor gradually encases part or all of the lung as a thick, yellowish gray mass involving both parietal and visceral pleurae. An attempt to strip the tumor from underlying parenchyma leads to tearing of the lung (Fig. 2-49); if decortication is attempted during thoracotomy, air leaks may ensue. In uninvolved areas, parietal, pleural, and diaphragmatic plaques may be recognized (Fig. 2-50). Their reported frequency is probably related to assiduity of search (see Table 2-7).

Most authors state that mesotheliomata do not arise through malignant degeneration of a pleural plaque, although there has been a report of a malignant mesothelioma arising by a stalk from a pleural plaque. This is most likely coincidental.[21]

Fig. 2-47 C, D. *PA and RAO views 1 year later. The patient had severe chest pain, nonpleuritic in nature. Preliminary diagnosis was dissecting aneurysm of thoracic aorta with hemorrhagic effusion. The pleural "peel" was misinterpreted as hemorrhagic effusion and the widening of the aortic shadow as dissection. The "peel" did not layer out on decubitus views as is usual with effusion. Pain due to mesothelioma is typically nonpleuritic in nature.*

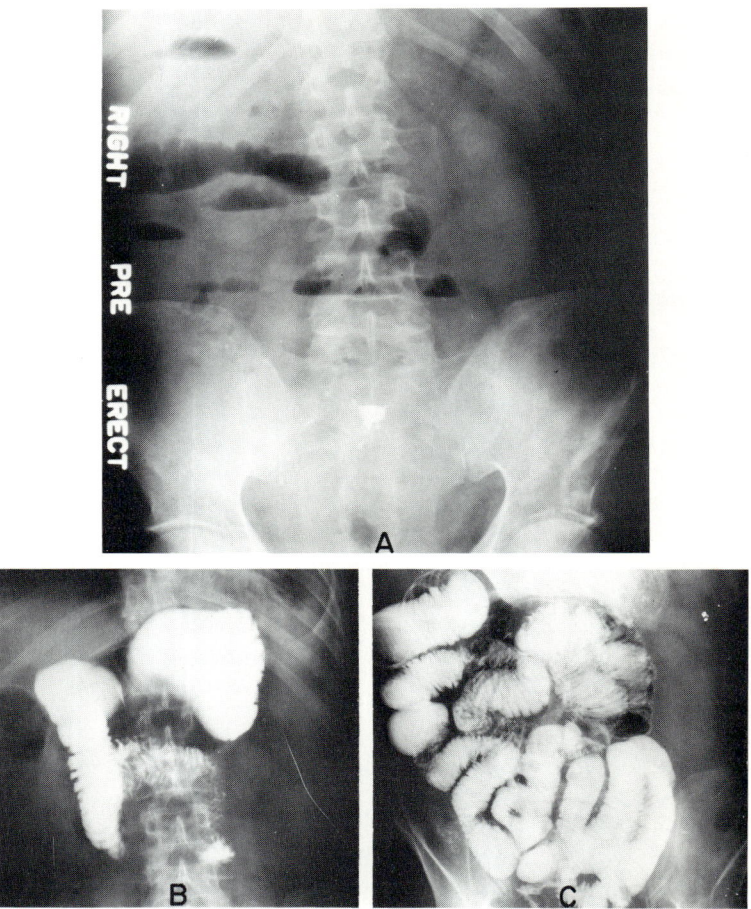

Fig. 2-48. Pleural mesothelioma invading the abdomen and obstructing the small bowel. (A) The erect film of the abdomen shows moderately dilated loops of small bowel in the upper abdomen and a paucity of gas in the left side of the abdomen and pelvis. A mesothelioma arising in the left lung had penetrated the diaphragm and spread along the peritoneal surfaces of the small and large bowel as well as the parietal peritoneum. Most of the tumor mass was in the left side of the abdomen. A bony metastasis is present in the left ilium above the acetabulum (compare left and right acetabular cortices). A prior myelogram was done because of metastases to the midthoracic vertebrae. (B and C) Barium examination shows involvement of transverse duodenum and displacement of the ligament of Trietz. The proximal small bowel loops are dilated from incomplete obstruction, they are slightly separated because of involvement of their peritoneal surfaces, and they are displaced from the left side of the abdomen where the bulk of the tumor mass lies.

Table 2-7
Radiographically Visible
Pleural Plaques Accompanying
Mesothelioma

Author	Percent
Elmes[40]	18%
Harris[20]	34%
Edge[19]	86%

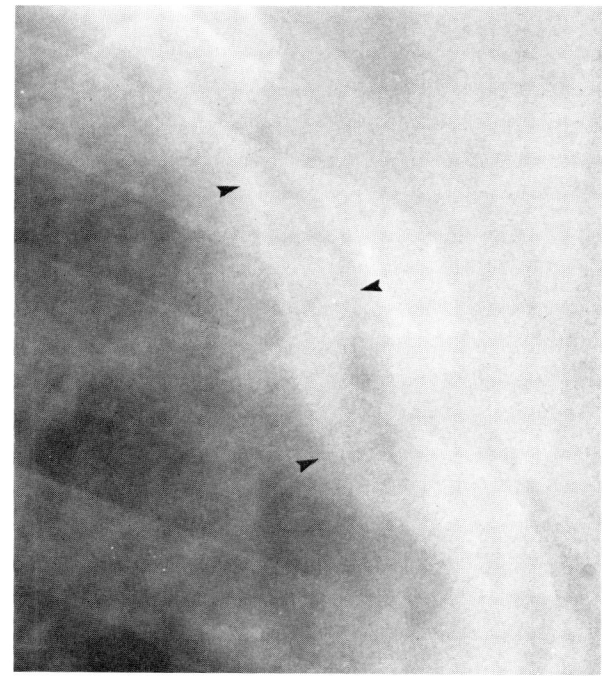

Fig. 2-49. Mesothelioma. Iatrogenic pneumothorax (arrow) outlines irregularly thickened visceral pleura. Air escaped from the lung when decortication was attempted during thoracotomy for tissue diagnosis. If mesothelioma is suspected, decortication should not be attempted. It may lead to a troublesome pneumothorax.

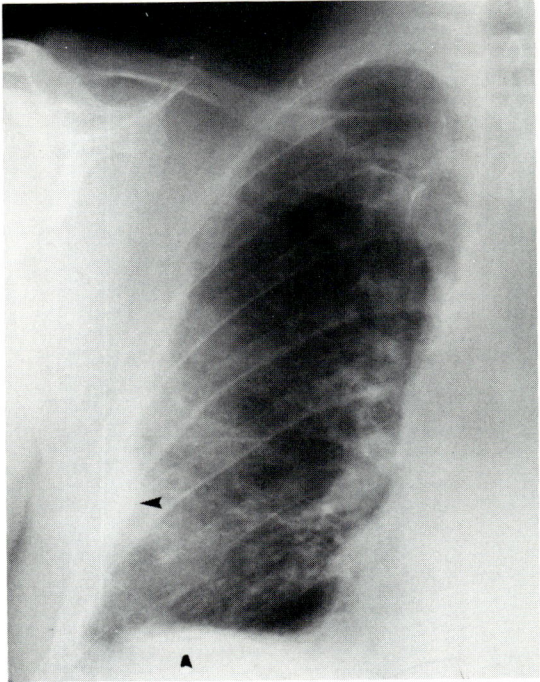

Fig. 2-50. Mesothelioma present in contralateral pleura. There are noncalcified lateral pleural plaques (horizontal arrow) and calcified diaphragmatic plaques (vertical arrow). A search for these biological markers should be made whenever mesothelioma is a diagnostic possibility. Note the irregular destruction of the outer end of the clavicle from metastatic disease.

Since most pleural plaques are never visualized during life, there is insufficient evidence to assume that mesotheliomata do not originate from malignant degeneration of a pleural plaque. In view of the large numbers of patients with pleural plaques and the low incidence of mesothelioma, however, the possibility of malignant degeneration must be slight.

Besides spreading to encase part or all of the lung, the tumor reaches into the interlobar fissures and lung septae and invades the pericardium. Deep in the tumor there is usually some parenchymal interstitial fibrosis, even though this may not be evident radiographically. Once through the pericardium, further penetration usually involves the atria rather than the ventricles, but involvement of the interventricular septum has been known. Involvement of the pericardium may produce constrictive pericarditis with an effusion demon-

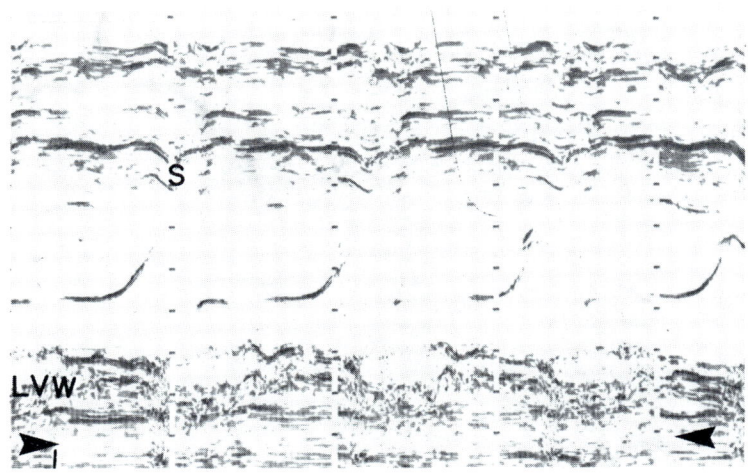

Fig. 2-51. *Mesothelioma. Echocardiogram of a patient with an extensive mesothelioma encasing the pericardium. There was a diminished cardiac output. The small anterior and posterior (arrow) pericardial effusions were believed insufficient to produce cardiac tamponade as an explanation of the low cardiac output. Pericardial restrictions due to malignant invasion was postulated. The septum (s) moves paradoxically, which is seen with large effusion, and the posterior left ventricular wall (LVW) contraction pattern is abnormal. It begins with a slow and sustained contraction, but there is an abrupt relaxation at the end. The catheterization data showed elevated pressures in the right atrium (17/5 mmHg mean 12), the right ventricle, (41/10 mmHg), and the pulmonary artery (27/12 mmHg), while the pulmonary capillary wedge pressure was 12 mmHg. Two Cope needle biopsies of the pleura were productive of fibrous tissue only; a subsequent "minithoracotomy" and open biopsy indicated hemothorax and pleural fibrosis. A further definitive thoracotomy was needed to provide sufficient histological material for the diagnosis of mesothelioma. This sequence of events underlines the difficulty of diagnosis of mesothelioma based on small amounts of tissue obtained by biopsy techniques whether open or closed. (Courtesy of N. Schiller, M.D., U.C.S.F.)*

strable by echocardiography (Fig. 2-51). The cardiac chambers may be compressed. If the pericardial effusion develops rapidly, cardiac tamponade may ensue. Diffuse mediastinal spread may involve the anterior, middle, and posterior mediastinal compartments. The aorta and esophagus may be encased. Primary esophageal cancer is more common in asbestos workers than in the general population, but differentiation from secondary spread of a mesothelioma is usually obvious. Spread may involve the axillary nerves or the lowest part of the brachial plexus and sympathetic ganglia and produce a Pancoast and Hornerlike syndrome. Posterior mediastinal spread may reduce the spinal cord's blood supply and result in paraplegia,[11] or this may result from

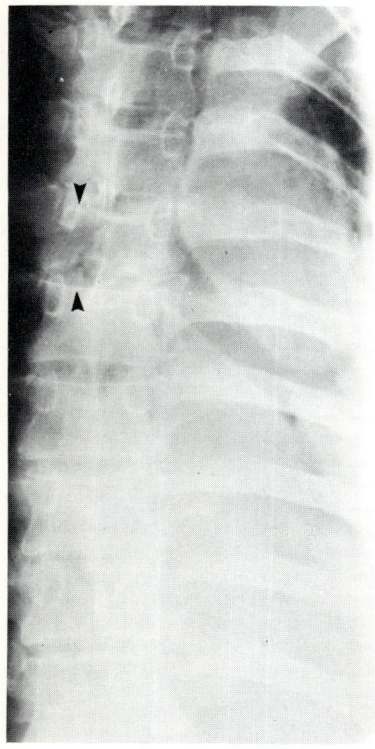

Fig. 2-52. Mesothelioma metastatic to the T5 vertebral body and encasing the left side of the mediastium. A myelogram did not show any macroscopic extradural mass. The patient's paraparesis was believed to result from thrombosis of the spinal cord vessels by microscopic deposits.

direct or bloodborne spread to vertebral bodies with subsequent cord compression (Fig. 2-52).

Mediastinal and hilar lymph nodes may be involved by encasement or by direct spread. Axillary, cervical, and abdominal nodes are involved less frequently. In general, the sarcomatous (fibrous type of mesothelioma) involves the regional lymph nodes by encasement rather than by lymphatic invasion. A hilar mass is not seen in uncomplicated asbestosis (pleural plaques, benign asbestos pleurisy, pulmonary fibrosis, and probably visceral pleural thickening), unlike some other forms of pneumoconiosis where hilar enlargement is a constituent of the uncomplicated disease. Despite about 50 percent incidence of hilar involvement in mesothelioma, its detection by x-ray is difficult because of mediastinal pleural involvement by tumor and associated pleural thickening and fluid.

Direct spread to involve superior and inferior venae cavae may ensue, impeding the entry of blood into the right atrium. Right ventricular dilation may

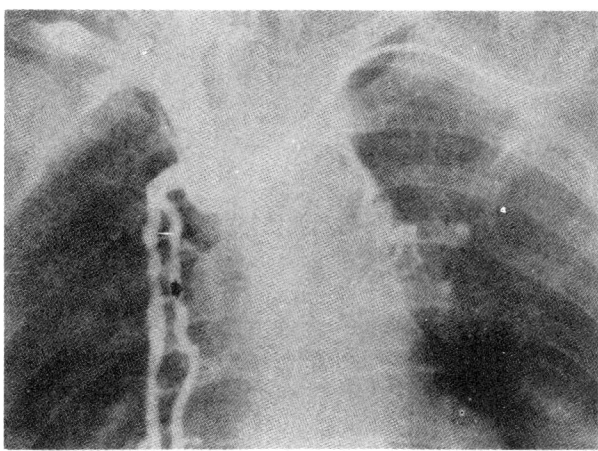

Fig. 2-53. *Localized mesothelioma arising in the superior mediastinum and causing the superior vena cava syndrome demonstrated by venography (Courtesy of D. E. Sanders, M.D., and the editors of the Journal of the Canadian Association of Radiologists.)*

occur. Lower limb edema and ascites may result from inferior vena cava compression; rarely does a full-blown superior vena cava syndrome of facial, neck, and upper thoracic congestion with collateral vein formation develop. (Fig. 2-53).

Direct spread through the chest wall occurs. In individual cases this has been preceded by percutaneous biopsy, thoracotomy, or deep x-ray or gamma ray treatment, but a causal effect is uncertain.[11] Destruction of adjacent ribs may occur. The mass may extend into the supraclavicular fossa.

Direct spread through the diaphragm and the aortic and esophageal hiatuses occurs as the disease advances but may be a relatively early complication with an appropriately sited tumor. Organs in the peritoneal cavity become encased with tumor, so that a thick peel may cover liver and spleen. Infiltration of the omentum and the visceral and parietal peritoneums occurs, so that, similar to the displacement of the esophagus that occurs in the chest, the stomach, duodenum, and small and large bowel may be displaced, adherent to each other or to the abdominal wall. Direct extension through the wall of the gastrointestinal tract develops but is usually minimal because death ensues. Spread is occasionally confined to one side of the peritoneal cavity. Direct spread into the retroperitoneal space is limited but may be sufficient to induce a severe desmoplastic reaction that may obstruct the ureters. The lumbar spine and lumbosacral plexus may be infiltrated.

There is a varying degree of pleural effusion accompanying thoracic mesothelioma. The effusion is usually large and bloody and reaccumulates rapidly. However, in Elmes' series, 43 of 89 patients had serous effusion.[22] Loculation of fluid may result in only a small pleural aspirate. A clue may be the thickness and relative impenetrability of the involved pleura by the aspirating needle. About one-third of the patients will have a lobulated soft tissue mass and no effusion. Others may have an apparently "benign" asbestos pleural effusion for many months before a mesothelioma is discovered. A contralateral apparently benign pleural effusion may occasionally accompany a mesothelioma. In early cases, it may be possible to identify discrete nodules of mesothelioma arising from both the visceral and parietal pleurae. It is conjectural as to whether it is true early seeding or a multifocal origin.

By the time of death, as many as 50 percent of patients have distant bloodborne metastases. The sarcomatous type of mesothelioma is the most prone to such spread. The contralateral lung, and occasionally the ipsilateral one, will show multiple nodules, some of which are necrotic. The liver, spleen, kidneys, adrenals, thyroid, axial and appendicular skeleton, calvarium, and meninges may be involved.

Peritoneal Mesothelioma

A mesothelioma arising in the peritoneal cavity usually appears as multiple coalescing nodules, differing from pleural mesothelioma, which usually has a more diffused sheetlike appearance. The coalescence produces large tumor masses which obliterate free spaces in the coelomic cavity, making it difficult to assign a point of origin, especially in the female pelvis where differentiation from a primary ovarian cancer is often difficult. The omentum is infiltrated early in the course of the disease and appears thickened and contracted before there is diffuse involvement of the peritoneum. As with pleural mesothelioma, the tumor tends to extend over organ surfaces, compressing them, but with only minimal invasion through their walls. The tumor mass has a glistening white color, and its cut surface has a mucinous appearance.[10] There is a varying amount of clear or bloody ascitic fluid. Bowel loops may be matted together and fixed throughout the abdomen. In other cases, they may be fixed in one area, presumably at the site of origin of the tumor, and displaced by the advancing tumor mass in others. Direct spread may occur upwards through the diaphragm, its muscle being heavily infiltrated with tumor, or through the diaphragmatic hiatuses in advanced cases to infiltrate the pleura. Unlike most intra-abdominal neoplasms, there is a relative paucity of regional lymph node involvement. Bloodborne spread, especially to the liver, ensues eventually.

MICROSCOPIC FEATURES

For many years, mainly as a result of the efforts of Willis, the identity of mesothelioma as a separate tumor entity was questioned, and many thoracic mesotheliomata were considered peripheral pulmonary adenocarcinomas or metastatic. Mesotheliomata is now recognized as a specific tumor, but its cell of origin is still a question. As a result of the histological heterogeneity of mesothelioma, its histogenesis has been attributed to mesothelial cells, subpleural connective tissue, and lymphatic endothelium. Cultured mesothelial cells are capable of producing epithelial cells and fibroblasts, and this explains the heterogeneity of most mesotheliomata which contain epithelial and fibrosarcomatous elements. It may be that benign fibrous mesotheliomata differ in that there is evidence that they arise from subpleural connective tissue.[23]

A classification that is commonly used is (1) epithelial, (2) mixed epithelial and fibrous, and (3) fibrous or mesenchymal. The epithelial group includes tumors with tubulopapillary formation composed of epithelial and cuboid cells, as well as solid groups of cells without tubulopapillary formation. The fibrous group is composed of tumors made up of spindle cells arranged in bundles without much intervening hyalinized collagen. Occasionally, the fibroblasts may not follow a bundlelike pattern but may occur loosely or in solid sheets. The mixed type which is the most common is composed of epithelial cells and fibroblasts.[10,24] The tubulopapillary pattern is difficult to differentiate from metastatic adenocarcinoma, especially from prostate, lung, breast, stomach, and ovary, and Willis' earlier opinion that most mesotheliomata were actually metastatic adenocarcinomas is recalled. Even currently, tumors initially considered to be mesotheliomata are frequently thought to be otherwise when reexamined at mesothelioma registries. The initial diagnosis of mesothelioma was not confirmed in 34 percent of a Dutch series[25] and 40 percent of a British series.

The fibrous mesenchymal or sarcomatous type, when arising in the chest, needs to be differentiated from other sarcomas of the pleura, from fibrosarcoma of lung, and from metastatic fibrosarcoma. Most primary fibrosarcomas are clinically obvious. The very rare mesothelioma with osseous metaplasia may need differentiation from extraosseous osteogenic sarcoma.[26] Mesotheliomata associated with amosite exposure are unusual in that they contain large amounts of bone and cartilage.[27] Differentiation from an uncomplicated asbestos plaque may be difficult if there is an excess of collagen and very few cells. When the tumor is widely invasive, e.g., through the diaphragm into the liver, sarcomatous cellularity is usually obvious.

The mixed type may be difficult to differentiate from a primary carcinosarcoma of the lung, but this usually has a bronchial origin and contains squamous cells.

The epithelial polygonal cell types, if very undifferentiated, need to be differentiated from carcinoma; if differentiated, they may appear relatively benign and resemble benign pleural hyperplasia such as may overlay a pulmonary infarct.

Great difficulty is experienced in histological diagnosis of diffusely spreading mesothelioma, which is most often of the epithelial type but may be fibrous or mixed. Purely histological criteria cannot absolutely distinguish mesothelioma from certain metastatic carcinoma. Electron microscopic demonstration of characteristic vacuoles and microvilli in the epithelial cells favors the diagnosis of mesothelioma.*

Histochemical techniques are of limited use. An effusion accompanying a mesothelioma may contain large amounts of hyaluronic acid. Secondary pleural tumors contain this substance in only 10 percent of all cases. Effusions accompanying squamous cell and alveolar cell malignancies may contain hyaluronic acid.[28] Tissue may be examined for acid mucopolysaccharide substances elaborated by mesothelial cells.[29] There is no histochemical test specific for mesothelioma.

The variability of recorded plaque formation in patients with mesothelioma, based on either x-ray or necropsy series, has been discussed. A similar situation applies to the incidence of pulmonary fibrosis associated with mesothelioma. Although this is rarely very severe during life, either clinically or radiographically, it is seen at autopsy examination. Oels et al.[12] reported that 17 of 37 patients with pleural mesothelioma had necropsy-proven pulmonary fibrosis. The pulmonary fibrosis was unrelated to the histological type of mesothelioma. Severe pulmonary fibrosis is more common with peritoneal mesothelioma because this type of mesothelioma is usually associated with severe crocidolite exposure, and this fiber is strongly fibrogenic.

CLINICAL FEATURES

Pleural Mesothelioma

The incidence in males predominates over females by approximately 4 to 1.[30] Because of the long period needed following asbestos exposure, most patients are older than 50 years at death, with a mean age of about 55 to 65 in

---

*Ellis K and Wolff M: Mesotheliomas and secondary tumors of the pleura. Seminars in Roentgenology 12(4):303–311, 1977

Table 2-8
Presenting Complaints of Pleural Mesothelioma

Onset	
Acute	4%
Insidious	96%
Pain	56%
Breathlessness	36%
Fatigue and weight loss	6%
Diagnosis in course of investigation of some other illness or prior to occurrence of symptoms	5%

Abstracted from Elmes' data.[40]

most series for pleural mesothelioma and some 5 to 10 years less for peritoneal mesothelioma. Asbestos-related mesotheliomata in patients as young as 16 are known, however. Most of the patients have been cigarette smokers, but smoking has not been shown to have a multiplicative effect on the incidence of mesothelioma, unlike its effect on bronchogenic carcinoma. There is no predilection for involvement of one side of the chest in a current large series despite conflicting reports in earlier small groups. The onset of symptoms is usually insidious, but in the elderly, gradual weight loss and increasing dyspnea may go unnoticed, and only when a sudden accumulation of fluid or the development of pneumothorax is noted is an acute onset suggested. Presenting symptoms in descending order of frequency include pain, dyspnea, weight loss, fever, hemoptysis, and joint pain (see Table 2-8). Cough is often present but is rarely a presenting symptom. The pain is usually dull, gradually increasing in severity as the chest wall and nerve plexi are infiltrated, and may be located adjacent to the mass or referred to shoulder or abdomen. Sharp, severe pain may be related to a specific event, such as an acute increase in fluid or the development of pneumothorax. Pleuritic-type pain is less common, but there may be protracted episodes of pleurisy dating back many years, especially in those patients with a prior history of recurrent "benign" asbestos effusions. There may be contralateral pain if a "benign" asbestos effusion is present on the other side. The typical insidious nature of the pain is illustrated by the fact that some mesotheliomata are only diagnosed when patients seen for presumed hemothorax due to trauma or an acute pneumonia do not respond to appropriate therapy.[31] Hemoptysis is rare as a presenting symptom but may develop if there is much invasion of the lungs or if unwise attempts at decortication are made during thoracotomy before the true nature of the lesion is realized. Dyspnea may diminish temporarily if much fluid is aspirated. Dyspnea may also be related to the development of constrictive pericarditis (Fig. 2-54) or cardiac tamponade. Occasionally the patients have thrombophlebitis as a marker of a malignancy. *Painful* hypertrophic osteoarthropathy is

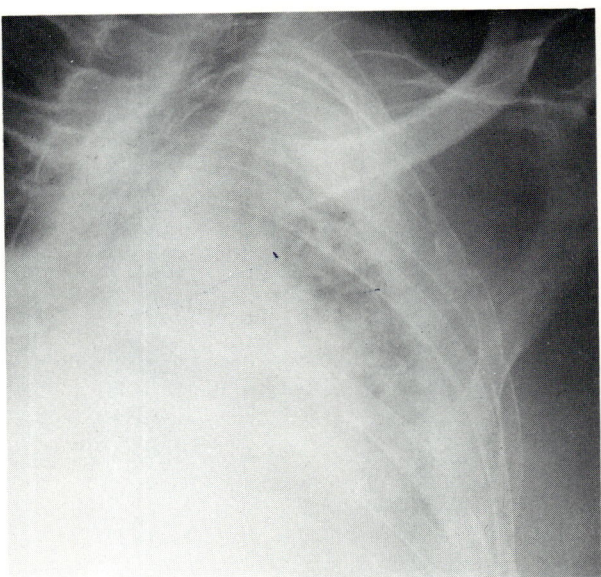

Fig. 2-54. Mesothelioma invading the pericardium to produce restrictive effusive pericardial disease (see Fig. 2-51).

rare. Direct upward spread may cause a Hornerlike syndrome. Symptoms resulting from superior vena cava obstruction are rare. Inferior spread through the diaphragm may cause gastrointestinal symptoms and complaints of abdominal distention (Fig. 2-55). Distant metastases to meninges, kidney, adrenals, thyroid, liver, opposite lung, and other organs cause appropriate symptoms. There is as yet no evidence that mesothelioma produces any paraendocrine effect, and no cases of hypoglycemia (as seen in some pleural benign solitary fibromata and fibrosarcomas) have been recorded in recent large series.

The clinical findings reflect the presence of a pleural mass and effusion. Extension of the tumor into the supraclavicular, chest wall, and abdominal areas may be palpable. Initially before the mediastinum is fixed, there may be displacement of the apex beat and trachea to the uninvolved side; this may eventually be reversed, and there may be physical signs of atelectasis on the involved side. Clubbing of fingers and, less commonly, of toes may be present.

Peritoneal Mesothelioma

Lassitude and weight loss accompanied by abdominal distention due to ascites occur. Pain and tenderness may be dull and diffuse or localized as a result of ascites or of localized fluid collection. Umbilical, inguinal, and

Organ Involvement in Asbestos-related Disease

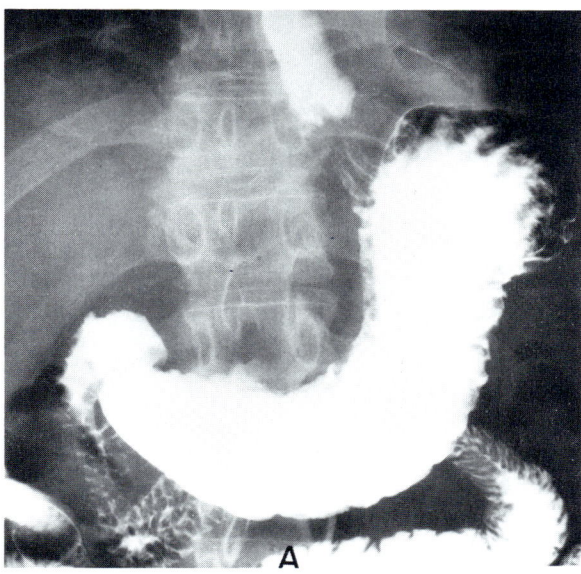

Fig. 2-55 A. *Mesothelioma invading the abdomen. Barium examination shows the irregular border of the lower esophagus and thickening of the mucosa of the descending duodenum. Only the latter was commented on. The patient had a prior decortication of the left lung with a tissue diagnosis of fibrothorax. Nine months later, development of a nodule in the thoracotomy scar led to diagnosis of mesothelioma. This sequence of events is not rare. The barium examination was prompted by complaints of epigastric pain.*

femoral hernias may develop secondary to ascitic distention. Physical signs relating to incomplete or complete bowel obstruction will develop.

INVESTIGATION

Although no form of treatment has been proven to be life extending for patients with mesothelioma, a correct tissue diagnosis is still necessary.

The accuracy of diagnostic procedures in a large series of pleural mesotheliomata is listed in Table 2-9 from Elmes[40]. The patients in this series died between 1960 and 1969. Current accuracy of cytological diagnosis is higher. Thus Butler and Berry[32] were able from appropriate aspirates to correctly diagnose by exfoliative cytological techniques 25 of 26 mesotheliomata, 28 of 30 metastatic pulmonary carcinomas, and 19 of 21 cases of mesothelial reaction.[32] Butler and Berry also examined aspirates from 6 patients believed to have "benign" and asymptomatic asbestos pleural effusion and in these found

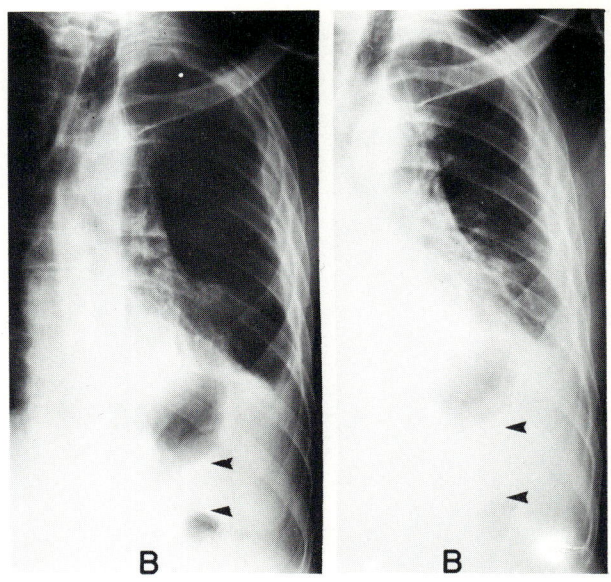

Fig. 2-55 B. *Deep x-ray therapy to the chest was given, but the epigastric pain continued. A control chest film showed widening of the space between the greater curvature of the stomach and adjacent bowel loops (between arrows) over a period of 5 months as a result of the mesothelioma penetrating the diaphragm and infiltrating the omentum.*

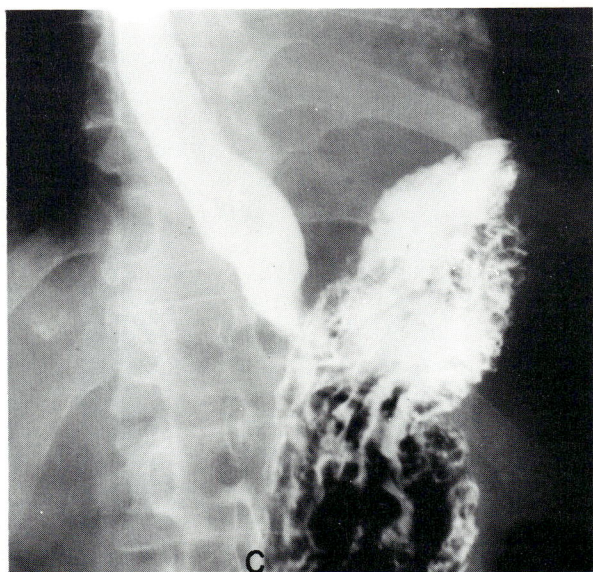

Fig. 2-55 C. *Repeat examination of the esophagus shows extrinsic involvement of both sides of the lower esophagus to a greater degree than in A and displacement of its lower half to the right by extension of the mesothelioma into the mediastinum.*

Organ Involvement in Asbestos-related Disease 141

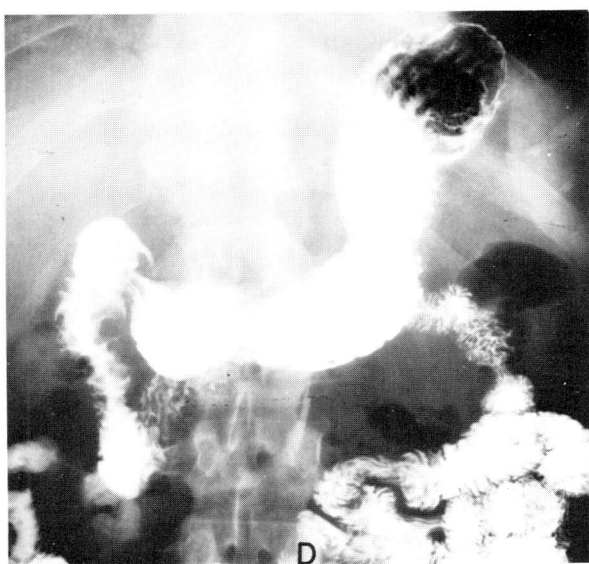

Fig. 2-55 D. *Repeat examination also shows more severe involvement of the mucosal folds of the descending duodenum and widening of the space between the greater curvature of the stomach and the first loop of the jejunum. The appearance confirms the impression obtained from plain films in B. There is also an extrinsic impression in the upper part of the greater curvature which was not apparent 6 months earlier in (A).*

atypical macrophages similar to those that accompany a mesothelioma effusion.[32] Two of these patients have subsequently developed clinical evidence of malignant mesothelioma, although tissue diagnosis is not yet available. Cytological diagnosis is difficult, and most pathologists need a large volume of tissue to ensure accuracy in diagnosis of mesothelioma.

Investigations other than radiographic examinations that may be of value in selective cases include computed tomography and ultrasonic examination to identify areas of fluid suitable for needle aspiration from pleural cavity and identification of solid masses in an ascitic abdomen. Echocardiography (Fig. 2-51) is helpful in identifying pericardial fluid or thickening. With constrictive

Table 2-9
Efficacy of Diagnostic Procedures

Method	Number Examined	Correct Diagnosis
Cytology of fluid	172	4%
Needle biopsy	69	26%
Open biopsy	115	38%
Excision	60	70%

disease the posterior left ventricular endocardium, epicardium, and parietal pericardium show a reduced diastolic excursion related to restricted ventricular filling. In addition, the anterior mitral valve may show abnormal diastolic closure, and septal motion may be abnormal. Pericardial effusions may be present both anteriorly and posteriorly, and with large effusions, there may be a swinging motion of the heart, the equivalent of electrical alternans on the ECG. This swinging motion may simulate paradoxical septal motion. Echocardiography is a simple noninvasive way of confirming cardiac tamponade and avoids the need of catheterizing those patients with a short life expectancy. Appropriate isotope examinations are useful for detection of skeletal and visceral metastases (see Figs. 2-56 to 2-60). Gray scale sonic and CT examinations are also of use in assessing extent of tumor.

TREATMENT

Treatment is essentially supportive and palliative. Interested readers are referred to a scientific but still compassionate survey of available modalities by Elmes.[40]

RADIOLOGY

Pleural Mesothelioma

The radiographic diagnosis of malignant pleural mesothelioma is based on the identification of appropriate radiographic findings and a compatible clinical history. Association with a history of asbestos exposure is helpful but not mandatory. The signs to be considered include pleural effusion; thickening of the parietal pleura, which may be diffuse or lobulated; thickening of the visceral pleura; solitary masses; hydropneumothorax; satellite lung lesions; and hilar adenopathy. In addition, evidence of prior asbestos exposure shown by calcified and noncalcified pleural plaques, pulmonary fibrosis, and visceral pleural thickening should be sought. A search for radiographic evidence of spread above the diaphragm to involve mediastinal structures, extrathoracic structures, and the diaphragm itself is made. Similarly examination of infradiaphragmatic areas is made, as well as a search for distant metastases.

Pleural Effusions

Radiographically detectable pleural effusion is a frequent initial sign (see Table 2-10). In Ratzer's series, 15 of 16 epithelial-type mesotheliomata and 8 of 15 fibrosarcomatous type had an initial pleural effusion.[35] The difference in

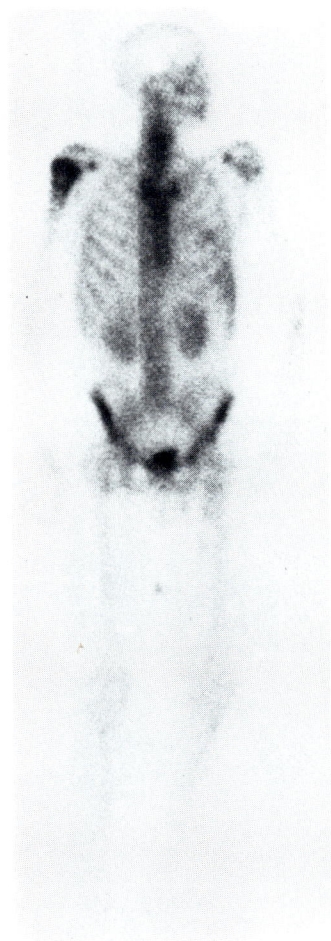

Fig. 2-56. Mesothelioma. Technetium 99m polyphosphate scintigram of a man who developed a cuboidal cell mesothelioma. He had worked for 20 years as a shipfitter and boilermaker. Anterior view shows metastatic deposits in the proximal part of the right humerus and in the left seventh and eighth ribs. Bloodborne metastases were present in both lungs, which also contained much pulmonary fibrosis and many ferruginous bodies. (Courtesy of Paul Hoffer, M.D., U.C.S.F.)

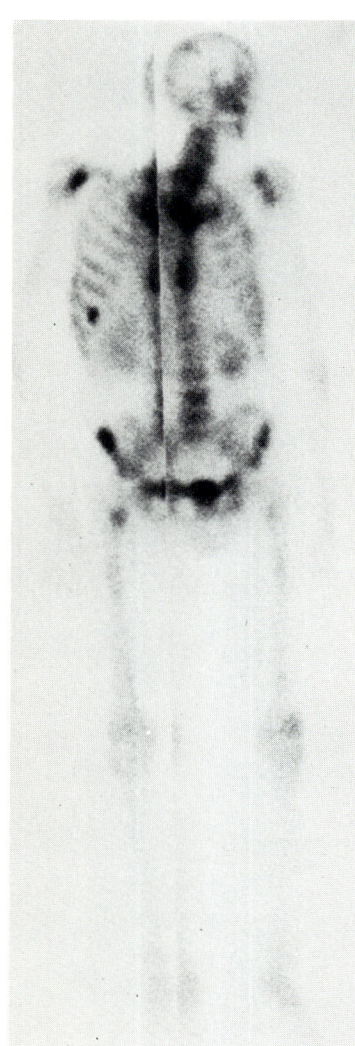

Fig. 2-57. Mesothelioma. Technetium 99m polyphosphate scintigram of a man who had developed a mesothelioma after working for 21 years in an asbestos insulating factory. Initial histological diagnosis was adenocarcinoma, which was later altered to mesothelioma after use of special staining techniques (mucicarmine, PAS, and mucopolysaccharide stains). Differentiation of mesothelioma from a peripheral adenocarcinoma is often difficult. Metastases are seen in the calvarium, the proximal right humerus, a right anterior rib, the thoracic and lumbar spine, and the proximal right femur. The tumor also invaded the abdomen. (Courtesy of Paul Hoffer, M.D., U.C.S.F.)

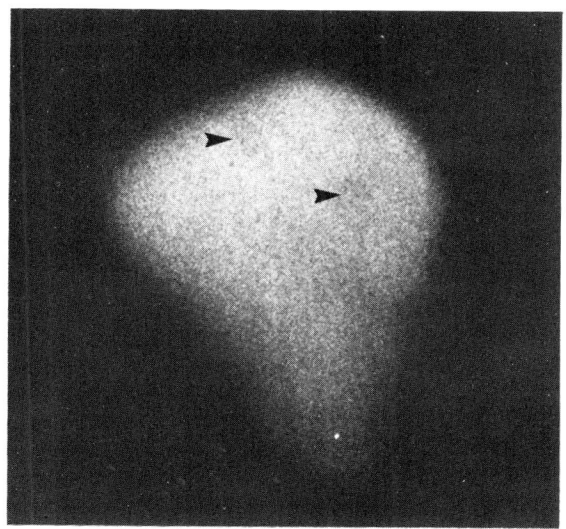

Fig. 2-58. Mesothelioma. Technetium 99m liver scintigram showing two bloodborne metastases in a man who was a shipyard worker in World War II. The initial diagnosis based on pleural biopsy was pleural fibrosis and chronic inflammation. A decortication procedure was done, and the diagnosis was unchanged after examination of removed tissue. Development of bony metastases prompted reexamination of the material at a mesothelioma referral center, and the diagnosis was changed to mesothelioma of mixed sarcomatous and carcinomatous type. The tumor invaded the retroperitoneal tissues, setting up a desmoplastic reaction around the ureters but not blocking them. (Courtesy of Paul Hoffer, M.D., U.C.S.F.)

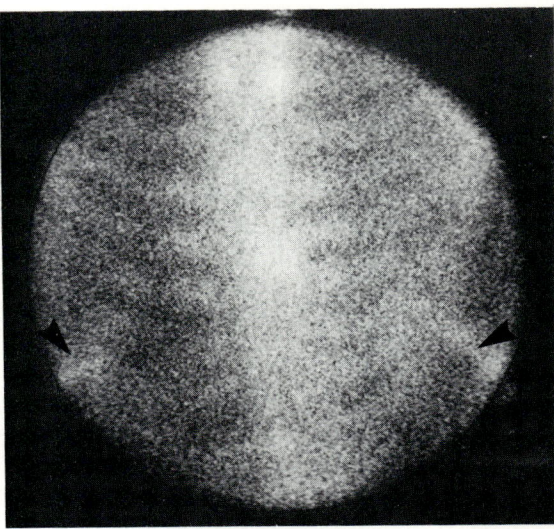

Fig. 2-59. Mesothelioma. Technetium 99 scintigram of a rib cage. The lesion in the right upper rib is a metastases from mesothelioma. The apparent left-sided lesion is secondary to thoracotomy for a diagnosis of an underlying mesothelioma. (Courtesy of Paul Hoffer, M.D., U.C.S.F.)

incidence of effusion may be related to the gross morphology. Epithelial mesotheliomata, which have a high incidence of accompanying effusion, are usually poorly demarcated areas of pleural thickening, while the fibrosarcomatous type, as elsewhere in the body, tends to more localized, discrete, and bulky. Nearly all patients will develop a pleural effusion as the disease progresses (Fig. 2-61). A frequent appearance is the irregular tumoral pleural thickening above the level of fluid (Fig. 2-62). Rarely the effusion may be large enough to produce x-ray signs of mediastinal shift; this may persist, or as the tumor enlarges and causes atelectasis or fixation, there may be shift of mediastinal structures to the affected side, as well as other signs of volume loss such as rib crowding or diaphragmatic elevation. It may be helpful for the radiologist to inquire about accompanying pain and friction rub. This is rarely typically pleuritic but more of a diffuse ache unrelated to breathing, and as the effusion increases, the pain increases. This is unlike pleurisy of an inflammatory nature in which the pain will diminish as the enlarging effusion separates inflamed parietal and visceral pleurae. Further, unlike most of the pleurisies resulting from inflammation, collagen disease, or pulmonary infarction, a friction rub is rarely heard, possibly because the layers of pleurae may be adherent or the effusion loculated. A certain amount of radiological caution is necessary in

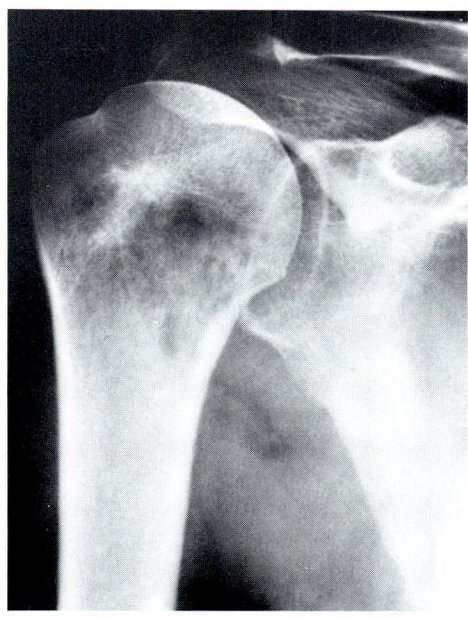

Fig. 2-60. *Mesothelioma. Patchy areas of increased and reduced density in the proximal right humerus due to bloodborne metastases from a mesothelioma of the left lung. Areas of reduced bony density in the upper extremity may be due to atrophy secondary to causalgia or disuse if they are on the same side as a mesothelioma and brachial plexus is invaded.*

Table 2-10
Percentage of
Pleural Mesothelioma
Accompanied by
Radiographically Identifiable
Pleural Effusion

Author	Percentage
Solomon[36]	61%
Elmes[22]	63%
Heller[34]	40%
Ratzer[35]	74%

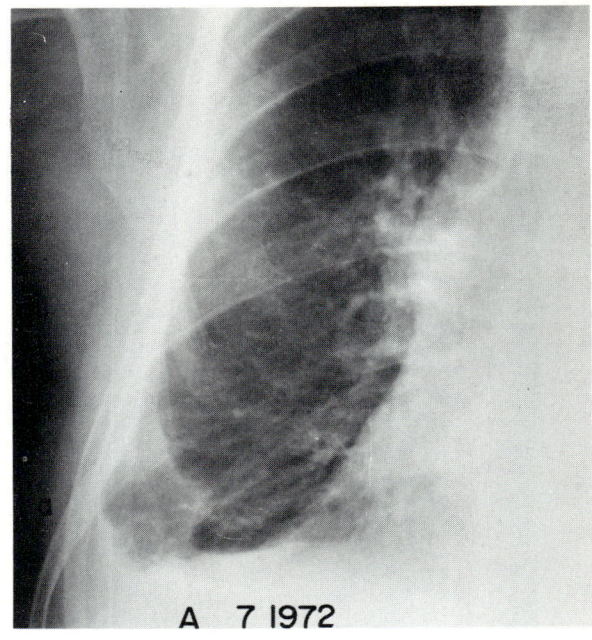

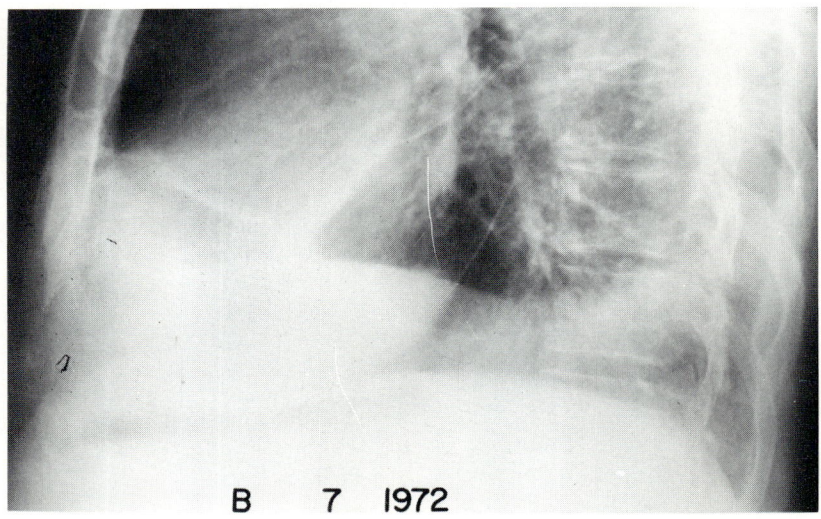

Fig. 2-61. Mesothelioma development, PA and lateral views. (A and B) There is a small pleural effusion and subaxillary noncalcified plaques in July 1972. (C) By April 1973, there is extension into the mediastinum. The hilus is enveloped by tumor (arrow), and the plaques are obscured by effusion. An erroneous diagnosis of hilar carcinoma would be suggested if the patient were first seen in this stage. (D) In April 1974, there is a pleural peel (seen toward apex), a huge tumor mass, and lung parenchymal invasion.

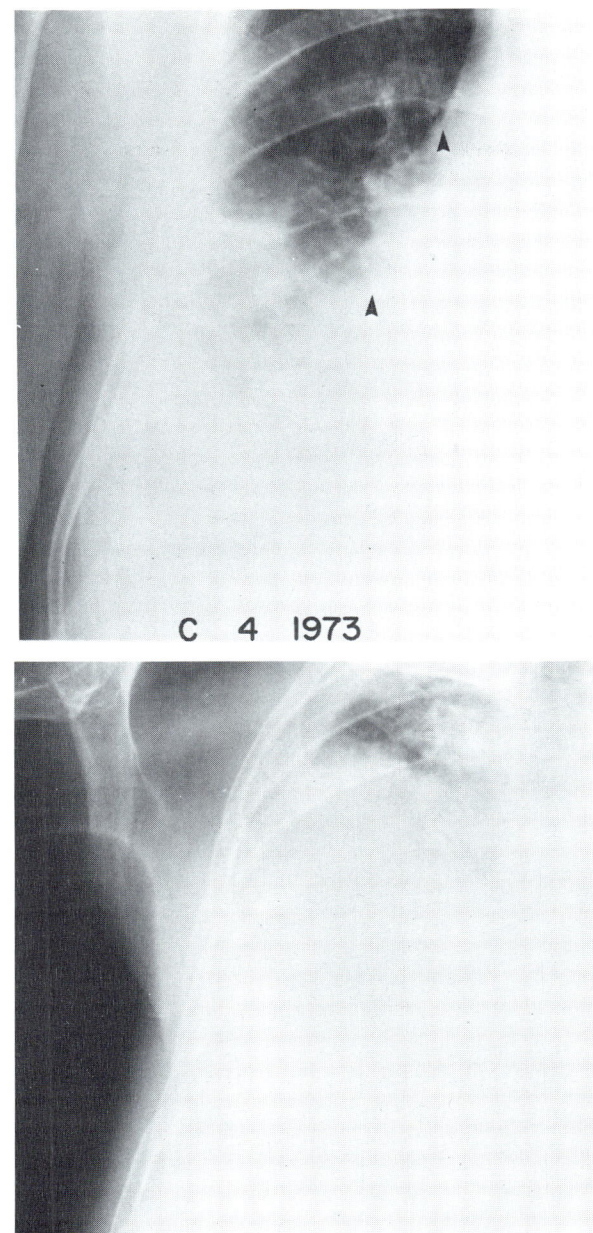

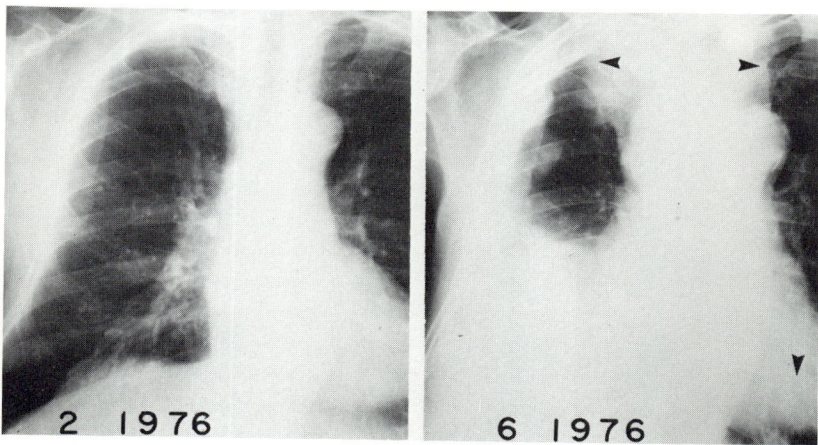

Fig. 2-62. *Rapid development of mesothelioma. In February 1976, the chest radiograph is normal, and there is some lobulation of the right hemidiaphragm. Four months later, a large pleural-based mass encases the right lung. Part of it is lobulated. There is involvement of both sides of the upper mediastinum (arrows) and a round bloodborne metastasis is seen at the base of the left lung (vertical arrow). The initial histological diagnosis was of anaplastic carcinoma from an unknown primary site; it was later revised to mesothelioma. The patient had been a shipfitter. This sequence of events is more rapid than most mesotheliomata. Conventional bedside teaching used to stress that where the clinical diagnosis was in doubt, the quickly spreading tumors were carcinoma and the more slowly spreading ones were mesothelioma.*

assessing effusion related to mesothelioma. A few patients may have a pleural effusion present for many months before clinical or cytological evidence of mesothelioma becomes apparent. An effusion may be present on the contralateral side, with no radiographic evidence of tumor spread from the side harboring the mesothelioma (Chapter 2, Section 5). Whatever the initial size of an effusion accompanying a mesothelioma, it usually reaccumulates rapidly when aspirated.

Pleural (Parietal, Visceral) Thickening

Pleural thickening may be diffuse or lobulated. Diffuse thickening is more frequent with the epithelial type (Fig. 2-63), and irregular lobular masses are more frequent with the fibrosarcomatous type. Since most tumors are mixed, this sign has its limitations. The malignant nature of diffuse pleural thickening may not be fully appreciated, because this may also occur as a nonmalignant response to asbestos exposure. Characteristically, hyaline pleural plaques, reasonably well circumscribed and either calcified or noncalcified, are a

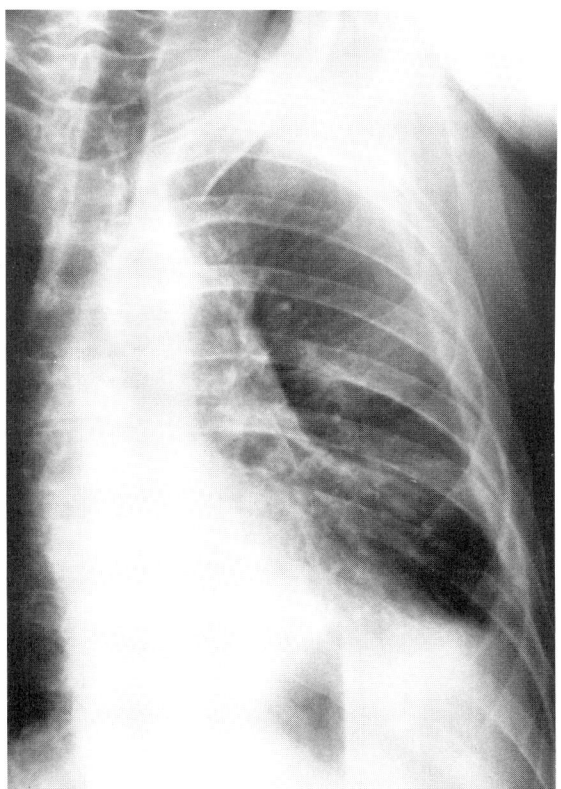

Fig. 2-63. *Mesothelioma. Thick pleural "peel" surrounds the lung from apex to base. This is a decubitus view (note gastric air bubble). The appearance in the erect view was identical with regard to the pleural peel. It is usually difficult to identify free pleural fluid accompanying a mesothelioma by conventional radiographic means, but decubitus CT sections are often helpful.*

frequent result of asbestos inhalation. Until recently, insufficient attention has been paid to the fact that diffuse thickening of the parietal pleura initially and the visceral pleura subsequently may occur.[36] Such diffuse areas of thickening of parietal and visceral pleurae do not calcify, unlike localized parietal pleural plaques. This benign thickening is progressive and has been reported up to 15 mm thick. It may therefore simulate mesothelioma, except that it is not lobulated. This benign thickening has to be differentiated from parietal and/or visceral pleural thickening residual from a prior benign asbestos effusion. The minor fissure is involved more frequently than is the major fissure in the dry type of diffuse benign pleural reaction.[36]

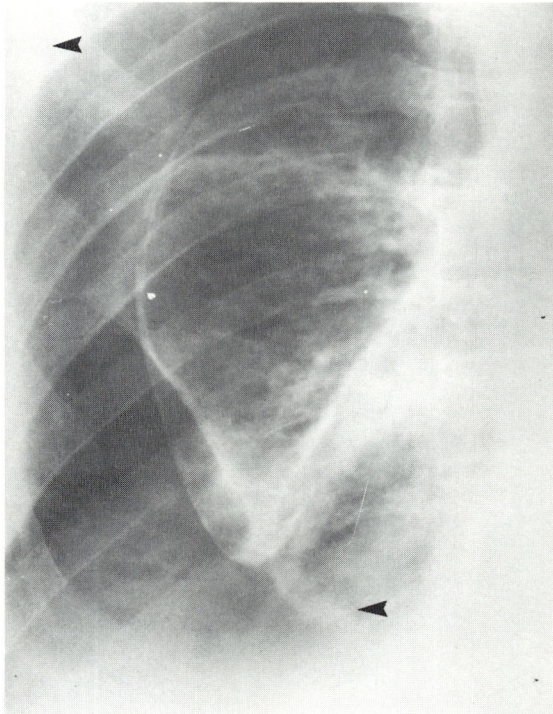

Fig. 2-64. *Mesothelioma. Pneumothorax accompanying mesothelioma. Mesothelioma may present with pneumothorax. The mechanism is unknown. Arrows indicate tumoral thickening of parietal and visceral pleurae.*

Lobular Thickening

Lobular thickening of the pleura may be apparent initially, or it may be apparent after an invasive diagnostic procedure if sufficient air remains to separate the pleural layers. A mesothelioma may occasionally present with or develop a spontaneous pneumothorax (Fig. 2-64) which permits visualization of these lobular masses. Tomography is helpful in showing the lobular areas. Lobular areas due to tumor are more frequent with the fibrosarcomatous than with the epithelial type. Some lobular areas result from pseudotumors, which occur in both the epithelial and fibrosarcomatous type. Pseudotumors are cavities within the thickened pleura filled with necrotic and fibrinous semiliquid material. They, too, are seen best with tomography and may sometimes appear to be within the lung parenchyma, their true site is not realized until surgical exposure or necropsy. Benign pleural tumors, especially fibrous mesothelioma may arise from a stalk. Although one malignant mesothelioma on a thin pedicle has been described, this is an exception. The radiographic appearance does not differ from other lobular pleural masses; differentiation from lymphangitic spread of carcinoma, malignant lymphoma, and pleural sarcoma (Fig. 2-65) is needed.

Most malignant mesotheliomata appear to originate from the lower portion of the pleura; very few are reported as arising near the apices. This is in contradistinction to benign cellular or fibrous mesotheliomata and other benign pleural tumors, lipomas, angiomas, fibromas, and chondromas that may arise in any pleural zone (see Figs. 2-66 to 2-68). Benign pleural tumors may also develop in the interlobar fissures, which is rarely the case with the malignant type. Diffuse thickening of the interlobar fissures, however, especially the minor fissure, is a recently reported sign of benign-type asbestos exposure.[36] Malignant mesothelioma due to asbestos exposure and arising from the pericardium has not been reported, but a study of Figure 2-47 suggests that this case may be an exception.

Solitary Mass

A solitary mass is a less common x-ray finding (Fig. 2-69). This presentation occurred in 2 out of 10 of Heller's patients and is more common in the fibrosarcomatous type. It may be indistinguishable radiographically, even with tomography, from a primary peripheral bronchogenic carcinoma. When it arises in the upper pleura, radiographic diagnosis is especially difficult, since most malignant mesotheliomata have a predilection for lower zones. Some fibrosarcomatous mesotheliomata may reach large dimensions, up to 30 cm, and still be confined to one lung zone. This radiographic appearance has not been stressed, since the more common appearance of a malignant mesothelioma encasing the lung is better known.

Hydropneumothorax

This may be an occasional rare form of presentation. It permits appreciation of the diffuse or lobular malignant thickening of the pleura and assessment of any benign calcified or noncalcified pleural plaques that may be present on the parietal pleura. It is conjectured that the limited invasion of underlying lung parenchyma that occurs with mesothelioma is sufficient to allow development of a pneumothorax. Spontaneous pneumothoraxes are seen with both the epithelial and fibrosarcomatous type. Parenchymal masses or infiltrates with a known association for spontaneous pneumothorax include peripheral rheumatoid nodules, cavitating pulmonary infarcts, cavitating osteogenic sarcoma and Hodgkin's disease, and pneumatoceles of varying etiology.

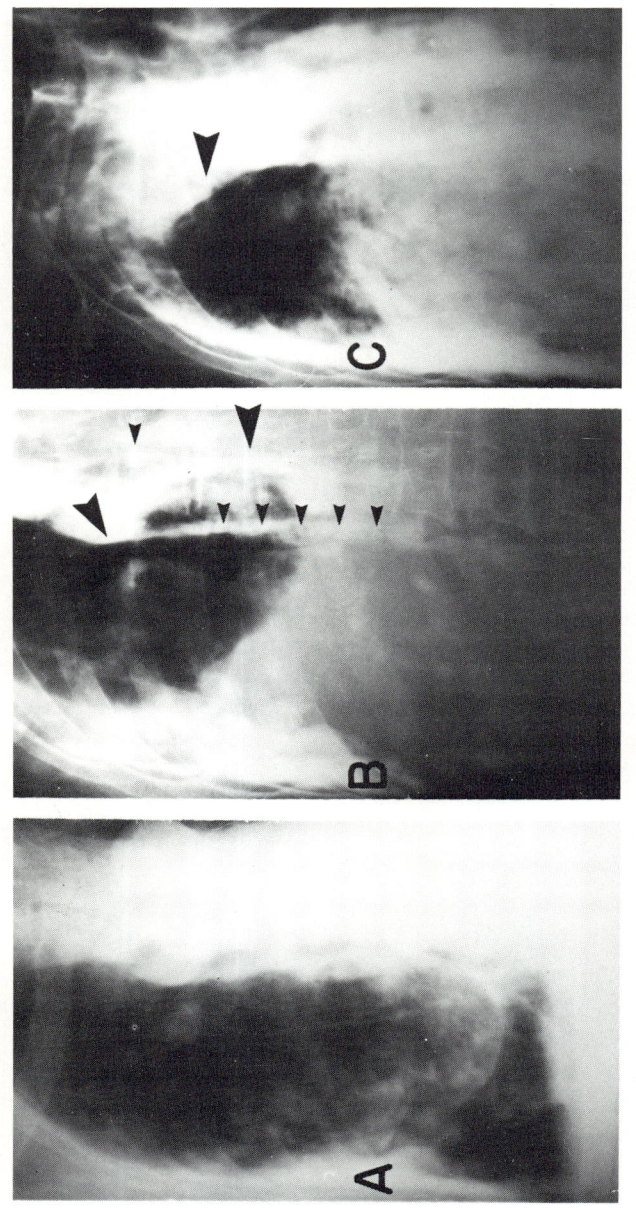

Fig. 2-65. Osteogenic sarcoma of pleura. (A) Hydropneumothorax showing involvement of parietal and visceral pleurae. (B) There are tumoral infiltrations along the anterior mediastinal line (large horizontal arrow), the posterior mediastinal line (small single horizontal arrow), the right paratracheal line which is bulbously enlarged (oblique arrow), and the lateral margin of the superior and inferior venae cavae (multiple small arrows). (C) Five months later than A and B, the paraspinous line (arrow) is grossly widened by tumor. The tumor has also widened more than in B, the other mediastinal lines both to left and right of midline. (Courtesy of Howard L. Steinbach, M.D. and W. H. Moncrief, Jr., M.D.)

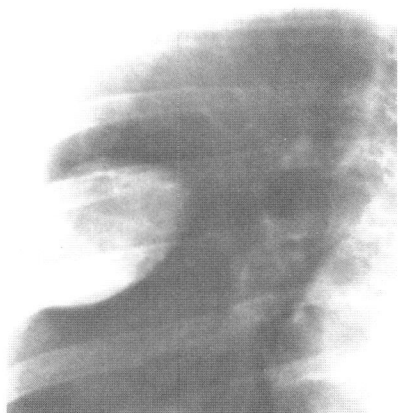 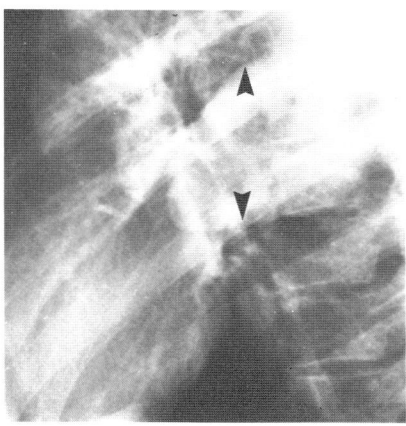

Fig. 2-66. *PA and lateral views of lipoma arising from parietal pleura. There is an accompanying iatrogenic pneumothorax. The elongated shape may be due to its position partly within the major fissure. (Compare Fig. 2-67.)*

Satellite Lung Lesions

This is a nonspecific term and may include metastatic deposits in the same or contralateral lung (Fig. 2-70), areas of local lung invasion, and the pseudotumors described above, which may appear on tomography to lie within the lung but are in fact areas of degeneration within the thickened pleura. Metastases to the opposite lung and/or pleura are common as a late finding, but occasionally, as in Solomon's series,[33] they may be present at first examination, making radiographic differentiation from metastatic carcinoma difficult. Although superficial invasion of the lung is common, localized deep invasion may occur to present as a satellite nodule.

Hilar Adenopathy

Hilar enlargement may be seen as a result of regional lymph node involvement. More frequently, a large mass in the region of the hilus results from the direct spread of the mesothelioma to this area (Fig. 2-71) or to primary involvement of the mediastinal pleura (Fig. 2-72).

To help substantiate the diagnosis of an asbestos-related mesothelioma, a search should be made for the other stigmata of asbestos exposure—pleural and diaphragmatic plaques and/or visceral pleural thickening and pulmonary fibrosis.

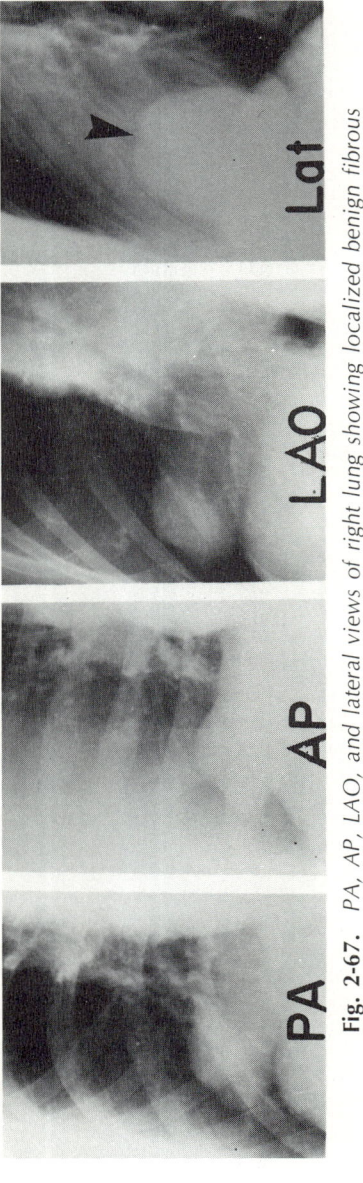

Fig. 2-67. PA, AP, LAO, and lateral views of right lung showing localized benign fibrous mesothelioma lying in a major fissure and attached to the visceral pleura overlying the middle lobe. The elongated shape is related to interlobar position; the small "dimple" seen on lateral view is helpful in differential diagnosis of this entity. It is extremely rare for a localized mesothelioma to metastasize, but such instances are known. Mesothelioma may invade the lung or chest wall. Although the cell nuclei show very little mitotic activity, absolute differentiation between benign and malignant mesothelioma may not be possible histologically. The majority of benign mesotheliomas are pedunculated; the blood supply entering via the pedicle is demonstrable by arteriography of bronchial, intercostal, or diaphragmatic vessels, according to the site of tumor origin. *Over 75 percent originate in visceral pleura. When the tumor is large there may be an accompanying pleural effusion, which makes radiographic identification of benign disease more difficult.

---

*Ellis K and Wolff M: Mesotheliomas and secondary tumors of the pleura. Seminars in Roentgenology 12(4):303–311, 1977

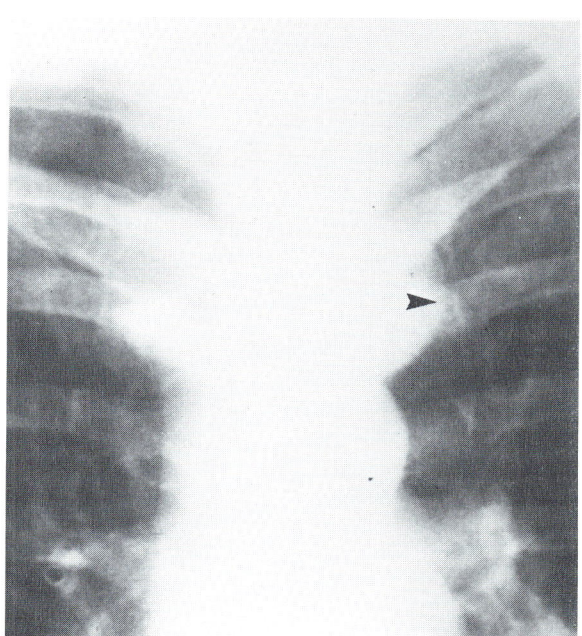

Fig. 2-68. AP view of the upper mediastinum. Above the aortic knob the rounded density (arrow) is a simple cyst of the pleura (arrow) containing clear fluid. (Courtesy of D. Cline, M.D., U.C.S.F.)

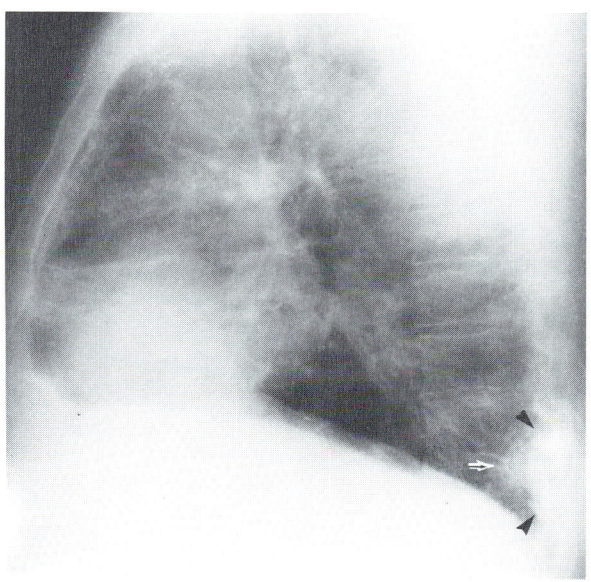

Fig. 2-69. A small mesothelioma is closely applied to the posterior ribs (oblique arrows), directly anterior in an area of direct lung parenchymal invasion (white arrow).

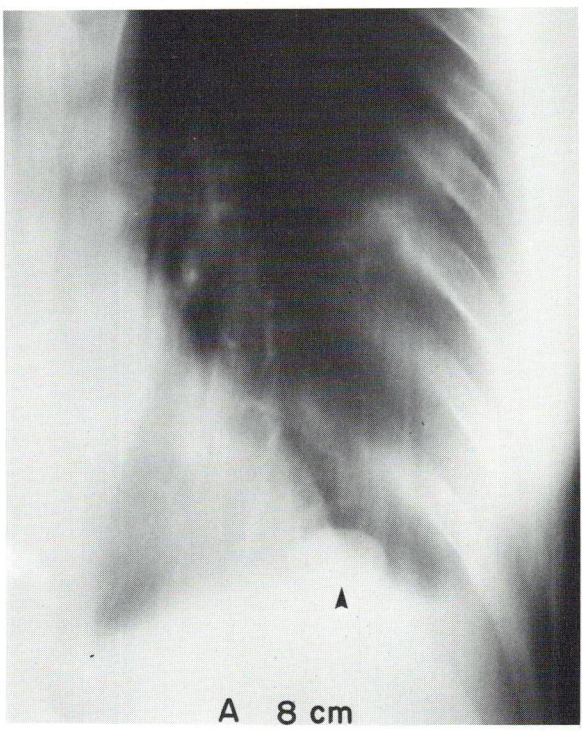

Fig. 2-70 A. *Mesothelioma. Tomographic section, 8 cm from back, shows an egg-shaped mass of metastatic mesothelioma (arrow). The main tumor lies along the lateral chest wall and is not seen well in this section. The egg-shaped mass could be construed as a primary peripheral malignancy with metastases to peripheral pleura, and a decade ago this might be the preferred diagnosis. Rib metastasis is also present.*

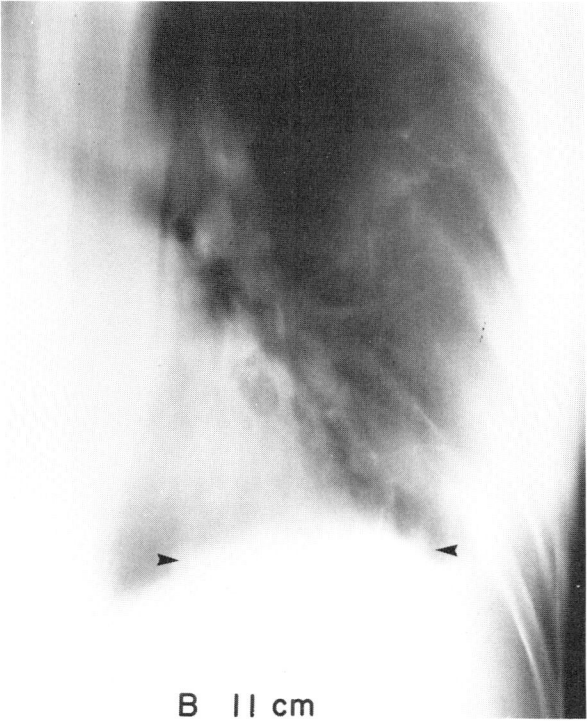

Fig. 2-70 B. *Tomographic cut, 11 cm from back, shows typical plateau-shaped noncalcified diaphragmatic plaque (arrows). The mesothelioma lies along the lower left chest wall.*

Pleural and Diaphragmatic Plaques

These should be searched for in the uninvolved areas of the pleura and diaphragm and on the contralateral side (Figs. 2-73 to 2-75). Solomon, finding only 2 of 33 mesothelioma patients to have calcified and 7 of 23 to have noncalcified plaques, postulated that a pleura with calcified plaques is less susceptible to malignant generation.[33] This appears improbable; more likely the number of calcified plaques found reflects assiduity of search and sophistication of radiographic techniques used. Thus, Edge found 20 of 28 mesothelioma patients to have pleural plaques, both calcified and noncalcified, on x-ray.[19] Since most mesotheliomata arise in lower zones, it is rare to be able to identify plaques adjacent to the ipsilateral diaphragm, but these are occasionally seen on tomograms (Fig. 2-70*B*).

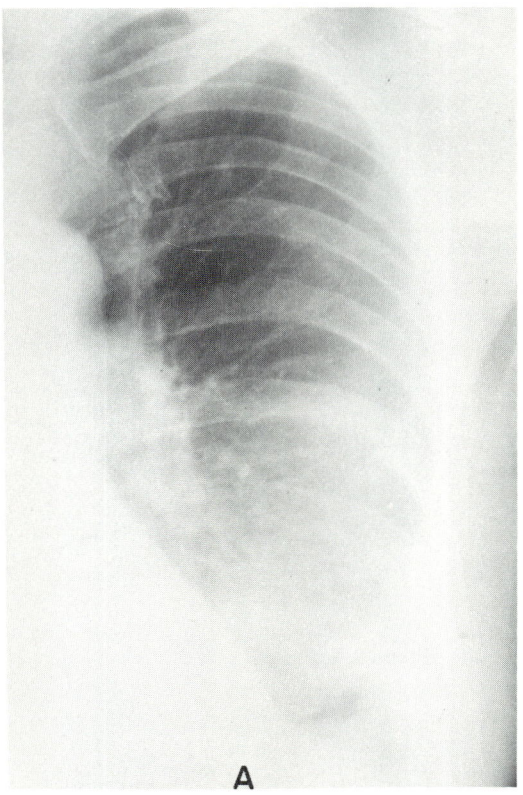

Fig. 2-71. Mesothelioma prior to thoracotomy. (A) There is as yet only slight invasion of underlying lung, and the mediastinum appears uninvolved. (B) Four months later, after thoracotomy. There is diffuse invasion of the mediastinum and underlying lung and metastases to scapula and ribs (horizontal arrow). Mesotheliomata tend to infiltrate along connective tissue planes associated with bronchovascular bundles. A small calcified plaque is still visible (vertical arrow).

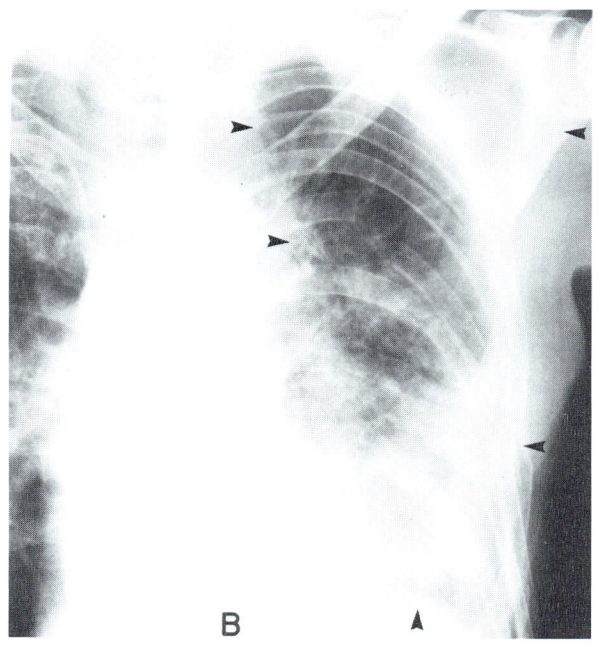

Pulmonary Fibrosis

Pulmonary fibrosis is seen histologically in about 50 percent of patients with asbestos-related pleural mesothelioma but is of sufficient degree to be apparent radiographically in only about 20 percent (Fig. 2-76). Severe pulmonary fibrosis is more common in association with peritoneal mesothelioma.

Diffuse Parietal and Visceral Pleural Thickening

Direct extension of the tumor may be above or below the diaphragm or by bloodborne spread to distant organs.

Above diaphragm. Fluoroscopy identifies fixation of the diaphragm as a result of direct involvement or extension into the phrenic nerve. The absence of clavicular companion shadows indicates extension into supraclavicular nodes, but a prior scalene fat pad biopsy may produce a false-positive sign. Enlargement of the axillary nodes is best seen by xerographic techniques. Extension through the chest wall may produce a soft tissue shadow with obliteration of fat planes; although it has been recorded in the literature, this

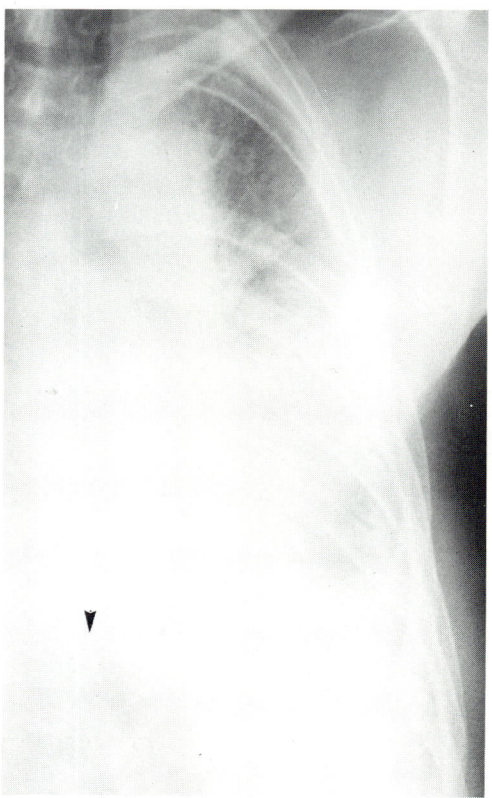

Fig. 2-72. Mesothelioma arising from mediastinal pleura. There is very little involvement of the lateral chest wall pleura. The tumor spread through the left side of the diaphragm to produce small bowel obstruction. Note the absence of bowel gas in the left upper quadrant of the abdomen and the dilated loop of small bowel.

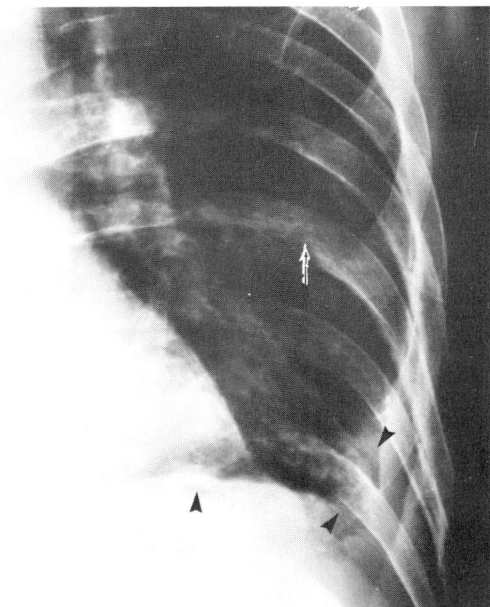

Fig. 2-73. *Mesothelioma in a boilermaker. In the left costophrenic angle is a pleural-based shadow extending over two costal interspaces; more medially (between oblique arrows) is a less defined density that arises in the pleura but whose radiographic appearance could be that of a parenchymal lesion; more laterally there is a pathological fracture through a rib involved in continuity. The undersurface of a midrib is destroyed by bloodborne spread (black and white arrows), there is a dense diaphragmatic pleural calcification (vertical arrow), and above it a small, plateaulike plaque that acts as a biological marker to suggest the diagnosis of mesothelioma.*

sign appears quite rarely. More easily assessed is rib destruction. The middle and posterior mediastinal structures are encased. The esophagus may be displaced (Fig. 2-55) or circumferentially narrowed. Differentiation from a primary esophageal cancer, of which there is an increased incidence in asbestos workers, is usually not difficult. Mucosa of the esophagus is usually not involved when there is direct extension. Involvement of the aortic wall by mediastinal extension obliterates the radiolucent line of the mediastinal pleural periaortic reflection and may simulate a dissecting aneurysm of the descending aorta, so that aortograms have occasionally been needed.[23] Venography may be needed[43] if involvement of the superior vena cava or the thoracic portion of the inferior vena cava occurs (Fig. 2-53). Involvement of the pericardium leads to enlargement of the cardiac silhouette, and if there is much pericardial effusion, tamponade with dilatation of the azygous vein width may occur. The

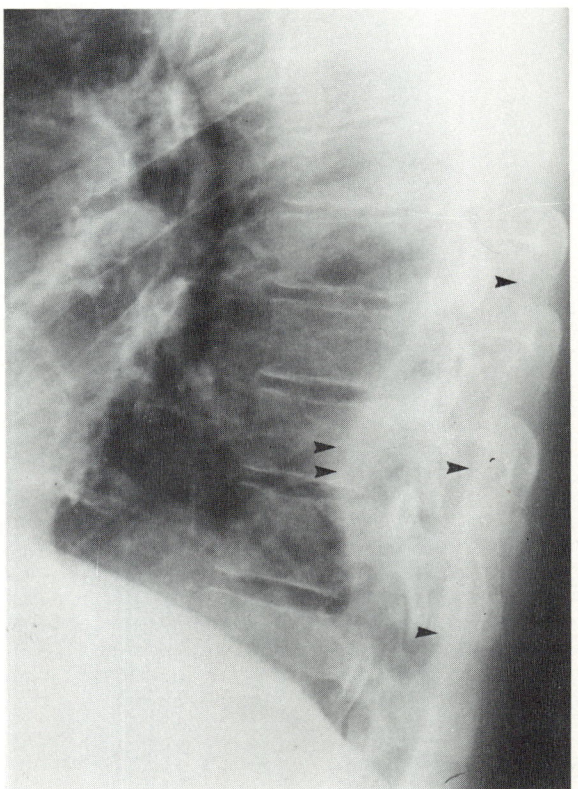

Fig. 2-74. Early mesothelioma. The localized pleural mass closely applied to the lower left ribs (double arrow) is a mesothelioma. Adjacent to the right ribs (3 arrows) there is a lesser degree of, but more diffuse, pleural thickening due to a noncalcified plaque. The patient died 12 months later. He also had a bowel resection some years previously for adenocarcinoma of the colon. There is evidence of approximately double the normal incidence of colon cancer in patients who have had heavy asbestos exposure.

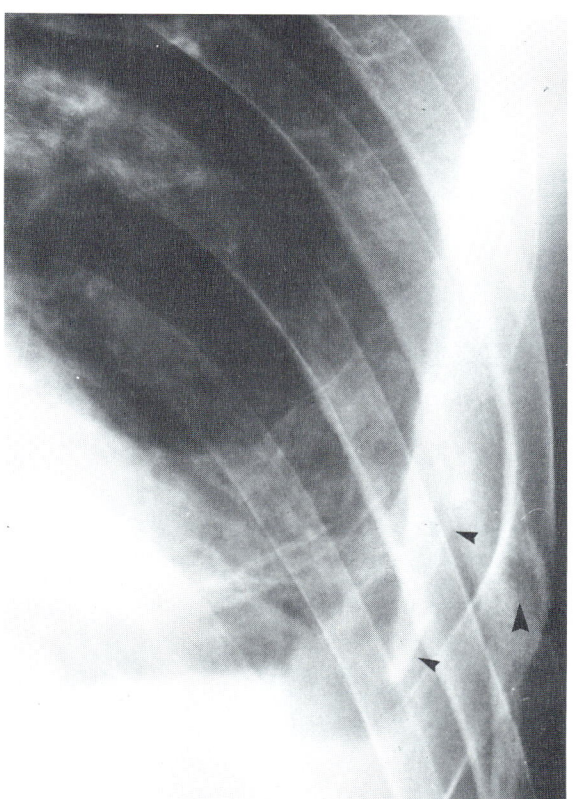

Fig. 2-75. Mesothelioma. Several calcified pleural plaques are seen at the lower border of the mesothelioma mass (oblique arrows). Noncalcified plaques are usually obscured by the tumor mass. Calcified plaques may be visible, depending on their size. Note direct rib invasion (vertical arrow).

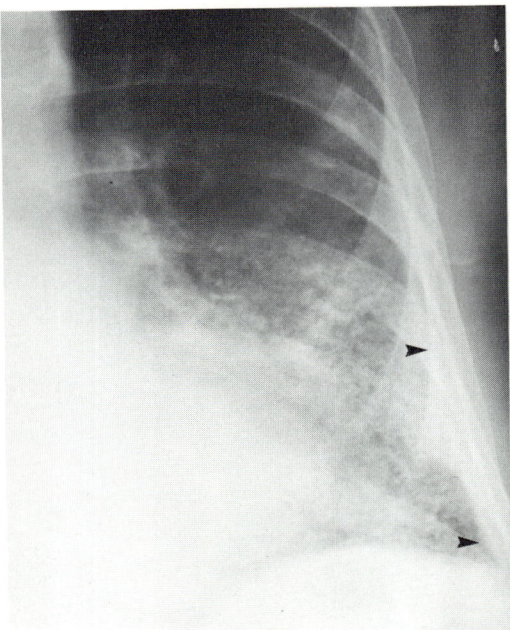

Fig. 2-76. *Mesothelioma. Arrows indicate an early pleural mesothelioma in a patient with severe lower lobe and lingular fibrosis. Fibrosis is more commonly associated with peritoneal mesothelioma.*

upper limit of the azygous vein in normal nonpregnant patients has been assessed variously as lying between 6 and 10 mm[37] on an upright 6-ft PA view. In many patients seriously ill with mesothelioma, only a supine portable film at a distance of 40 in. is available. For this group of patients, an azygous vein width greater than 15 mm is associated with a raised central venous pressure. The linear relationship between the two is (azygous vein width in millimeters × 1.4) − 3 = CVP millimeters of water.[33] Conventional radiography may suggest signs of pericardial effusion or thickening. These signs may be summarized as marked nonspecific cardiac enlargement, especially if lung fields are clear; encroachment of cardiac shadow on retrosternal space; asymmetric enlargement of cardiac silhouette produced by uneven distensibility of pericardial space or by loculation; sudden change in heart size, especially in absence of heart failure; and widening of the pericardial stripe.[38] In the lateral chest film, especially when coned-down and centered on the lower anterior chest wall, the thin radiolucent black line of epicardial fat is visible. Anterior to it is a radiopaque white stripe composed of the layers of the pericardium, and more anterior is the radiolucent mediastinal fat. Widening of the white pericardial

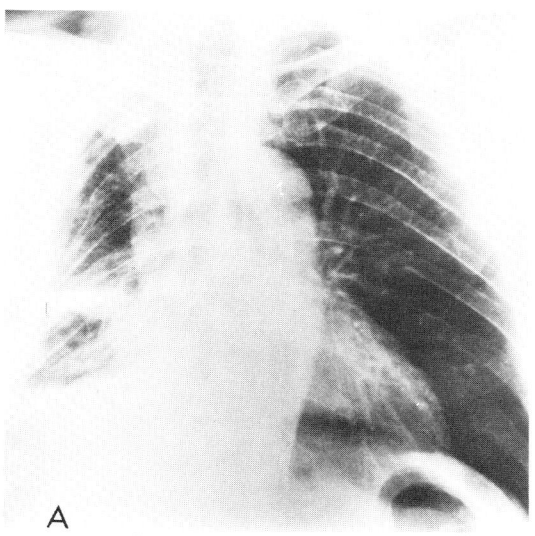

Fig. 2-77 A. Mesothelioma. A 55-year-old man with decortication of right lung 3 years previously for recurrent pleural effusion. Chest film showing decreased volume of right lung, thickened pleura, and a mass at the lung apex.

stripe is suggestive of pericardial effusion or thickening. This sign has its limitations in women, in whom breast shadows may obscure the area. The hilar overlay sign, in which an enlarging pericardial effusion obscures the origin of the pulmonary arteries, unlike an enlarging heart which displaces them, is very useful but may be difficult to assess on portable films, especially if there is a slight apical-lordotic tilt of the tube. Echocardiography[41] has replaced fluoroscopy. Positive and negative contrast examination and radioisotopic scanning in which the blood pool is labeled with ^{131}I, iodine-tagged albumin, or technetium-labeled albumin were other useful techniques prior to the advent of echocardiography.

CT has a part in the assessment of mesothelioma because of its ability to identify adjacent areas with only a slight difference in the attenuation coefficient. There may be insufficient radiographic contrast from surrounding air to visualize some mesotheliomata, peripherally located carcinomata, lymphomata, and sarcomata with conventional radiography. The transverse sections are ideally suited to the display of the circumferential or localized involvement of the lung, encasement or actual involvement of the hilar nodes, involvement of the pericardium and the myocardium of the atria and ventricles, encasement of the aorta and penetration of the intercostal muscles and the diaphragm. (Fig. 2-77). Scans at upper levels in the thorax may show spread to axillary and

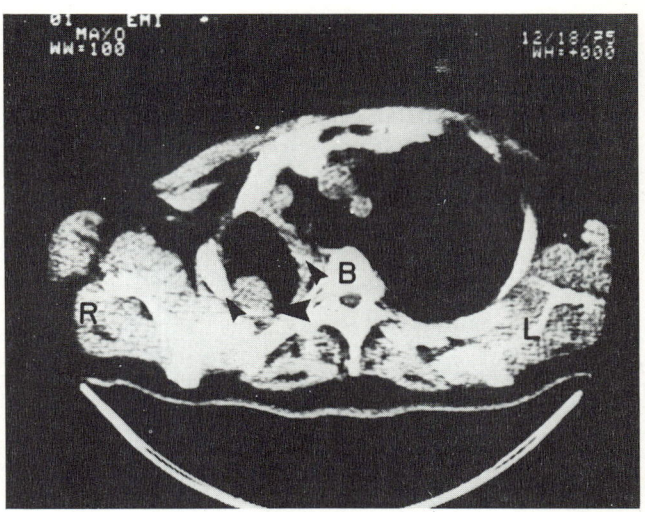

Fig. 2-77 B. *CT section through lung apices showing peripheral mediastinal pleural thickening (oblique arrows) and rounded mass posteriorly (large horizontal arrow). The innominate and left carotid arteries are seen in cross section anterior to vertebral body.*

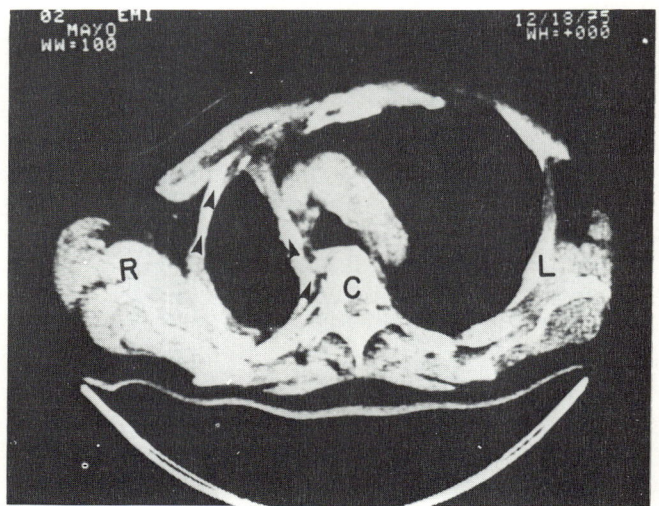

Fig. 2-77 C. *CT section at lower level showing a large rind of thickened pleura completely encircling the right lung (arrow). The arch of the aorta lies anterior to the vertebral body.*

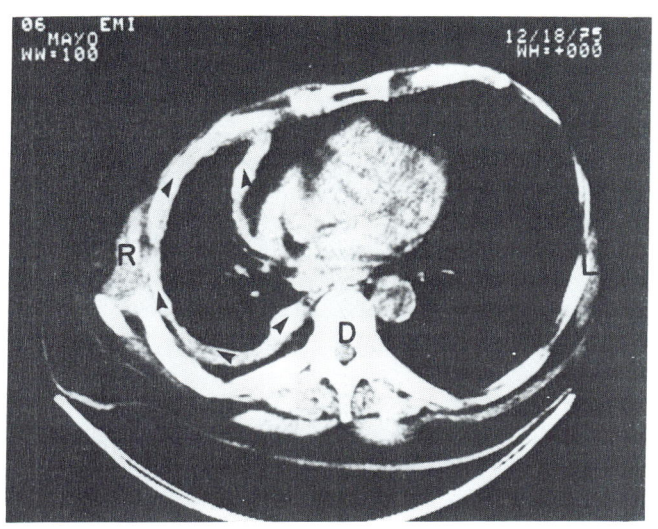

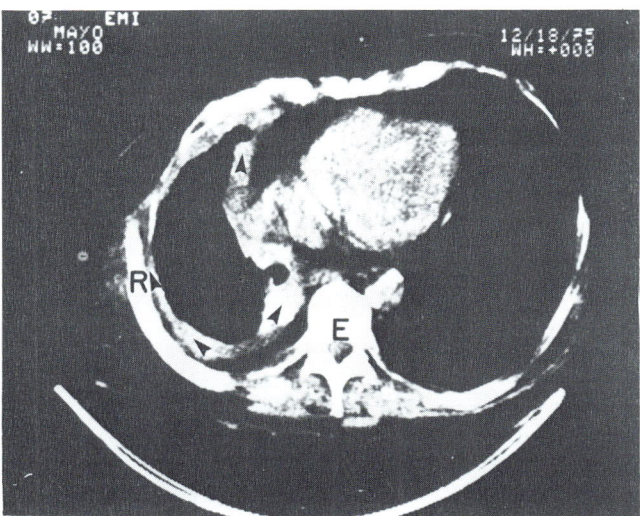

Fig. 2-77 D, E. *CT sections at lower levels below the right hilus show extensive pleural rind (arrow) due to mesothelioma. (Courtesy of Drs. P. F. Sheedy II, D. H. Stephens, R. H. Hattery, J. R. Muhm, G. W. Hartman, and the publishers of the American Journal of Roentgenology.*

retrosternal nodes. The place of CT in the differentiation of mesothelioma from widespread pleural involvement by anaplastic carcinoma has not yet been determined. Use of appropriate window widths and heights will differentiate secondaries in the bony thorax, however. The thickness of a mesothelioma varies, and CT may indicate the optimal site for aspiration biopsy. Utilizing CT in the decubiti positions, an accompanying effusion may be separated from mesothelioma tumor mass, which is an additional aid in planning percutaneous biopsy. CT in individual cases has been shown to be of value in following reduction of mesothelioma bulk during treatment.[39]

Below diaphragm. Plain films may show signs of intestinal obstruction. Barium examination may be used to confirm this and show extrinsic pressure on bowel. Mucosa usually shows only minimal changes. With large masses, it is difficult to separate intraperitoneal and extraperitoneal extension of the mesothelioma; both occur, although intraperitoneal extension is more common. Separation of bowel loops may be due to free fluid or serosal thickening. Infiltration of the omentum may displace gastric air bubble (Fig. 2-55B). Ureteric obstruction should be sought for by pyelography.

Peritoneal Mesothelioma

The radiographic findings[42] are similar to those found in thoracic mesothelioma extending into the abdomen and so will not be detailed. A greater amount of ascites may be present, and depending on the site of origin, distortion of the pelvic colon may be greater than when a thoracic mesothelioma has extended inferiorly. Occasionally, pleural and peritoneal mesothelioma appear to have originated concurrently.

REFERENCES

1. Wagner JC, Sleggs CA, Marchand P: Diffuse pleural mesothelioma and asbestos exposure in the Northwest Cape Province. Br J Ind Med 17:260–271, 1960
2. Rossiter CE: Discussion summary, in Bogovski P, Gilson JC, Tembrill V, et al (eds): Biological Effects of Asbestos. Lyon, IARC Scientific Publications, 1973, pp 226–227
3. Baginsky E: Occupational illness and accidents reported from California shipyards. Environ Res 11:271–279, 1976
4. Webster I: Malignancy in relation to crocidolite and amosite, in Bogovski P, Gilson JC, Tembrill V, et al (eds): Biological Effects of Asbestos. Lyon, IARC Scientific Publications, 1973, pp 195–198

5. Selikoff IJ, Hammond EC, Seidman H: Cancer risk of installation workers in the United States, in Bogovski P, Gilson JC, Tembrill V, et al (eds): Biological Effects of Asbestos. Lyon, IARC Scientific Publications, 1973, pp 209–216
6. Newhouse ML, Berry G, Wagner JC, et al: A study of the mortality of the female asbestos worker. Br J Ind Med 29:134–141, 1972
7. Milne JEH: 32 Cases of mesothelioma in Victoria, Australia: A retrospective survey related to occupational asbestos exposure. Br J Ind Med 33:115–122, 1976
8. Greenberg M, Davis Lloyd TA: Mesothelioma register 1967–1968. Br J Ind Med 31(2):91–104, 1974
9. Webster I: Biological effects of asbestos. Ann NY Acad Sci 32:1–761, 1965
10. Borow M, Conston A, Livornese L, et al: Mesothelioma following exposure to asbestos: A review of 72 cases. Chest 64 (5):641–6, 1973
11. Elmes PC: The epidemilogy and clinical features of asbestos and related disease. Postgrad Med J 42:623–635, 1966
12. Oels HC, Harrison EG, Carr DT, et al: Diffuse malignant mesothelioma of the pleura: A review of 37 cases. Chest 60(6):564–570, 1971
13. Magner D, McDonald AD: Malignant mesothelioma tumors—histological types and asbestos exposure. N Engl J Med 287:570–1, 1972
14. Anderson HA, Lilis R, Daum S, et al: Household-contact asbestos neoplastic risk. Ann NY Acad Sci 271:311–23, 1976
15. Hall SA: Occupational exposure to pollution. J R Coll Physicians Lond 5:379–384, 1971
16. Newhouse ML: Cancer among workers in asbestos textile industry, in Bogovski P, Gilson JD, Tembrill V, et al (eds): Biological Effects of Asbestos. Lyon, IARC Scientific Publications, 1973, pp 203–208
17a. Poole FD: Mesothelioma in relation to exposure, in Bogovski P, Gilson JD, Tembrill V, et al (eds): Biological Effects of Asbestos. Lyon, IARC Scientific Publications, 1973, pp 222–225
17b. Poole FD: Electron microscopic charteristics of inhaled chrysotile asbestos fibers. Br J Ind Med 29:146–153, 1972
18. Lawther, PJ: Asbestos. Some nonradiological aspects. Proc R Soc Med 64:833–834, 1971
19. Edge JR: Asbestos related disease in Barrow-in-Furness. Environ Res 11:244–247, 1976
20. Harris PG: Experience with asbestos disease and its control in Great Britain's naval dockyards. Environ Res 11:261–267, 1976
21. Lewinsohn HC: Early malignant changes in pleural plaque due to asbestos exposure. Br J Dis Chest 68(2):121–7, 1974
22. Elmes PC: The natural history of diffuse mesothelioma, in Bogovski P,

Gilson JD, Tembrill V, et al (eds): Biological Effects of Asbestos. Lyon, IARC Scientific Publications, 1973, pp 267–272
23. Taryle DA, Lakshminarayan S, Sahn SA: Pleural mesothelioma-An analysis of 18 cases and review of the literature. Medicine 55:153–162, 1976
24. Whitwell F, Rawcliffe RM: Diffuse malignant pleural mesothelioma and asbestos exposure. Thorax 26:6–22, 1971
25. Zielhus RL, Versteeg JPG, Planteudt HT: Pleural mesothelioma and exposure to asbestos. Int Arch Occup Environ Health 36:1–18, 1975
26. Pearson KD, Rubin D, Szemes GC, et al: Extraosseous osteogenic sarcoma of the chest. Br J Dis Chest 63:231–234 1969
27. Webster I: Quoted in Discussion Summary by C.E.Rossiter, in Bogovski P, Gilson JD, Tembrill V, et al (eds): Biological Effects of Asbestos. Lyon, IARC Scientific Publications, 1973, pp 226–227
28. Boersma A, Degand P, Havez R: Diffuse mesothelioma: Biochemical stages in the diagnosis, detection and measurement of hyaluronic acid in pleural fluid, in Bogovski P, Gilson JD, Tembrill V, et al (eds): Biological Effects of Asbestos. Lyon, IARC Scientific Publications, 1973, pp 65–67
29. Kannerstein M, Churg J, Magner D: Histochemical studies of mesothelioma, in Bogovski P, Gilson JD, Tembrill V, et al (eds): Biological Effects of Asbestos. Lyon, IARC Scientific Publications, 1973, pp 62–64
30. Elmes PC: Therapeutic openings in the treatment of mesothelioma, in Bogovski P, Gilson JD, Tembrill V, et al (eds): Biological Effects of Asbestos. Lyon, IARC Scientific Publications, 1973, pp 277–280
31. Hochberg LA: Endothelioma (mesothelioma) of the pleura. Am Rev Tuberculosis 63:150–175, 1950
32. Butler EB, Berry AV: Diffuse mesotheliomas: Diagnostic criteria using exfoliative cytology, in Bogovski P, Gilson JD, Tembrill V, et al (eds): Biological Effects of Asbestos. Lyon, IARC Scientific Publications, 1973, pp 68–73
33. Solomon A: Radiological features of diffuse mesothelioma, in Shapiro HA (ed): Pneumoconiosis. Proceedings of the International Conference, Johannesburg, 1969. Capetown, OUP, 1970, pp 261–265
34. Heller RM, Janower ME, Weber AL: The radiological manifestations of malignant pleural mesothelioma. Radiology 108:53–59, 1973
35. Ratzer ER, Pool JL, Melmamed MR: Pleural mesothelioma. Clinical experience with 37 patients. Am J Roentgenol 99:863–880, 1967
36. Solomon A, Webster I: The visceral pleura in asbestosis. Environ Res 11:218–234, 1976
37. Preger L, Hooper TI, Steinbach HL et al: Width of azygous vein related to central venous pressure. Radiology 93:521–523, 1969

38. Ellis K, Latham DK: Pericarditis and pericardial effusion, radiologic and echocardiographic diagnosis. Radiol Clin North Am XI (2):393–413, 1973
39. Kreel L: Personal communication
40. Elmes PC, Simpson MJC: The clinical aspects of mesothelioma. Q J Med 45:427–49, 1976
41. Goldberg BB, Kotler MN, Ziskin MC, et al: Diagnostic Uses of Ultrasound. New York, Grune & Stratton, 1975, Chap 5, pp 146–201
42. Roberts GH, Irvine RW: Peritoneal mesothelioma: A report of 4 cases. Br J Surg 57:645–650, 1970
43. Sanders DE: Pleural mesothelioma. J Can Assoc Radiol 19:64–73, 1968
44. Selikoff IJ, Hammond EC, Churg J: Mortality experience of asbestos insulation workers, in Shapiro HA (ed): Pneumoconiosis. Proceedings of the International Conference, Johannesburg, 1969. Capetown, OUP, 1970, pp 180–186

SECTION 5
LUNG CANCER

Asbestos is one of many substances incriminated in lower respiratory tract carcinogenesis, as shown in Table 2-11. In the assessment of the role of asbestos and other industrial agents in carcinogenesis, a multifactorial approach is necessary because these agents are not restricted to industrial workers congregated at work sites; these noxious agents may spread far from industrial areas. Lung cancer mortality is increased in patients with high ferruginous body counts without known asbestos exposure[1] other than that of urban living. Similarly, there is an excess lung cancer mortality in those living in the vicinity of arsenic-emitting smelters[10] or in heavily industrialized areas with much air pollution from benzo(a)pyrene and other polycyclic aromatic hydrocarbons.[5,6,15] The role of hydrocarbons contained in vehicular exhaust gases in respiratory tract carcinogenesis is controversial.[16]

Synergistic and multiplicative effects need to be considered. In male and female asbestos workers, cigarette smoking increases the lung cancer burden;[17,18] this is discussed more fully below (see Table 2-12).

A similar relation exists in uranium miners inhaling radon daughter products. An excess of alcohol predisposes to cancer of the larynx, oropharynx, and esophagus, all of which are more prevalent in asbestos workers.[20] Experimental[21] and epidemiological data[22] indicate that an excess of lung cancer is associated with a lower vitamin A intake.

The drug history of asbestos workers needs to be considered. Leukemia is said by some to be more common in asbestos workers (see references in Chapter 2, Section 6), and to this risk there is the additive one from the use of myeleran (busulphan) in myeloid leukemia. This agent produces precancerous cytological changes in the lung and, in one reported patient, an apparent progression to bronchiolar cell carcinoma. Bronchogenic carcinoma is more common in patients with leukemia than in the general population. There is an excess of adenocarcinoma of the lung, as well as histiocytic lymphoma following immunosuppressive therapy.[16]

Immunologic susceptibility may be responsible for some lung cancers in asbestos and other workers. Abnormally high levels of inducible aryl hydrocarbon hydroxylase activity in cultured lymphocytes is present in those who smoke[23] and in some lung cancer patients[24] but not in others.[23] This genetically regulated defect affects hydrocarbon metabolism and may be related to the

Table 2-11

Occupational Lung Carcinogens	References
Asbestos	1
Radon	2
Halo ethers	3
Mustard gas	4
Polycyclic hydrocarbons	6, 7
Chromates	8
Arsenic and arsenic trioxide	9, 10
Iron (hematite)	11
Printing ink	12
Vinyl chloride	13
Nickel	14

multiplicative effect of cigarette smoking and the risk of asbestos-induced lung cancer.[16] There is insufficient data accumulated to know if patients with easily inducible aryl hydrocarbon hydroxylase are susceptible to certain histological types of lung cancer. The inducibility of the enzyme system in cultured lymphocytes parallels that in lung tissue and may be a way of distinguishing asbestos workers at greatest risk of lung carcinogenesis. The increased incidence of certain antigens and antibodies in some patients with asbestos-related pulmonary fibrosis is described in Chapter 1 and Chapter 2, Section 2. The mechanism of transition of pulmonary fibrosis to lung cancer and the reason for the increased incidence of lung cancer in asbestos-induced pulmonary fibrosis

Table 2-12

Bronchogenic Carcinoma in:	Incidence per Million	Relative Risk Ratio
Nonsmokers (30% population)	8	1
General population	60	7
All smokers (70% population)	85	10
Heavy smokers (25% population)	130	15
Nonsmoking asbestos workers	8	1
Smoking asbestos workers	560	70

Modified from Higginson[19]; The percentage estimates of smoking population are Higginson's.

The incidence of lung cancer in nonsmoking asbestos workers is not greater than that in the *general* population (smokers and nonsmokers), but there are very few asbestos workers with long exposure who do not smoke. There is insufficient data to be certain that there is no lung cancer excess as compared with *nonsmokers* in the general population.

Table 2-13
Epidemiologic Data of Lung Cancer Risk in Asbestos Workers

Author	Exposure	Increased Incidence of Lung Cancer	Comments
Kogan[34,35]	Chrysotile workers (Russia)	× 1.9 for miners × 3.1 for millers × 2.3 factory workers	Based on mortality figures, 1948–1967.
McDonald[36]	Chrysotile mines and mills (Quebec)	× 1.45	Effective dust control began early 1950. 45% is overall increase incidence in those exposed to high dust index, i.e., greater than 800 mppcf-years.[a] Rate was 5 times those with dust index of less than 10 mppcf-years.
Vigliani (quoted by McDonald)[36]	Chrysotile mines and mills (Italy)	× 1.3	Increased burden of lung cancer deduced from mortality rate.
Webster[37]	Cape blue crocidolite mines; Transvaal blue crocidiolite mines Amosite Chrysotile (South African)	2.8% of autopsy material 9.8% of autopsy material 3.4% of autopsy material 4.1% of autopsy material	Note high incidence of lung cancer in Transvaal crocidolite and South African Chrysotile.
Meurman[38]	Anthophylite mines (Finland)	× 1.4[b] (asbestos workers assumed to be nonsmokers) × 17.0 (smoking asbestos workers) × 12.0 (smoking without asbestos exposure)	Based on smoking habits of current asbestos workers and autopsies of prior asbestos workers.
Newhouse[39]	Asbestos textile industry using crocidolite, amosite and chrysotile	Men × 4.0 less than 2 years on job, heavy exposure × 6.3 more than 2 years on job, heavy exposure. × 2.5 less than 2 years on job, low to moderate exposure × 4.3, more than 2 years on job, low to moderate exposure Women × 3.0 less than 2 years on job, heavy exposure × 2.2 more than 2 years on job, heavy exposure.	By adjusting this data for smoking habits, no significant excess of lung cancer was found in low-exposure workers, but the excess remains for those with heavy exposure. The data is from workers followed for 25 years since first exposure.

Selikoff[40]	New York and New Jersey insulation workers using chrysotile and amosite	× 8.3	Follow-up more than 20 years since first exposure.
			Follow-up less than 20 years since first exposure.
	U.S. and Canadian asbestos workers using chrysotile and amosite	× 3.1	Follow-up more than 20 years since first exposure.
	Amosite asbestos workers	× 3.5	
		× 6.4	First employed during World War II and followed until 1971.
	U.S. and Canadian insulation workers	Lapsed time since onset of exposure	Excess lung cancer appears as early as 10–14 years after first exposure, increased to 30–40 years after exposure.
		10–14 years × 2.4	
		15–19 years × 3.7	
		20–24 years × 3.3	
		25–29 years × 4.8	
		30–34 years × 7.1	
		35–39 years × 6.5	
		40–45 years × 5.9	
		45–49 years × 4.6	
		50+ × 4.5	
Edge[41]	Shipyard workers U.K.	× 2.4	
Fletcher[42]	Shipyard workers U.K.	× 2.5	Compared registration of lung cancer in dockyard workers with age-related controls living in same geographical area but not employed in dockyards.
Lumsley[43]	Shipyard workers	No increased incidence detected	
Enterline[44]	Asbestos production workers	× 1.7	Includes pleural mesothelioma. Is an average for all intensities of exposure; with heavy exposure, increased incidence is × 5.0.
	Asbestos maintenance workers	× 2.5	

[a] mppcf—million particles per cubic foot years is an index determined from the products of asbestos fibers in the air at the place of work and years of exposure.

[b] This value of × 1.4 increased incidence of lung cancer in "nonsmoking" asbestos workers is at variance with most series in which no detectable excess burden of lung cancer is found in nonsmoking asbestos workers. The "nonsmoking" status is an assumption attributed to those who died from lung cancer and was based on smoking habits of current workers. The assumption may be unjustifiable.

are less clear. Adenocarcinoma and alveolar cell carcinoma are seen in patients with systematic sclerosis (scleroderma),[25] and sarcoidosis patients with impaired cellular immunity are prone to lung cancer;[26] both these diseases are characterized by pulmonary fibrosis. Subclinical immune defects have been found in familial sporadic cases of lung adenocarcinoma,[27,28] and some patients with asbestosis tend to have impaired cellular immunity and histocompatibility antigens[29,30] that may affect subsequent carcinogenesis. There is a reduction in T-cell immunocompetence in patients with pulmonary asbestosis. It is suggested that these factors may play a part in fibrogenesis and carcinogenesis. In a pilot study of asbestos workers,[30] HLA W27 antigen was three times more common than among controls. Those with HLA W27 antigen appeared to have more severe pulmonary fibrosis, and a shorter and more recent period of exposure to asbestos. More recent reports have not confirmed this finding (see Chapter 2, Section 2). The influence of race has not been investigated in asbestos-related cancers; there is an increased incidence of lung cancer in black men and Mexican Americans irrespective of asbestos exposure.[31,32] In a survey of counties with known natural asbestos deposits, which were matched with those without known deposits, no great hazard to the general population of counties with asbestos deposits was noted.[33] Table 2-13 presents a survey of epidemiologic data on lung cancer risk in asbestos workers.

CELL TYPE OF ASBESTOS-RELATED LUNG TUMOR

A peripheral lower lobe adenocarcinoma is typical of an asbestos-related lung tumor (see Fig. 2-78). Based on U.K. workers with certified asbestosis who died of cancer of the lung, an analysis by Whitwell et al.[45] of 88 male cases in which there was adequate tumor tissue yielded the data listed in Table 2-14. One patient with alveolar cell carcinoma was included in the adenocarcinoma group. The female group was small, 9 patients, and in females, histological cell types in controls differ from that of men, but 3 of 9 patients had adenocarcinoma and a further 3 of 9 had oat cell carcinoma. A preponderance of adenocarcinoma is present in some, but not all, other series (see Table 2-15 and Fig. 2-79).

Accepting an incidence of about 35 percent adenocarcinoma in the asbestos-related groups, what is the percentage of this cell type in unselected controls? For autopsy material, Whitwell et al. state 27 percent.[45] Much depends on the source of pathological material. Bronchial biopsy specimens

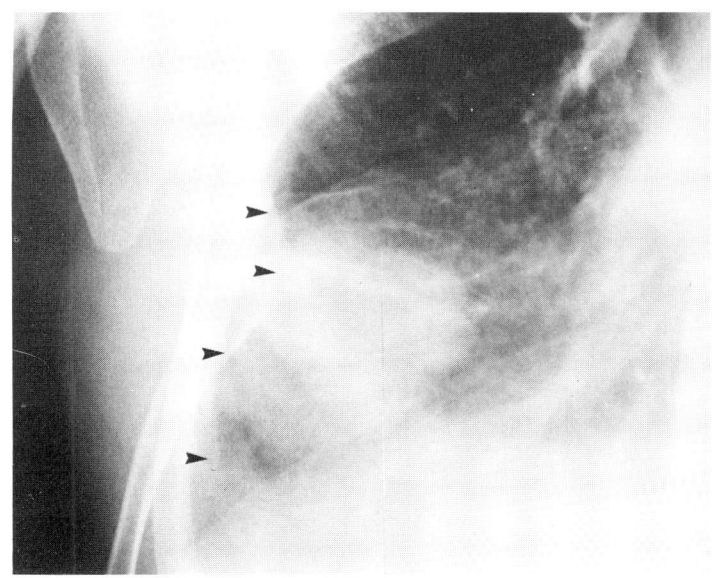

Fig. 2-78. Bronchogenic cancer in an asbestos worker. Note the typical lower lobe and peripheral location. Tissue type was adenocarcinoma, which predominates in asbestos workers, even in those with a smoking history. The subaxillary noncalcified parietal pleural plaques act as biological markers of prior asbestos exposure (horizontal arrows).

Table 2-14

Histological Type	%
Adenocarcinoma	34.1
Oat	26.1
Squamous	21.6
Other	18.2

Table 2-15

Author	Number of Patients with Asbestos Exposure and Lung Cancer	% Adenocarcinoma
Heuper[46]	104	19
Hourihane[47]	17	35
Kannerstein[48]	50	22
Warnock[49]	30	43

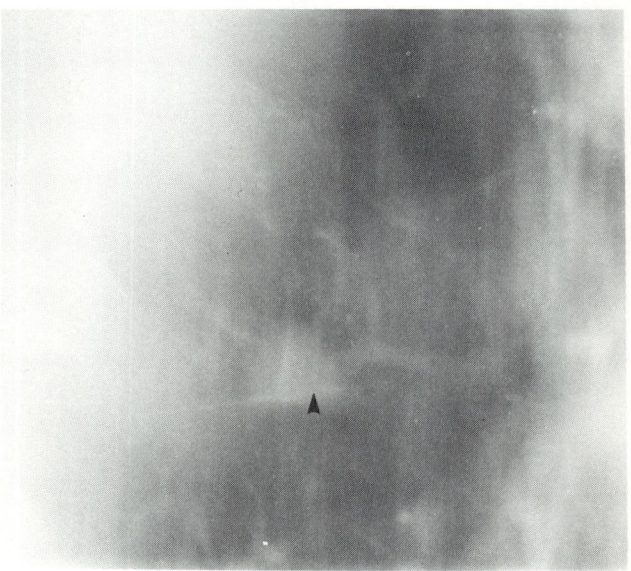

Fig. 2-79. Upper lobe adenocarcinoma demonstrated by tomography. The adjacent minor fissure is thickened by invasion (arrow). This patient had small parietal pleural plaques. His occupational exposure to asbestos was 30 years previously.

Table 2-16

Cell Type	% Bronchial Biopsy Series	% Operative Series	% Necropsy Series
Adenocarcinoma	2	9	27
Oat	34	13	37
Squamous	41	57	17
Others	23	20	19

obtained with a rigid bronchoscope reflect the high incidence of oat cell and squamous tumors in the larger, more accessible proximal airways. Transbronchial lung biopsy with a fiberoptic bronchoscope with fluoroscopic visualization samples peripheral masses. A high proportion of squamous cell and a low proportion of oat cell and adenocarcinomas are seen in surgical series, since squamous cell carcinomas are more likely to be resectable, and adenocarcinoma and oat cell are frequently inoperable. Conversely, a higher percentage of adenocarcinoma is present in autopsy series, since autopsies are more frequently done when the diagnosis is in question. This is more common in peripheral adenocarcinoma, which may be inoperable when first seen, compared with more central carcinoma, e.g., squamous or an oat cell types, where a cytological or histological diagnosis is more easily made. The experience of Whitwell et al.[45] along these lines is summarized in Table 2-16. The percentage is expressed to the nearest percent and is based on 1841 male lung cancer patients seen from 1950 to 1960 at an acute general Liverpool hospital. These patients did not show lung parenchymal evidence of asbestosis, but in this area, about 10 percent of males have pleural plaques at autopsy. Thus the observed adenocarcinoma (2 percent in biopsy series, 9 percent in operative series, and 27 percent in necropsy material) probably includes some asbestos-related tumors. A reasonable estimate of frequency of adenocarcinoma in an unselected population is therefore about 15 to 20 percent of all lung tumors, while in asbestos workers it is about double.

LOCATION OF ASBESTOS-RELATED LUNG TUMORS

A peripheral location in one of the lower lobes is typical (see Table 2-17 and Fig. 2-80). In a large autopsy series without special attention to the history of evidence of asbestos exposure and regardless of cell type, the incidence of lower lobe tumors is about 24 percent. Kannerstein and Churg[48] did not find a

Table 2-17

Author	% Lower Lobe Cancer
Whitwell[45]	78
Kannerstein[48]	53
Hueper[46]	87
Control group	24

greater proportion of peripheral location or pleural involvement in their asbestos-associated group as compared with controls.

The tendency to a lower lobe and peripheral location may be explained by the effect of gravity on asbestos fibers and the fact that respiratory mechanics ensure a greater degree of ventilation in the lower zones. It is these areas that contained the highest concentration of ferruginous bodies in earlier series, although more recently uniform distribution has been reported, and the more severe fibrotic disease. The peripheral predilection is explicable if asbestos dust acts as a cocarcinogen with cigarette smoke or other atmosphere pollutants and so exerts its carcinogenic effect at the place of deposition.

RELATION OF LUNG CANCER AND PULMONARY FIBROSIS

Lung carcinoma is about twice as common in asbestos workers with moderate or severe pulmonary fibrosis as in asbestos workers with only mild fibrosis or otherwise normal lungs[45] (see Figs. 2-81 and 2-82). In addition, the proportion of adenocarcinoma increases with moderate and severe pulmonary fibrosis. Whitwell et al.'s[45] data are summarized in Table 2-18. Additional data relates ferruginous body counts in the lung with tumor type and position[49] (see Table 2-19). The ferruginous body counts were per gram of wet lung tissue; all the patients had low asbestos exposure. The apparent increase in proportion of adenocarcinoma with increasing ferruginous body counts is, however, not statistically significant, since the total number of patients was only 30. This is not surprising, because in asbestosis there is a relation between asbestos load in the lung and mild fibrosis, but in severe fibrosis there is no correlation with a further increase in asbestos fiber concentration. It is in the more severely fibrotic lungs that the excess of adenocarcarcinoma develops. In systemic sclerosis in which, like asbestosis, lower lobe pulmonary fibrosis is frequent, adenocarcinoma, together with alveolar and bronchiolar carcinoma, occurs relatively frequently.[25,50] In sarcoidosis, lung cancer has been reported to occur three times more frequently than in the general population.[26] In this disease,

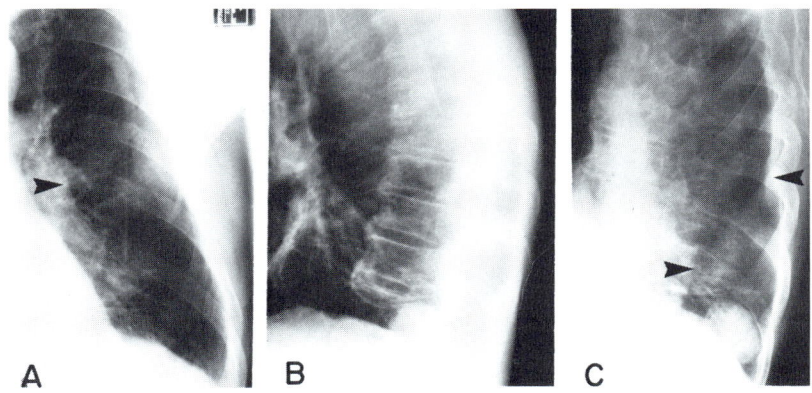

Fig. 2-80. Peripheral adenocarcinoma hidden by diaphragm in PA view (A) and better seen in lateral and LAO views (B and C). Hilar involvement (A), fibrosis, and plaques (C) are indicated by arrows. This is a 71-year-old male who smoked, with occupational exposure to asbestos.

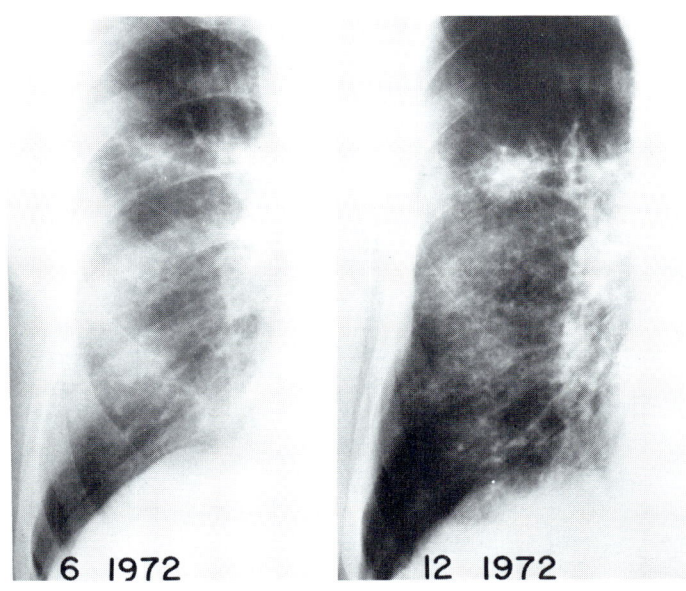

Fig. 2-81. Alveolar cell carcinoma (scar carcinoma) developing in an area of pulmonary fibrosis. In June 1972, the multiple densities were thought to be focal areas of fibrosis. In December 1972, the malignant nature of one of the densities is apparent. The interstitial fibrotic change in the remainder of the lung is more apparent in later, more heavily exposed film.

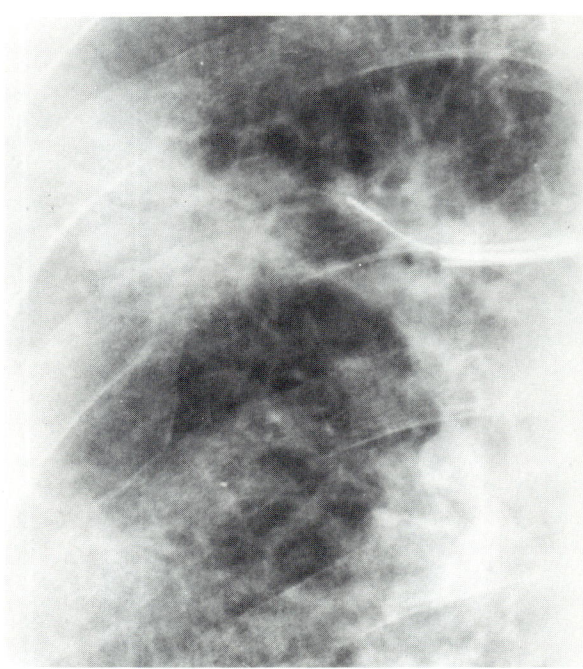

Fig. 2-82. *Alveolar cell carcinoma in a fibrotic lung in an ex-asbestos worker. An unsuccessful attempt at brush biopsy was made. Penetration of peripheral bronchi in fibrotic lungs is difficult. Percutaneous needle biopsy may be a wiser choice.*

Table 2-18

Cell Type	Normal Lung or Mild Asbestosis	Moderate or Severe Asbestosis
Adenocarcinoma	25%	38%
Oat	25%	28%
Squamous	29%	19%
Other	21%	15%

Table 2-19

Ferruginous Body Count	Adenocarcinoma	Lower Lobe Location
Low	33%	14%
High	58%	33%

pulmonary fibrosis is characteristic. The sequence of events may be different, however, since in sarcoidosis the increased lung cancer burden may be related to an immunologic deficiency;[26] furthermore, since many of the patients are treated with steroids, ease of inducibility of aryl hydrocarbon hydroxylase may be relevant, because steroids increase levels of this enzyme (see Chapter 2, Section 2).

RELATION OF LUNG CANCER AND PLEURAL PLAQUES

There is a 2.5-fold increase of bronchial carcinoma in shipbuilders with plaques but no radiographic evidence of pulmonary fibrosis compared with controls from a neighboring area whose x-rays were strictly normal but who may have had some degree of asbestos exposure.[51] The significance of this very recent report is difficult to assess. One inference is that patients with plaques should be followed for detection of lung cancer; but in some urban areas, about 10 percent of persons coming to autopsy will have pleural plaques, no clear-cut history of asbestos exposure, and the cause of death attributed to some disease unrelated to asbestos exposure.

RELATION OF SMOKING AND LUNG CANCER IN ASBESTOS WORKERS

Lung cancer in male asbestos workers is mainly confined to those who have smoked cigarettes (see Fig. 2-83). If there is a risk of lung cancer in nonsmoking asbestos workers, the increase over the control population of nonsmoking workers not exposed to asbestos is slight or none (see Table 2-12). Hammond[52] reports a 5.3-fold increased risk of lung cancer in asbestos insulation workers who smoke cigarettes compared with age-specific U.S. mortality per white males, disregarding smoking. The number of nonsmoking insulation asbestos workers was too small to be statistically significant. These insulation workers had been exposed to both chrysotile and amosite but not to crocidolite. The effect of smoking could be additive or multiplicative to the risk of carcinogenesis from asbestos. Studying a group of asbestos textile workers who had been exposed to chrysotile, amosite, and crocidolite, Newhouse's data suggests a multiplicative rather than an additive effect.[39] Death from lung cancer was 2.5 times greater for male asbestos workers who smoked than for a group of male smokers without asbestos exposure; for women the rate was 11

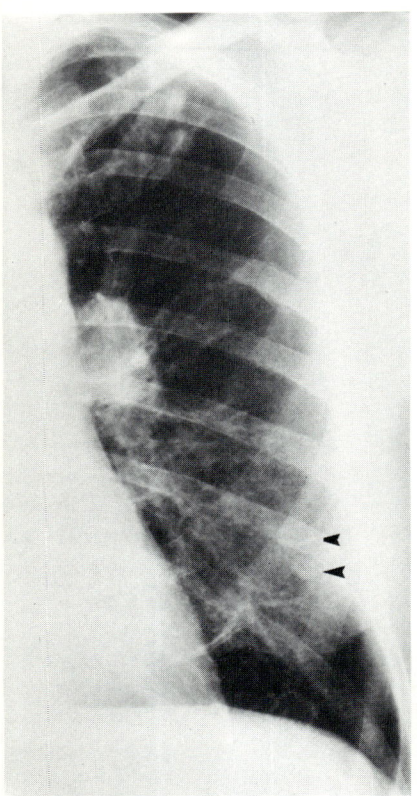

Fig. 2-83. Hilar oat cell carcinoma in an asbestos worker who was a heavy smoker. Apex contains old tuberculous foci with scarring and calcifications. Faint parietal pleural ringlike densities are present (horizontal arrow). Cigarette smoking tends to produce oat cell carcinoma proximally and adenocarcinoma distally. By absorbing carcinogenic pollutants in cigarette smoke, asbestos fibers may effect carcinogenesis at the site of fiber deposition in the airways.

times the rate in a control group. The difference between incidence of lung cancer death for smoking asbestos workers and other smokers only became significant for those with severe asbestos exposure. It thus appears that there is no proof that asbestos exposure in the absence of a smoking history is carcinogenic to the lungs. In accepting this concept, two series that appear contradictory must be mentioned. First, in Finland, miners of anthophyllite who smoke have a 17-fold burden of lung cancer in comparison to nonsmoking nonasbestos workers; compared to nonsmoking anthophyllite miners, there is a 40 percent excess of lung cancer. A possible explanation to explain the 40 percent burden, when compared to the insignificant excess burden in other series of nonsmoking asbestos workers, is that anthophyllite is relatively insoluble in human lungs as compared to the chrysotile.[38] Second, Quebec chrysotile miners and millers who developed lung cancer have a higher proportion of nonsmokers and light smokers than do controls in general population. The reason is unclear, but the burden of excess lung cancers in Canadian chrysotile workers only becomes apparent with heavy exposure.

Mesothelioma-related death is described in Chapter 2, Section 4. One may note, however, that for death due to mesothelioma, the rate is 50-fold greater for those exposed to crocidolite during production of filter pads for military gas masks in World War II compared to that associated with chrysotile production.[54]

It is probable that the type of tumor induced by an inhaled carcinogen may depend on which part of the respiratory tract is affected.[55] With cigarette smoke, which contains a higher proportion of carcinogens while it is in the proximal airways, squamous and oat cell cancers are produced proximally and adenocarcinomas peripherally. When the multiplicative effect of asbestos dust is added, the cocarcinogen reaches the distal airways, and peripheral adenocarcinomas become common.[45]

RELATION OF INTENSITY AND DURATION OF EXPOSURE TO LUNG CANCER

Accepting the increased risk of bronchial carcinoma associated with asbestos use, how is this related to intensity and duration of exposure? The data show increasing risk with intensity and duration of exposure. The various study groups are not comparable in that not only are there fiber differences but, in addition, age at first exposure and period of follow-up vary. Also, the comparison group is derived variously from national mortality data and mortality data from nonexposed groups in the same geographical area, and matching for age, sex, and smoking habits is nonuniform. Tables 2-20A to 2-20D present data from the various study groups.

The lung cancer excess manifests itself with a dust exposure index of more than 200 mpcc-years. The dust exposure index reflects two components, duration and intensity of exposure. These may be examined separately (Table 2-20B).

The almost quadrupling of the lung cancer mortality when the follow-up is extended from 15 to 25 years is seen in Table 2-20B. A similar trend is seen in U.S. asbestos workers (Table 2-20C).

There is no great difference in mortality based on age at which asbestos exposure began (Table 2-20D).

Table 2-20A
Quebec Chrysotile Miners (Male)

Death from Lung Cancer per 1000 Men	Dust Exposure Index (million particles per cubic foot–years)
10.3	< 10
13.1	10–100
13.4	100–200
15.5	200–600
21.4	600–800
32.1	800 +

Data from McDonald[36]

Table 2-20B
British Male Asbestos Textile Workers

	Deaths from Lung Cancer: Ratio of Deaths from Lung Cancer: Observed to Expected:	
	15 Years After First Exposure	25 Years After First Exposure
Low intensity of exposure and short duration less than 2 years	2.5	0.5
Low intensity of exposure and long duration more than 2 years	4.3	1.3
Severe intensity of exposure and short duration less than 2 years	4.0	1.4
Severe intensity of exposure and long duration more than 2 years	6.4	1.8

Data from Newhouse.[38]

Table 2-20C
Deaths from Lung Cancer in U.S. Male Asbestos Insulation Workers

Observed to expected ratio less than 20 years from first exposure	1.9
Observed to expected ratio more than 20 years from first exposure	3.5

Data from Webster.[37]

Table 2-20D
Deaths from Lung Cancer in U.S. Male Asbestos Insulation Workers

Age at Onset of Exposure	Observed to Expected Ratio of Death
< 25	5.6
25–30	4.3
35–44	4.3
45 +	3.1

Data from Webster.[37]

FIBER TYPE IN RELATION TO LUNG CARCINOGENESIS

Crocidolite is the most potent initiator of mesothelioma. So far, however, a definite statement on the importance of fiber size in the production of bronchogenic carcinoma cannot be made.[56] This situation is unlike that regarding mesothelioma, in which studies of cohorts of workers exposed to a certain type of fiber (e.g., fine fiber Western Australian crocidolite) have enabled the formulation a statement relating risk of mesothelioma induction with fiber length and diameter (see Chapter 2, Section 4). The morphology of fibers from a single source varies with processing; currently used chrysotile is finer than that used previously. Transvaal crocidolite and amosite contain a larger portion of large fibers, which are less likely to penetrate deeply into the lungs than those obtained from the NW Cape Province of South Africa. Despite this, one may deduce from data published by McDonald,[36] Webster,[37] and Meurman[38] that crocidolite and amosite are more carcinogenic than anthophyllite and chrysotile. This opinion is based on recent epidemiologic surveys, and the author has not read any confirmatory experimental data.

Lung cancer follows inhalation of asbestos fibers by experimental animals, but the data do not correlate well with clinical experience. Carcinogenicity data are given in Table 2-21. Squamous cell and adeno (alveolar cell) carcinoma were produced, always in a peripheral location and in areas of severe fibrosis. Adenocarcinomas were slightly more common than squamous cell carcinomas.[57]

The relation between the aerodynamic qualities inherent in various fiber shapes and the consequent degree of airway penetration and retention within the lung is discussed in Chapter 2, Section 2.

Table 2-21
Cancer in Rates Following
Asbestos Inhalation

Fiber	Percent of Animals Developing Cancer
Chrysotile	59
Anthophyllite	50
Amosite	43
Crocidolite	22

CHEMICAL FACTORS AND TRACE AGENTS IN CARCINOGENESIS

The discrepancy between the high incidence of lung cancer in asbestos workers who smoke compared with those who do not suggest that bronchogenic carcinoma induction in humans is not directly related to fiber shape (unlike pulmonary fibrosis and mesothelioma), or to the metals that are an intrinsic part of asbestos fibers, or to trace elements such as chromium, lead, and nickel which are known to be carcinogenic in other circumstances. The inference is that the carcinogenic effect may be due to asbestos fibers concentrating on their surface, carcinogenic hydrocarbons, or other substances found in cigarette smoke that have entered the lung by other means.[58] The trace metals may play an indirect role.[59] These trace metals may be eluted from asbestos trapped in the lung and may inhibit metabolism of carcinogenic benzo(a)pyrene, so that it remains biologically active in the lung for a longer period. This hypothesis, suggesting that the fibers are inert carriers of the cancer-potentiating trace metals, is unproven; in the case of Canadian chrysotile, carcinogenicity is unrelated to content of iron, chromium, and nickel.

Asbestos fibers contain various oils in small amounts. There is no evidence that the small amounts present are carcinogenic. Previously, oil in jute bags used for transfer and storage of asbestos fibers was found to be absorbed onto the fiber surface, and since this oil is weakly carcinogenic, jute bag use has been discontinued in the asbestos industry. Polyethylene bags were substituted, primarily to reduce the release of fibers to the environment. Unfortunately, antioxidants incorporated into polyethylene may be converted by asbestos into carcinogenic quinones. The problem of the precise mechanism of asbestos carcinogenesis is far from a solution, and current work is centered on effect of asbestos on DNA and RNA synthesis.

RADIOLOGY

The radiological technique and assessment of pulmonary neoplasia is described in many current texts and is omitted here in favor of a discussion of the problems encountered in the assessment of lung cancer associated with asbestos exposure. The early detection of lung cancer may be difficult, even when one is on the alert. Two problems confront the radiologist. Identification of a tumor may be difficult if it develops in an area of severe pulmonary fibrosis and if it lies near a large or dense pleural plaque.

Detection of Lung Cancer in Fibrotic Lungs

The presence of pulmonary fibrosis of any etiology, not just from asbestos, should indicate the need for periodic assessment to identify an early scar carcinoma. If the interstitial fibrosis is slight, no great difficulties should ensue; in areas of severe or conglomerate fibrosis the development of an additional homogenous opacity may be undetected until the tumor is large. Figure 2-84 illustrates a patient with a working lifetime exposure to asbestos as an asbestos scraper in a boiler factory. Despite the presence of hemoptysis as a warning sign, a right lung neoplasm was not detected until it had reached a large size. Hemoptysis is not a sign of uncomplicated pulmonary fibrosis, and its occurrence, or a change in symptoms such as increasing cough or dyspnea, should initiate a search for an occult lung malignancy as well as exclusion of other causes such as bronchiectasis, mitral stenosis, infarcts, and infections. Similarly, an effusion is unusual in uncomplicated pulmonary fibrosis; rheumatoid lung in men is an exception. The presence of an effusion should initiate a search for an associated malignancy. The older techniques of tomography and bronchography have their limitations. Conventional tomography may reveal a homogeneous localized density in an area of diffuse fibrosis, but on two occasions the author was content to assume erroneously that these were areas of nodular fibrosis when, in fact, they eventually proved to be adenocarcinoma (see Fig. 2-81 and Fig. 2-85). Bronchography may reveal distorted bronchi due to pulmonary fibrosis, and any additional distortion due to neoplasia may be undetected. Many asbestos-related lung cancers are peripheral, and the bronchographic signs of bronchial tumor encasement and occlusion may not be present. Peripheral bronchi may be unfilled with contrast material as a result of distortion by fibrosis.

It should be stressed that the fibrosis of asbestosis is usually diffuse and not nodular as it is in silicosis. Large fibrotic nodules (Progressive Massive Fibrosis) and necrobiotic nodules are very rare in asbestosis and exclusion of malig-

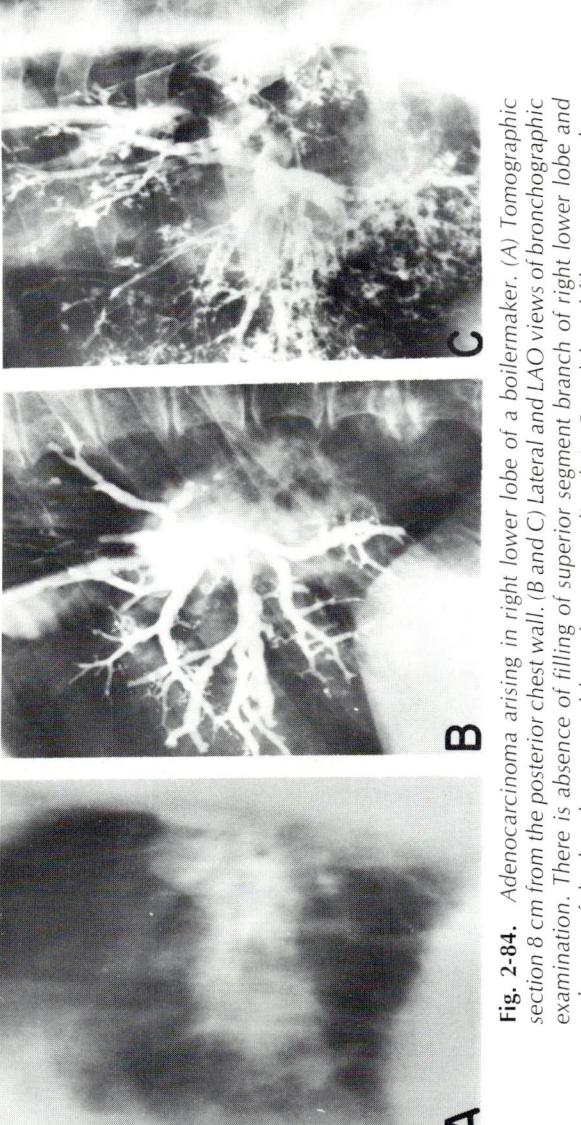

Fig. 2-84. Adenocarcinoma arising in right lower lobe of a boilermaker. (A) Tomographic section 8 cm from the posterior chest wall. (B and C) Lateral and LAO views of bronchographic examination. There is absence of filling of superior segment branch of right lower lobe and only two of the basal segmental branches are outlined. In C, a delayed film, an anomalous downward-pointing branch of posterior segment right upper lobe gives a false impression of contrast in the superior segment of the right lower lobe.

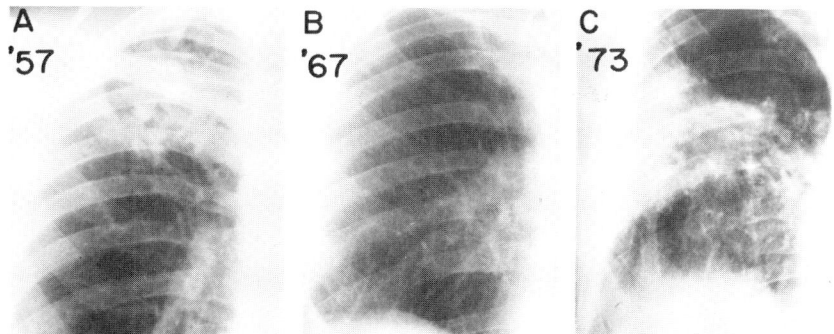

Fig. 2-85. Adenocarcinoma. Part A, (1957) shows tuberculous infection in right upper lobe. In Part B (1967), there is a residual fibrothorax with some parenchymal fibrosis. In Part C (1973), a large infiltrative adenocarcinoma is seen. The patient had been a boilermaker with heavy asbestos exposure. He is alive and well 4 years later after cobalt therapy, the tumor being unresectable.

nancy is necessary. There is a tendency for the masses of progressive massive fibrosis to be bilateral and migrate slowly by fibrotic retraction towards the hila. If only one mass migrates, the possibility that the controlateral mass is a malignant tumor needs consideration.

Pleural Plaques Obscuring or Simulating Lung Cancer

On occasions, the author has found CT (computed tomography) useful in making the diagnosis of a parenchymal mass, separate from an adjacent large pleural plaque when this was not apparent from plain radiographs and conventional tomograms (see Figs. 2-86 to 2-88). Prior to the introduction of CT, the author has missed the diagnosis of lung cancer when its image was masked by an adjacent plaque.

Rarely, some plaques are quite rounded and not of the typical flat shape. They are usually noncalcified, unlike the flatter plaques. In addition, these rounded plaques occur more frequently near the diaphragms, arising from either the diaphragmatic parietal pleura or the parietal pleura near the costophrenic angle (see Fig. 2-89). Their uncalcified nature and lower zone of location make them quite indistinguishable from an asbestos-related tumor, which also typically occurs in the lower zone and peripheral in position. Computed tomography may have a potential in their assessment, but their differentiation from a circumscribed mesothelioma (a rare type most are diffuse) would still be difficult.

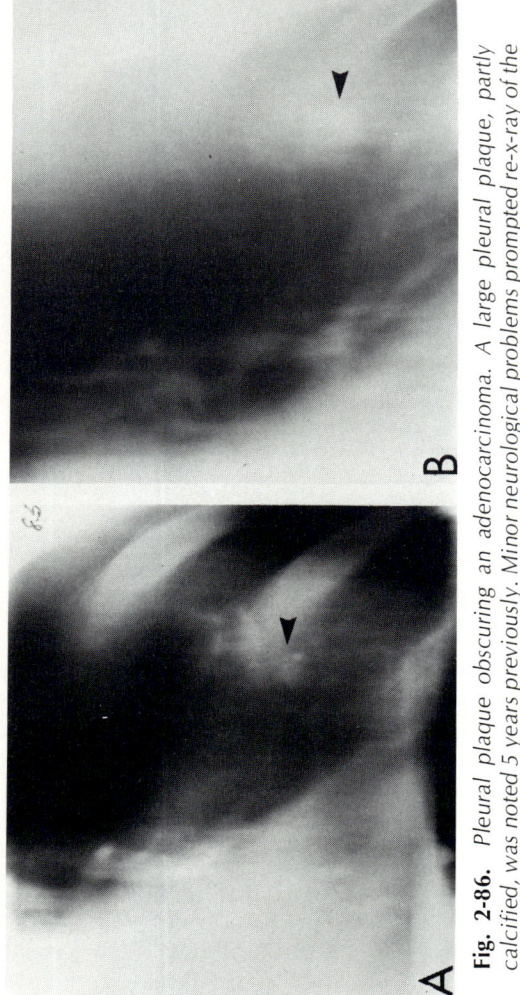

Fig. 2-86. Pleural plaque obscuring an adenocarcinoma. A large pleural plaque, partly calcified, was noted 5 years previously. Minor neurological problems prompted re-x-ray of the chest to exclude pulmonary neoplasm metastatic to the brain. The 1975 tomogram (A) was misinterpreted as confirming the presence of posterior parietal pleural plaque only. Neurological symptoms a few months later prompted retomography (B). The lesser exposed later tomogram (B) film demonstrate a primary lung cancer (arrows) which on the earlier film is seen to coalesce with the lower border of the pleural plaques (arrow in A).

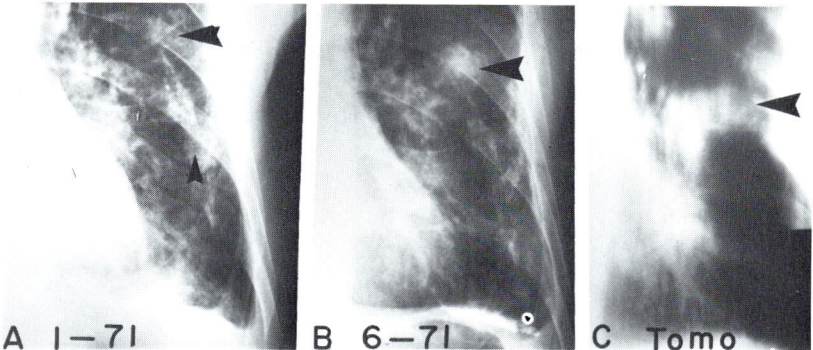

Fig. 2-87. Poorly differentiated squamous cell carcinoma (horizontal arrow) that was initially not differentiated from adjacent plaques (vertical arrows). Part A is 5 months before B and C. C is a tomogram. Note the dense diaphragmatic and pleural plaques. The patient is a 78-year-old male smoker and ex-shipyard worker.

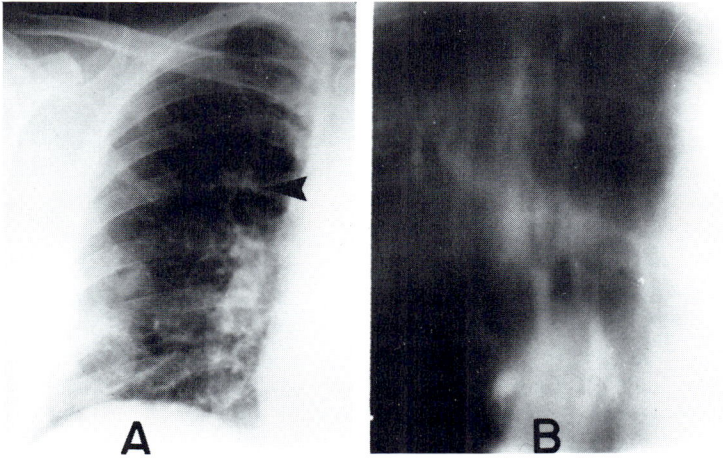

Fig. 2-88. (A) Barely visible parenchymal density in the right upper lobe of a nonsmoking insulator. Note larger subaxillary plaques. (B) Tomogram (photographic enlargement). Bronchoscopy and cytological examination showed no abnormality. The probability of an asbestos-related lung tumor seems probable. Prior film from 5 years earlier was eventually obtained, however, and no change had occurred.

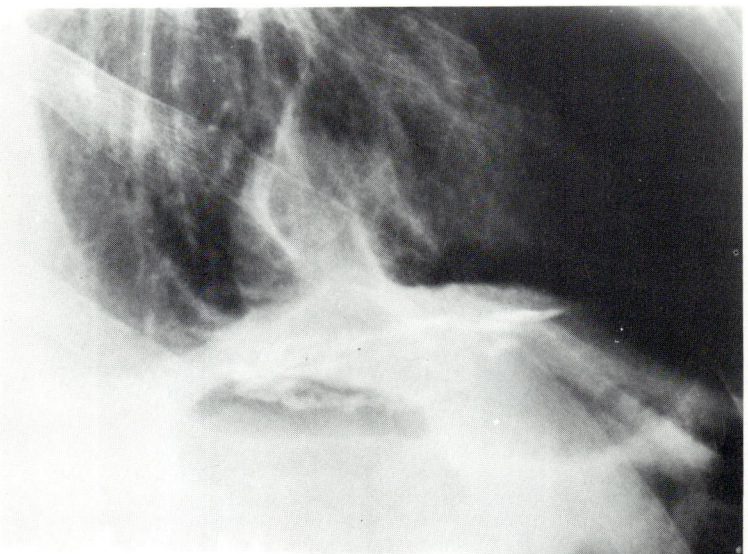

Fig. 2-89. *Rounded peripheral plaque merging with diaphragmatic pleural surface. Calcification is present within the depth of the diaphragm. The rounded shape did not alter significantly in various projections. Differentiation from lung tumor was impossible until prior films showing constant size became available. The linear density projected through the lesion might otherwise suggest a scar or alveolar cell carcinoma.*

Rounded pleural plaques may develop quite rapidly, over a period of about a year, and simulate peripheral lung masses (see Fig. 2-90). The problem is compounded if the patient has a history of asbestos exposure. These plaques were known to prior generations of physicians. They occurred as fibrin balls in patients with therapeutic pneumothoraces for antituberculous therapy. These fibrin balls became adherent to the parietal pleura and occasionally remained as localized densities on the chest radiograph when the lung was allowed to reexpand.[60] The author has noted a similar radiographic appearance following a transthoracic incision for repair of a hiatus hernia (Fig. 2-90).

An additional problem may occur when several plaques are present. A false impression of multiple tumors may be obtained, and a fruitless, time-consuming (and expensive) search for a primary tumor may ensue. Here again, computed axial tomography may have an important but yet unproven role.

Computed Tomography

Accuracy of detection of peripheral tumors is greater with CT than with conventional radiographic techniques.[61] For central lesions or hilar deposits from peripheral masses, differentiation from normal mediastinal structures may

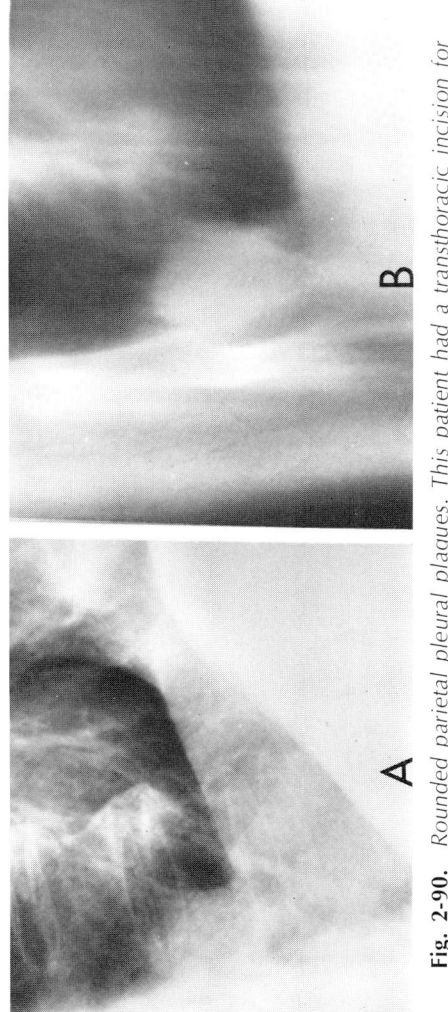

Fig. 2-90. Rounded parietal pleural plaques. This patient had a transthoracic incision for repair of a hiatus hernia. Nine months later, a density was noted in the costovertebral angle (see lateral radiograph (A) and steep oblique tomogram (B). It was erroneously diagnosed as a peripheral lung or pleural neoplasm. Exploration revealed a dense parietal pleural plaque. The patient had no occupational asbestos exposure.

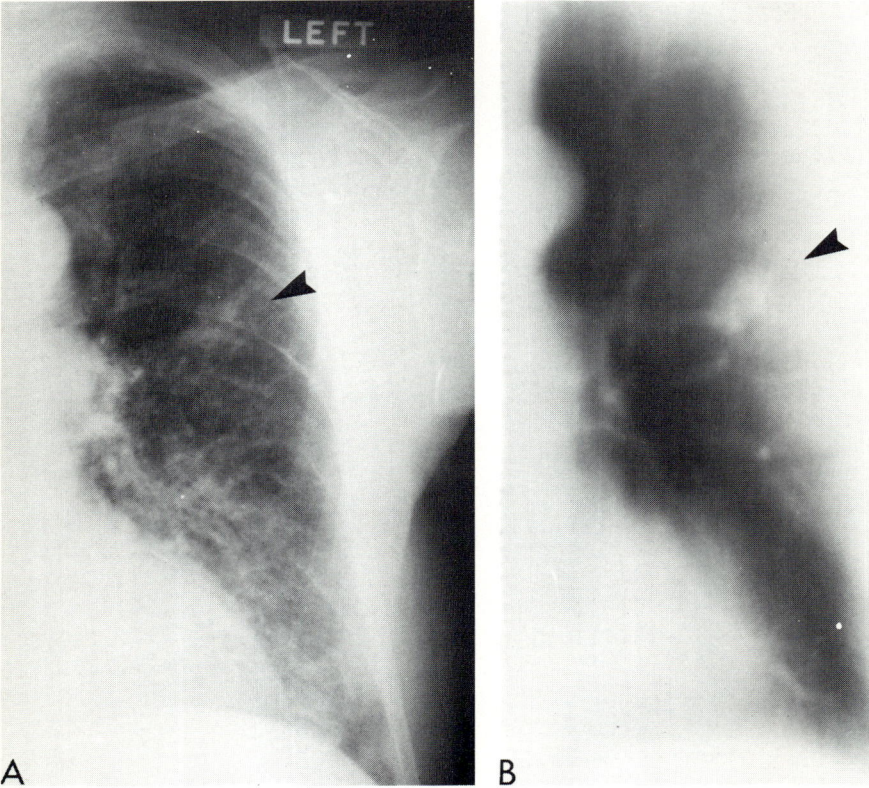

Fig. 2-91. *(A and B) PA and tomographic views of left upper lobe carcinoma in an ex-insulator (oblique arrows). Fibrosis is seen in lower lung fields. (see facing page for C and D. (C) CT view. Homogeneous density due to carcinoma in the left lung. (D) Subpleural metastasis in right lung.*

be made if there is much mediastinal fat which, because of its lower attenuation coefficient, will enhance the visibility of denser structures. The author has not seen a critical analysis of the value of CT in the detection of central malignancy. The use of intravenous contrast material will enhance the aortic density and should make for easier assessment of central tumors or mediastinal spread, but again no critical assessment has been documented. There is a growing tendency with some clinicians to perform fiberoptic bronchoscopy and bronchial washings on patients with severe asbestos-related pulmonary fibrosis. In some instances, class III-V cells are found, despite the absence of any discernible masses on conventional radiographic examinations. In these circumstances, CT is extremely helpful in suggesting areas of the lung that may

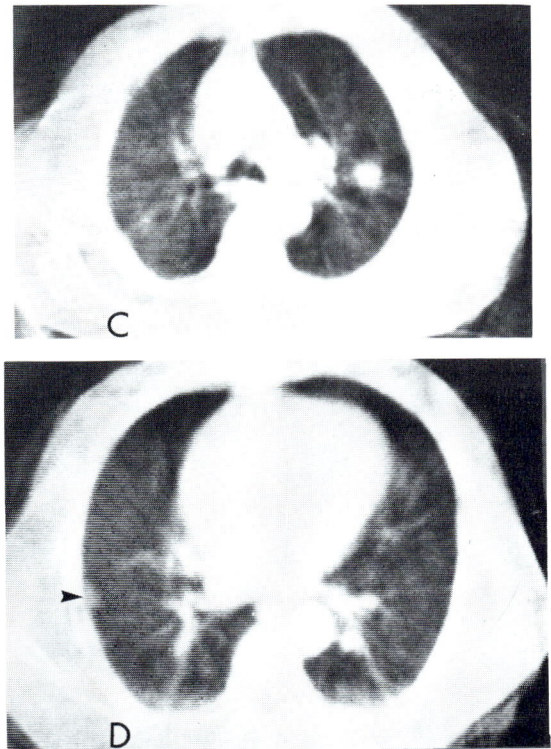

be subsequently examined by conventional tomography to gain additional data so that an intelligent decision concerning thoracotomy may be made. Aspiration needle biopsy of lung masses is made easier with CT. Currently, with conventional techniques, a combination of fluoroscopy and triangulation is used; with CT, accurate measurements along the X and Y axes may be made either directly from the CRT image if a graticule is available or from the Polaroid or film image by utilization of the appropriate minification factor.

Although metastasis of bronchogenic carcinoma to the opposite lung is rare (Fig. 2-91), and even rarer to the ipsilateral lung, it is expected that the ability of CT to identify subpleural deposits,[61] the common site for such metastases, will shorten the time spent on investigations, diminish the number of resections without hope of cure, and hasten the introduction of palliative radiation and chemotherapy when appropriate. Similarly, CT identifies small pleural effusions more readily than do conventional techniques but at greater expense. Metastases may be detectable in the bony thorax by CT: the appropriate window width and height for bone must be utilized. The author has not read a critical comparison of CT to isotopic methods. Central bronchogenic carcinomas commonly invade the pericardium to produce an effusion; this too is detectable by CT. Identification of calcification is made easy by CT, provided the appropriate window width and height is used. CT will show more widespread plaques than will conventional radiography, especially when sections are made to include the upper abdomen, since plaques may grow through diaphragm and extend on its undersurface. Mediastinal plaques become more evident on CT examination.

Radiographic Differentiation of Peripheral Cancer and Mesothelioma

Radiographic differentiation of an asbestos-related peripheral primary lung cancer from a circumscribed mesothelioma is impossible with current radiological methods. Both may be accompanied by pleural effusion. Fortunately, circumscribed mesotheliomata are rare. The differentiation is important, since a peripheral primary lung cancer may be resectable, while no methods of treatment are currently known to produce much prolongation of life in patients with mesothelioma.[62] More frequent is the problem associated with the presence of pseudotumors in mesothelioma masses. These pseudotumors are rounded masses of necrotic and pseudomucinous material of a slightly different tissue density than the adjacent mesothelioma mass. The difference is often apparent with conventional tomography. The radiographic problem is then to appreciate that the appearance is not due to a peripheral primary lung cancer with diffuse peripheral involvement but rather to a pseudotumor in a mesothelioma. A third problem in the differentiation of lung cancer from mesothelioma arises when a lobulated pleural mass, extending over a wide area, with or without accompanying effusion, is present. This is a common finding in metastatic pleural disease from an extrathoracic primary cause, and it is not rare with an anaplastic, rapidly developing peripheral lung cancer. A mesothelioma may have an identical appearance; however, most mesotheliomata produce a diffuse peel-like appearance, enveloping the lung, rather than a diffuse polycyclic contour.

In all cases of suspected lung cancer in those previously exposed to asbestos, a careful search for other stigmata such as pulmonary fibrosis, pleural plaques, and pleural effusion should be made. The presence of pulmonary fibrosis may indicate the need for lung function assessment prior to thoracotomy. An accompanying effusion must not be considered a "benign" asbestos effusion, even if the lung tumor is small. The author has seen no reports, or had personal experience, of a pleural effusion accompanying a lung tumor that resolved during the observed biological life of the tumor.

REFERENCES

1. Warner ML, Churg AM: Association of asbestos and bronchogenic carcinoma in a population with low asbestos exposure. Cancer 35:1236–1242, 1975
2. Lundin FE Jr., Lloyd JW, Smith EM, et al: Mortality of uranium miners in relation to radiation exposure, hard rock mining and cigarette smoking—1950 through September, 1967. Health Phys 16:571–578, 1969
3. Figera WG, Raszkowski R, Weiss W: Lung cancer in chloromethyl methyl ether workers. N Engl J Med 288:1090–1097, 1973
4. Wada Mijoniski M, Nishimoto Y, et al: Cancer of the lung in iron ore (haematite) miners. Br J Ind Med 27:97–105, 1970
5. Menck HR, Casagrande JT, Henderson BE: Industrial air pollution: Possible effect on lung cancer. Science 183:210–312, 1971
6. Carnow BW, Meier P: Air pollution and pulmonary cancer. Arch Environ Health 27:207–218, 1973
7. Doll R, Vessey MP, Beasley RW, et al: Mortality of gas workers—final report of a prospective study. Br J Ind Med 29:394–406, 1972
8. Langard S, Norseth T: A cohort study of bronchial carcinomas in workers producing chromate pigment. Br J Ind Med 36:62–65, 1975
9. Ohm G, Holder BB, Gordon HL: Respiratory cancer and occupational exposure to arsenicals. Arch Environ Health 29:250–255, 1974
10. Blott WJ, Fraumeni JF Jr: Arsenical air pollution in lung cancer. Lancet 2:142–144, 1975
11. Boyd JT, Doll R, Faulds JS, et al: Cancer of the lung in iron ore (haematite) miners. Br J Ind Med 27:97–105, 1970
12. Moss E, Scott TS, Atherley GR: Mortality of newspaper workers from lung cancer and bronchitis, 1952–1956. Br J Ind Med 31:224–232, 1974
13. Monson RR, Peters JM, Johnson MN: Proportional mortality among vinyl chloride workers. Lancet 2:397–398, 1974
14. Doll R, Morgan LG, Speizer FE: Cancer of the lung and nasal sinuses in nickel workers. Br J Cancer 24:623–632, 1970
15. Caston JG, Finklea JF, Sandifer JH: Cancer of larynx and lung in three urban counties in South Carolina. South Med J 65:753–756, 1972
16. Fraumeni JF Jr: Respiratory carcinogenesis: An epidemiologic appraisal. J Natl Cancer Inst 55:1039–1046, 1975
17. Hammond EC, Selikoff IJ: Relation of cigarette smoking to risk of asbestos associated disease among insulation workers in the United States, in Bogovski P, Gilson JC, Timbrell V, et al (eds): Biological Effects of Asbestos. Lyon, IARC, 1973, pp. 312–317
18. Berry G, Newhouse ML, Turok M: Combined effect of asbestos exposure

and smoking on mortality from lung cancer in factory workers. Lancet 2:476–479, 1972
19. Higginson J: Importance of environmental factors in cancer in Environmental Pollution and Carcinogenic Risks. Lyon, IARC Scientific Publication No. 13, 1976, pp 15–23
20. Rothman K, Keller A: The effect of joint exposure to alcohol and tobacco on risk of cancer in mouth and pharynx. J Chronic Dis 25:711–716, 1972
21. Saffiotti V: Metabolic host factors in carcinogenesis, in Doll R, Vodopija I (eds): Host Environmental Interaction in the Etiology of Cancer In man. Lyon, IARC 1973, pp 243–252
22. Bjelke E, Dutey V: Vitamin A and human lung cancer. Int J Cancer 15:561–565, 1975
22. Min KW, Gyoakey F: Interstitial pulmonary fibrosis, atypical epithelian changes and bronchial cell carcinoma following busulphan therapy. Cancer 22:1027–1032, 1968
23. Jett JR, Taylor WF, Fontana RS, et al: An evaluation of aryl hydrocarbon hydroxylase and lymphocyte transformation in lung cancer patients and in smoking and nonsmoking controls. Am Rev Resp Dis 115(4) part w:125, 1977
24. Kellerman G, Shaw CR, Luyten-Kellerman M: Aryl hydrocarbon hydroxylase inducibility in bronchogenic carcinoma. N Engl J Med 289:934–937, 1973
25. Tomkin GH: Systemic sclerosis associated with carcinoma of the lung. Br J Dermatol 81:213–216, 1969
26. Brincker H, Wilber E: The incidence of malignant tumors in patients with respiratory sarcoidosis. Br J Cancer 29:247–251, 1974
27. Fraumeni JF Jr., Wertelechi W, Blatner WA: Varied manifestations of familial lymphoproliferative disorder. Am J Med 29:145–151, 1975
28. Gross RL, Latty A, William EA, et al: Abnormal spontaneous rosette formation and rosette inhibition in lung carcinoma. N Engl J Med 292:439–443, 1975
29. Kang K-Y, Sera Y, Okochi T, et al: T lymphocytes in asbestosis. N Engl J Med 291:735–736, 1974
30. Merchant JA, Klouda PT, Soutar CA, et al: The HL-A system in asbestos workers. Br J Med 1:189–191, 1975
31. Burbank F, Fraumeni JF Jr.: U.S. cancer mortality: Nonwhite predominance. J Natl Cancer Inst 49:649–659, 1972
32. Buell PE, Mendez WM, Dunn JE Jr.: Cancer of the lung among Mexican immigrant women in California. Cancer 22:186–192, 1968
33. Fears TR: Cancer mortality and asbestos deposits. Ann J Epidemiol 104:523–526, 1976

34. Kogan FM, Troitsky SK, Guleuskaya MR: On the carcinogenic effect of asbestos dust. Gigiena Truda: Professional'nye Zabolevaniya, 8:28–33, 1966
35. Kogan FM, Guselnikova NA, Guleuskaya MR: On the causes of death in patients with asbestos. Gigiena Truda: Professional'nye Zabolevaniya, 15:43–46, 1971
36. McDonald JC: Cancer in chrysotile mines and mills, in Bogovski P, Gilson JC, Timbrell V, et al (eds): Biological Effects of Asbestos. Lyon, IARC, 1973, pp 189–194
37. Webster I: Malignancy in relation to crocidolite and amosite, in Bogovski P, Gilson JC, Timbrell V, et al (eds): Biological effects of asbestos. Lyon, IARC, 1973, pp 195–198
38. Meurman LO, Kiviluoto R, Hakama M: Mortality and morbidity of employees of anthophyllite asbestos mines in Finland, in Bogovski P, Gilson JC, Timbrell V, et al (eds): Biological Effects of Asbestos. Lyon, IARC, 1973, pp 199–202
39. Newhouse ML: Cancer among workers in the asbestos textile industry, in Bogovski P, Gilson JC, Timbrell V, et al (eds): Biological Effects of Asbestos. Lyon, IARC, 1973, pp 203–208
40. Selikoff IJ, Hammond EC, Seidman H: Cancer risk of insulation workers in the United States, in Bogovski P, Gilson JC, Timbrell V, et al (eds): Biological Effects of Asbestos. Lyon, IARC, 1973, pp 209–216
41. Edge JR: Asbestos related disease in Barrow-in-Furness. Environ Res 11:244–247, 1976
42. Fletcher DE: A mortality study of shipyard workers with plaques. Br J Ind Med 29:142–145, 1972
43. Lumsley KPS: A proportional study of cancer registrations of dockyard workers. Br J Ind Med 33:108–114, 1976
44. Enterline P, Decoufle P, Henderson V: Mortality in relation to occupational exposure in the asbestos industry. J Occup Med 14:897–903, 1972
45. Whitwell F, Newhouse ML, Bennett DR: A study of the histological cell types of lung cancer in workers suffering from asbestosis in the United Kingdom. Br J Ind Med 31:298–303, 1974
46. Hueper WC: Occupational and Environmental Cancer of the Respiratory Tract. Recent Results in Cancer Research, vol 3. Berlin, Springer, 1966, p 43
47. Hourihane D O'B, McCaughey WTE: Pathological aspects of asbestosis. Postgrad Med J 42:613–622, 1966
48. Kannerstein M, Churg J: Pathology of carcinoma of the lung associated with asbestos exposure. Cancer 30:1:14–21, 1972
49. Warnock ML, Churg AM: Association of asbestos in bronchogenic carci-

noma in a population with low asbestos exposure. Cancer 35:2:1236–1242, 1975

50. Twersky J, Twersky N, Lehr C: Scleroderma and carcinoma of the lung. Clin Radiol 27:203–209, 1976
51. Edge J: Asbestos related lung disease in a British shipbuilding population with particular regard to the incidence of bronchial carcinoma in men with pleural plaques. A mortality study. Am Rev Resp Dis 115 (4) part 2: 211, 1977
52. Hammond EC, Selikoff IJ: Relation of cigarette smoking to risk of death of asbestos associated disease among insulation workers in the United States, in Bogovski P, Gilson JC, Timbrell V, et al (eds): Biological Effects of Asbestos. Lyon, IARC, 1973, pp 312–317
53. Meurman LO, Kiviluoto R, Hakama M: Mortality and morbidity among the working population of anthophyllite asbestos mines in Finland. Br J Ind Med 31:105–112, 1974
54. McDonald AD, McDonald JC: Mesothelioma, asbestos fiber type. Am Rev Resp Dis 115 (4) part 2: 229, 1977
55. Ashley DJ, Davis HD: Cancer of the lung histology and biological behavior. Cancer 20:165–174, 1967
56. Gilson JC: Asbestos cancers as an example of the problem of comparative risks, in Environmental Pollution and Carcinogenic Risks. Lyon, IARC Scientific Publication No. 13, 1976, p 107–116
57. Wagner JC, Berry G, Skidmore JW, et al: The effects of inhalation of asbestos in rats. Br J Cancer 29:252–289, 1974
58. Harington JS: Chemical factors (including trace elements) as etiological mechanisms, in Bogovski P, Gilson JC, Timbrell V, et al (eds): Biological Effects of Asbestos. Lyons, IARC, 1973, pp 306–311
59. Holmes A, Morgan A, Sandells FJ: Determination of iron, chromium, cobalt, nickel and scandium in asbestos by neutron activation analysis. Am Ind Hyg Assoc J 32:281–286, 1971
60. Parkes RW: Personal communication
61. Muhm JR, Brown LR, Crowe JK: Use of computer tomography in the detection of pulmonary nodules. Mayo Clin Proc 52:345–348, 1977
62. Wanebo HJ, Martini N, Melamed MR, et al: Pleural mesothelioma. Cancer 38:241–2488, 1976

SECTION 6
EXTRATHORACIC EFFECTS OF ASBESTOS

The extrathoracic effects of asbestos are summarized in Table 2-22.

ASBESTOS WARTS

In the past, asbestos warts were common in persons who handled asbestos fibers and textile. They occurred on the knuckles, fingertips, and forearms. Asbestos fibers, especially amphiboles rather than chrysotile, are responsible. The warts are tender and may persist for years unless the asbestos fiber is removed. They are rare today because manual handling of fibers is no longer done.[1]

GASTROINTESTINAL CANCER

Some disorders such as ulcerative colitis, familial polyposis, and to a lesser extent, regional enteritis predispose to the development of gastrointestinal malignancy. Exogenous effects such as diet and constipation also play a part. Asbestos may be an additional exogenous factor. Epidemiologic studies of cohorts of asbestos workers have shown an increased risk for gastrointestinal cancer. Data from recent series are summarized in Table 2-23. It may be that the true incidence of gastrointestinal cancer is understated, since some cancer patients will die from unrelated causes.

With the exception of the Finnish group exposed to anthophyllite, an excess of gastrointestinal malignancies is indicated in the other series. To gain further detailed information, the American Cancer Society has underway a prospective study of 16,000 asbestos workers.[11] The study will follow the workers for many years, and in the event of development of colon or rectal cancer, the surgical or autopsy specimens will be examined for the presence of asbestos fibers in the bowel epithelium and wall at the site of the lesion and in adjacent areas.

There are occasional observations of an excess of pancreatic, kidney,

Table 2-22
Extrathoracic Effects of Asbestos

1. *Known to be due to asbestos exposure*
   Asbestos warts
   Peritoneal mesothelioma
2. *Probably due to asbestos exposure*
   Gastrointestinal cancer
   Laryngeal cancer (only in smokers)
   Splenic and hepatic capsular hyaline sclerosis
3. *Sporadic reports suggesting relationship with asbestos exposure*
   Hemopoetic system malignancy
   Breast cancer
   Ovarian cancer
   Renal cancer

Modified from Parkes.[1]

prostate, and brain cancers in communities occupationally or environmentally exposed to asbestos. Because of sex and exposure differences in the observed excesses of some of these cancers, a cause-and-effect relationship for asbestos has not yet been accepted.* In vitro experiments have not demonstrated a teratogenic effect for chrysotile.**

Source of Ingested Asbestos

Asbestos Workers

Some 99 percent of inhaled dust is passed back to the oropharynx by the tracheobronchopulmonary clearance mechanism and subsequently swallowed. Thus, about 100 times the amount of dust stored in the lungs will end up in the gastrointestinal tract. The significance is clear for those living or working in an asbestos-contaminated atmosphere.

General population. Asbestos fibers may reach the gastrointestinal tract from contaminated water, beverages, food, and air. Industrial waste containing asbestoslike fibers has been emptied into Lake Superior since 1955. The adjacent population of Duluth has shown an increasing incidence of rectal carcinoma but not of cancer of the esophagus, stomach, and colon.[12] The

*Wigle DT: Cancer mortality in relation to asbestos in municipal water supplies. Arch Environ Health 32:185–190, 1977
**Schneider U, Maurer RR: Asbestos and embryonic development. Teratology 15:273–280, 1977

Table 2-23

Author	Date	Site	Standardized Mortality Ratio (Observed/Expected)	Comment
Enterline and Weill[2]	1973	Digestive tract	1.5	No difference between asbestos cement pipe workers (crocidolite exposure) and asbestos shingle and sheet workers (no crocidolite exposure).
McDonald[3]	1973	Digestive tract	Not given	Data suggested probable link with chrysotile exposure in Quebec miners and millers. Risk is probably dose-related. In the earlier deaths, increased risk for colorectal carcinoma was apparent; in later deaths, cancer of the esophagus and stomach became more common.
Meurman, Kiviluoto, and Hakama[4]	1973	Digestive tract	No increased risk	Group too small and follow-up too short to be of definite statistical value. Exposure was to anthophyllite only.
Newhouse[5]	1973	Gastrointestinal tract	1.4	Exposure had been to crocidolite, amosite and chrysotile. Histological verification of cause of death was poor.
Selikoff, Hammond and Seidman[6]	1973	Esophagus, colon, and rectum	4.0	(a) Data based on 623 New York–New Jersey insulators. Cause of death when dying 20 or more years after first

Table 2-23 continued

Author	Date	Site	Standardized Mortality Ratio (Observed/Expected)	Comment
				exposure. Standardized mortality ratio increased with elapsed time since first exposure, being approximately 1.7 in first decade after exposure and 4.0 more than 20 years after exposure. These workers had amosite and chrysotile but no crocidolite exposure.
		Esophagus stomach colon and rectum	4.4 2.6 1.5	(b) Data based on 17,800 asbestos insulation workers in U.S. and Canada exposed to chrysotile and amosite only. Standardized mortality ratios when dying 20 years or more after first exposure. Risk of GI malignancies was slightly less if dying earlier than 20 years after first exposure.
		Esophagus stomach rectum	No increase 3.1 2.8	(c) Data based on 933 amosite insulation workers in eastern U.S. Standardized mortality ratios when dying 20 or more years after first exposure. The absence of increased risk of esophageal cancer is striking when compared with (b).

Enterline, Decoufle, and Henderson[7]	1972	Digestive tract	1.3	Data based on 1404 retired asbestos workers, average length of service 25 years. Some had very high exposures, i.e., more than 50 million particles per cubic foot of air. The standardized mortality ratio was dose-related, ranging from 1.23 to 1.8 according to calculated cumulative dust exposure. There was little difference in standardized mortality ratio between production and maintenance service workers. There was exposure to chrysotile, amosite, and crocidolite.
Anspach[8]	1974	Stomach, colon, rectum	2.3 (approx)	Data derived from 397 deaths among Dresden asbestos workers and extrapolated from author's data. Standardized mortality ratio not quoted in original article.
Doniach, Swettenham, and Hathorn[9]	1973	Stomach	1.6	East London workers with occupational exposure in shipping, insulation.
Lumsley[10]	1976	Digestive tract	Increasing SMR after 1960 onwards but not yet reached statistical significance	Data based on cancer registrations of dockyard workers, not cause of death.

209

predilection for a rectal site is at variance with what might be expected for an ingested carcinogen, but the period of follow-up is short. An average urban tap water supply may contain 2–9 million asbestos fibers per liter. Exceptions occur when, as in Thetford, Canada, the source is a lake in an asbestos-mining area and counts of 173 million asbestos fibers per liter are obtained.[13] Asbestos fibers may originate from asbestos-cement pipes used for water mains. Typical counts are 400–1400 fibers per liter, which are considered to be a "small, approaching zero, risk to health." Chrysotile filters are used in the filtration of beer, wines, spirits, and soft drinks because of the ability of asbestos to absorb bacteria, thus imparting a permanent clarity to the liquid. No health hazard is known to exist,[14] even though asbestos particle counts up to 4 million per liter (beer) and 12 million per liter (ginger ale) have been recorded.

Talc-treated rice has obtained notoriety as a cause of gastric cancer. Rice, especially when intended for Japanese consumers, may have talc added to it after the milling stage to increase its whiteness and to retain its flavor on storage. Although United Kingdom samples of talc are not reported to contain asbestos, many U.S. samples contain varying amounts of chrysotile and anthophyllite, since both minerals may be present in the same rock vein. The presence of asbestos is said to explain in part the high mortality from gastric cancer in Japan. The age-adjusted mortality resulting from this disease in Japanese males age 62–63 is 68 per 100,000 male population, about seven times the U.S. rate. Furthermore, the rate is less in those areas of Japan where cereals and soya beans are used as rice substitutes and in Japanese living in Hawaii or the continental U.S.A. who use fewer rice products.[15]

For most people, asbestos in the air is the more important than asbestos-contaminated water and rice.

Pathogenesis

Accepting that much inhaled asbestos may eventually find its way to the gastrointestinal tract and that there is an increase in incidence of gastrointestinal cancer in those working or living in an asbestos-contaminated environment, the actual method of induction of these neoplasms is obscure. If dust particles in general could penetrate gastrointestinal mucosa with any ease, one would expect that the wall would become anthracite-colored in coal miners and fibrotic in hard rock miners, while mesenteric lymph nodes would blacken or become stony hard, respectively. This is not the case with regard to the gut wall, although occasionally calcified mesenteric nodes are seen in upper abdomen in chest radiographs of miners. Asbestos fibers must act differently in entering the gastrointestinal mucosa and inducing carcinoma. In rats with an opened abdominal wall, intragastric injection of asbestos fibers has resulted in later accumulation of these fibers in lungs, brain, omentum, and other organs via the bloodstream. If one accepts that asbestos fibers reached these sources by penetration of the gastrointestinal mucosa (rather than by leakage through the injection site), then one needs to consider the mode of penetration. Long fibers might penetrate the gastrointestinal mucosa, but most of the fibers are small because gastric acidity will disintegrate chrysotile fibers into small fibers. Engulfment by plinocytosis would need to be postulated. The omentum had the highest proportion of asbestos fibers in this experiment, and since the omentum contained peritoneum and small lymph nodes, this may have a bearing on the induction of mesothelioma. Whether the omentum has a specific affinity for asbestos fibers or whether lymph nodes filter out and retain the fibers is conjectural.[12] In mice fed a diet containing 6 percent by weight of chrysotile, electron microscopy shows uncoated chrysotile fibers in the colonic mucosa.[16] Transmission electron microscopy has revealed the presence of amosite fibers in the jejunal epithelium and lamina propria of rats after three months of asbestos feeding (see Fig. 2-94C.)

In most experiments where asbestos has been given by natural feeding (not by injection), short-term tests have revealed no appreciable penetration of fibers through the gut wall (considered by most a prerequisite for peritoneal mesothelioma), and long-term feeding has not led to any gastrointestinal tract cancer.[14]

The poor correlations between these animal experiments and epidemiologic experience with asbestos fibers has posed many questions. Analogous to the multiplicative effect of smoking in asbestos and induction of lung cancer, organic additives such as nitroso compounds may play a synergistic role.[17] Another question relates to the difference in the mucosal barrier between species and individuals. Mucosal barrier differences are related to blood groups and susceptibility to gastric ulcer. Do certain mucosal barrier differences increase absorption of asbestos particles and lead to gastrointestinal neoplasm?

Pathology

Stimulated by the high incidence of gastric cancer in the Japanese, surgical specimens received from Japanese stomach cancer patients have been examined for asbestos fibers. Chrysotile and amphibole fibers (crocidolite or amosite) have been found in only three out of seven specimens in one series (one colloid cancer and two adenocarcinomas), but talc was present in all seven. A search for ferruginous bodies (as opposed to asbestos fibers) in U.S. colon

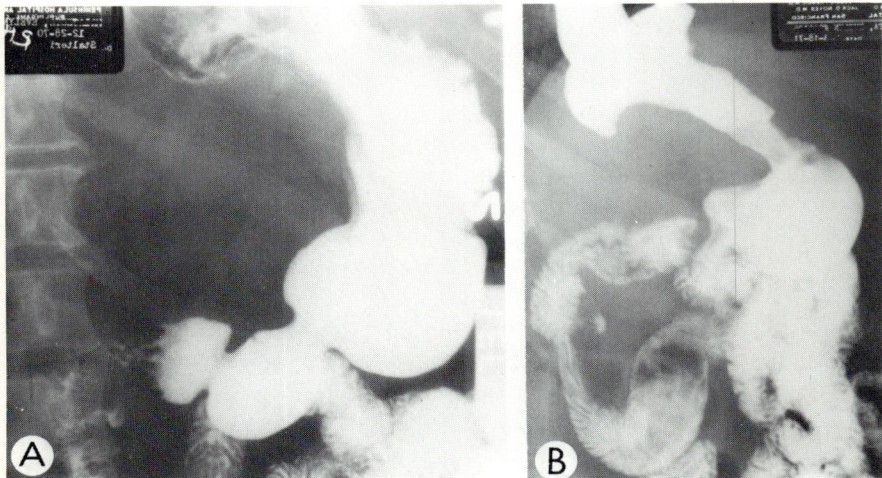

Fig. 2-92. *Adenocarcinoma of the stomach in a 49-year-old asbestos worker. (A) The flattening of the upper part of the lesser curvature was missed. (B) Three months later, the tumor was nonresectable. An incidental duodenal diverticulum is present; displacement of a duodenal diverticulum may be an early sign of cancer of the head of the pancreas.*

neoplasm specimens examined by light microscopy was unrewarding. In 16 patients, none had typical ferruginous bodies in their colonic mucosa. Eight patients, however, mainly those with cancer of the right colon, had atypical ferruginous bodies. It is conjectured that electron microscopy might yield greater counts, since chrysotile is broken up by an acid medium (such as stomach acid) into submicroscopic particles.[16]

Radiology

Examples of an esophageal and colonic cancer in prior asbestos workers are seen in Figures 2-92 to 2-94; there are no distinguishing features. Both patients had radiographic evidence of pleural plaques. Some patients with asbestosis may have multiple primary neoplasms developing synchronously or metachronously; two neoplasms in the same patient are not rare, and three neoplasms have been known to occur. The most frequent association is colorectal cancer and bronchogenic carcinoma, both in asbestos workers and in the control population.[19] With this possibility in mind, solitary masses or even two masses in the lung of asbestos-exposed patients with colorectal or other cancer need not be metastatic, and the possibility of synchronous or metachronous lung malignancy needs to be considered.

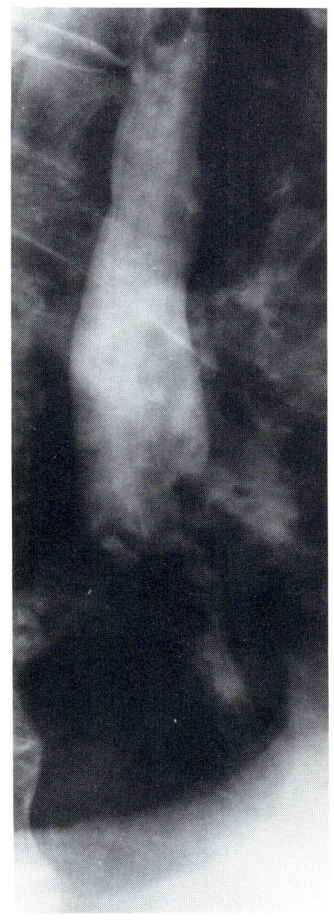

Fig. 2-93. *Esophageal cancer in a shipyard worker. Those exposed to chrysotile and amosite have a fourfold burden of cancer of the esophagus.*

LARYNGEAL CANCER

There is no conclusive evidence linking asbestos exposure and laryngeal cancer in those who do not smoke. Morgan and Shettigara concluded from a study of asbestos workers, matched for their smoking habits, that the risk of laryngeal cancer is confined to those who smoke.[20] It is postulated that carcinogens in smoke may be absorbed onto asbestos fibers and play a part in induction of laryngeal cancer.[21]

Earlier reports[8,22] which were not matched for smoking habits[23] did assert an increased susceptibility to laryngeal and other head and neck cancers. Of

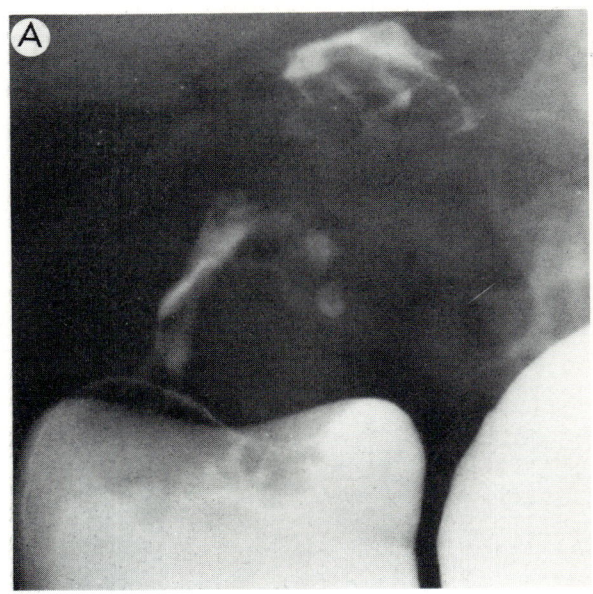

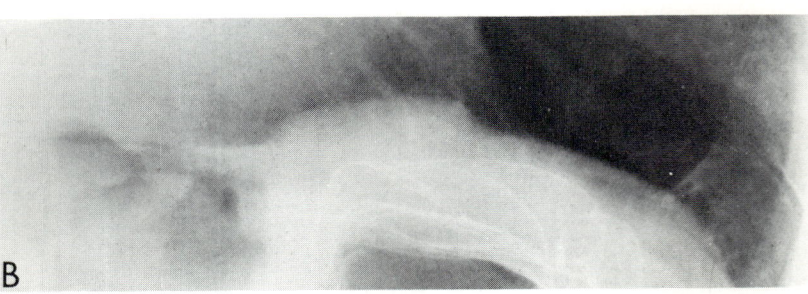

Fig. 2-94. (A) Apple core deformity due to cancer of the transverse colon. (B) Plateau-like diaphragmatic plaque in the same patient shown during air contrast barium enema examination. (C) Scanning electron micrograph. Amosite asbestos fiber penetrating epithelial cell of rat jejunal mucosa. Bar 1 μm long is shown at lower right (× 2,000) (see facing page). From penetration of the small intestinal mucosa by asbestos fibers, by Storeygard AR and Brown AL; Mayo Clinic Proc 52:809–812, 1977. Reproduced with permission of the author and the publisher.

Organ Involvement in Asbestos-related Disease

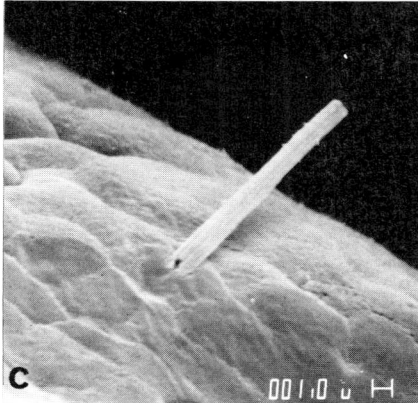

4000 asbestos factory workers, 2 developed laryngeal cancer compared with an expected incidence of 2 per 100,000 of the general population,[24] i.e., a 25-fold incidence. Libshitz et al. described 3 patients with laryngeal cancer, all smokers and all with a history of asbestos exposure, whose radiographs show typical pleural plaques and, in one instance, pulmonary fibrosis.[25]

HEMOPOIETIC SYSTEM MALIGNANCY

An association between asbestos exposure and subsequent development of malignant disorders of the hemopoietic system is suggested by the following observation. A fivefold incidence of such malignancies has been found in asbestos workers who had typical radiographic findings of plaques and pulmonary fibrosis. The malignancies include multiple myeloma, lymphosarcoma, polycythemia vera, and Waldenstrom's macroglobulin anemia.[26] Other surveys of asbestos workers have shown 2 leukemias in 58 neoplasms;[27] 1 lymphosarcoma in 96 neoplasms;[28] 3 leukemias, 1 lymphoblastoma, and 1 patient with multiple myeloma in 21 neoplasms;[29] and 2 lymphosarcomas and 1 leukemia in 380 consecutive deaths.[26]

Because of these epidemiologic findings, bone marrow aspirates have been examined in groups of otherwise healthy asbestos workers. In one group with long exposure to crocidolite, amosite, and chrysotile, there was a generalized hyperplasia in 16 out of 17 workers, especially of the myeloid series, reticulum cells, and plasma cells.[30] Despite this hyperplasia, peripheral blood samples showed a total leukocyte count in the low normal level or leukopenia. There is presumably a phagocytosis of the excess leukocytes in the reticuloendothelial system of the lungs. The marrow changes did not show any

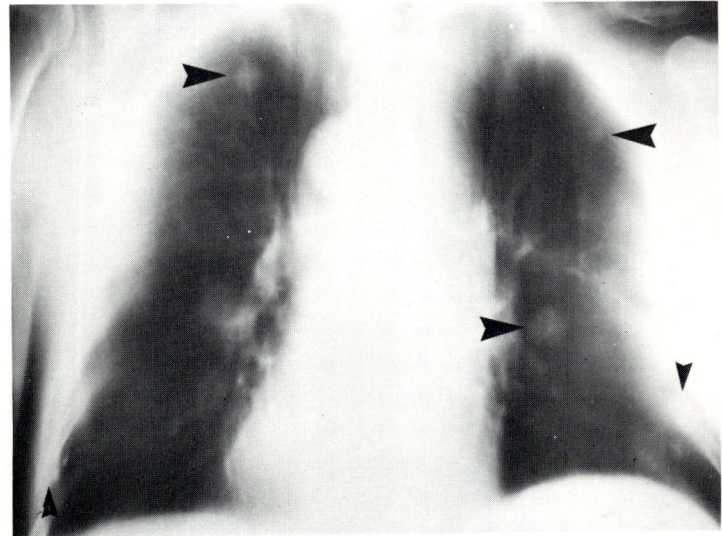

Fig. 2-95. *Illustration of metastatic lung disease from breast cancer in a male asbestos worker. Tomographic section shows multiple metastases (horizontal arrows) and calcified and noncalcified plaques (vertical arrows).*

correlation with the lung changes. Despite this data, a causal effect by asbestos in the induction of hemopoietic system malignancy is not yet accepted.

BREAST CANCER

In a study of East London necropsies of patients with known high occupational and/or environmental exposure, there was 1.4 times the expected incidence of breast cancer in women.[9] This report is the only one suggesting any association between asbestos exposure and breast cancer. If asbestos is incriminated the fibers would need to be carried into the breast by direct extension from pleural plaques or by lymphatics. The former would not be surprising when one remembers how deeply into the diaphragm and intercostal muscles calcified and noncalcified plaques penetrate.

Figure 2-95 illustrates metastic lung disease from breast cancer in a male asbestos worker. Carcinoma of the male breast differs from that in women by several features.[31] The stage of the disease is more advanced with some 65 percent of patients in TNM stage III or IV on presentation; a comparable figure for women is about 45 to 50 percent. The age of onset is on the average 5 to 10 years later in men than in women. Double primaries are more common in male patients with breast cancer than in women—13 percent in men compared with 3 percent in women; in men there is a disproportionate involvement of the large bowel and rectum. The histological pattern in male breast cancer compared with women shows a higher proportion of intraductal carcinoma, less comedocarcinoma, and no lobular medullary or mucoid carcinoma. An association exists between male breast cancer and Klinefelter's syndrome, and clinical assessment, together with a search for Barr positive cells and additional X chromosomes, is warranted. A causal effect by asbestos in induction of breast cancer is not yet accepted.

OVARIAN CARCINOMA

The role of asbestos in the induction of ovarian cancer is conjectural, and not yet accepted. There is experimental evidence that intraperitoneal injection of tremolite asbestos is associated with subsequent development of ovarian cancer in experimental animals.[32] Furthermore, in one group of 15 female asbestos workers, there was an increase in the incidence of ovarian malignancy.[33] This is not confirmed by other epidemiologists. It is often difficult to differentiate mesothelioma and papillary adenocarcinoma of the ovary on a microscopic basis. In addition, a large malignant mass arising from the pelvis of a female asbestos worker may present a problem in diagnosing the site of origin, which may not be apparent even on most careful palpation. Histological diagnosis may be in doubt even when specialized histochemical stains and assays for acid mucopolysaccharide are used.[33,34] The ovary is the most common origin of undifferentiated peritoneal carcinoma in females, and this organ is therefore frequently stated to be the primary site in carcinomatosis peritonei, while some such cases may be diagnosed as mesothelioma by other observers. Finally there is the fact that anthophyllite may be converted naturally to talc, and talc has been found in female genital malignancies. Talc crystals were found in 10 out of 13 ovarian cancers, in 12 out of 25 cervical cancers, and in 1 primary endometrial cancer but not in a secondary ovarian malignancy in the same patient.[35]

REFERENCES

1. Parkes RW: Asbestos-related disorder. Br J Dis Chest 67:261–279, 1973
2. Enterline PE, Weill H: Asbestosis in asbestos cement workers, in Bogovski P, Gilson JC, Timbrell V, et al (eds): Biological Effects of Asbestos. Lyon, IARC, 1973, pp 179–183
3. McDonald JC: Cancer in chrysotile mines and mills, in Bogovski P,

Gilson JC, Timbrell V, et al (eds): Biological Effects of Asbestos. Lyon, IARC, 1973, pp 189–194
4. Meurman LO, Kiviluoto R, and Hakama M: Mortality and morbidity of employees of anthophyllite asbestos in mines in Finland, in Bogovski P, Gilson, JC, Timbrell V, et al (eds): Biological Effects of Asbestos. Lyon, IARC, 1973, pp 199–202
5. Newhouse ML: Cancer among workers in the asbestos textile industry, in Bogovski P, Gilson JC, Timbrell V, et al (eds): Biological Effects of Asbestos. Lyon, IARC, 1973, pp 203–208
6. Selikoff IJ, Hammand EC, Seidman H: Cancer risk of insulation workers in the United States, in Bogovski P, Gilson JC, Timbrell V, et al (eds): Biological Effects of Asbestos. Lyon, IARC, 1973, pp 209–216
7. Enterline PW, Decoufle P, Henderson V: Mortality in relation to occupational exposure in the asbestos industry. J Occup Med 14:897–903, 1972
8. Anspach M: Extrathoracic asbestos cancer. Radiobiol Radiother (Berl) 15(2):253–257, 1974
9. Doniath I, Swettenham KV, Hathorn MKS: Prevalence of asbestos bodies in a necropsy series in East London: Association with disease, occupation and domicilary address. Br J Med 32:16–30, 1975
10. Lumsley KPB: A proportional study of cancer registrations of dockyard workers. Br J Ind Med 33:108–114, 1976
11. Hammond EC: Long range study of colonia and rectal cancer. Dis Colon Rectum 13:108–111, 1970
12. Masson TJ, McKay FW, Miller RW: Asbestos-like fibers in Duluth water supply. Relation to cancer mortality. JAMA 228(8):1019–20, May 1974
13. Cunningham HM, Pontefract RD: Asbestos fibers in beverages drinking water and tissues: Their passage through the intestinal wall and movement through the body. J Assoc Off Anal Chem 56(4):976–986, July 1973.
14. Selected written evidence submitted to the Advisory Committee on Asbestos, 1976–1977. Her Majesty's Stationery Office, 1977, London, pp 17–20
15. Henderson WJ, Evans DM, Davies JD, et al: Analysis of particles in stomach tumors from Japanese males. Environ Res 9(3):240–249, June 1975
16. Westlake GE, Spjut HJ, Smith MN: Penetration of colonic mucosa by asbestos particles. Lab Invest 14:2029–2033, 1965
17. Langer AM: Inorganic particles in human tissues and their association with neoplastic disease. Environ Health Perspect 9:299–232, 1974
18. Zaidi SH: Ingestion of asbestos. Environ Health Perspect 9:239–240, 1974

19. Dohner VA, Beegle RG, Miller WT: Asbestos exposure and multiple primary tumors. Am Rev Resp Dis 112:181–199, 1975
20. Morgan RW, Shettigara PT: Occupational asbestos exposure, smoking and laryngeal cancer. Ann NY Acad Sci 271:308–310, 1976
21. Gaston JC, Finklea JF, Sandifer SH: Cancer of the larynx and lung in three urban counties in South Carolina. South Med J 65 (6):753–756, 1972
22. Guidotti TL, Abraham JL, Denee PB: Letter: Asbestos exposure and cancer of the larynx. West J Med 122 (1): 75, 1975
23. Holmes S: Asbestos and cancer of head and neck. Lancet 1 (807): 75, 1975
24. Newhouse ML, Berry G: Asbestos and laryngeal carcinoma. Lancet 2 (829): 615, 1973
25. Libshitz HI, Wershba MS, Atkinson GW, et al: Asbestosis and carcinoma of the larynx. A possible association. JAMA 228 (12):1571–1572, June 1974
26. Gerber MA: Asbestos and neoplastic diseases of the haemopoietic system. Am J Clin Pathol 53:204–208, 1970
27. Mancusco TF and El-Attar AA: Methodology in industrial health studies. Arch Environ Health 6:210–226, 1973
28. Mancusco TF and Coulter EJ: Mortality patterns in a cohort of asbestos workers. J Occup Med 9:147–162, 1967
29. Lieben J: Malignancies in asbestos workers. Arch Environ Health 13:619–621, 1966
30. El Sewefy ZA, Shaheen H, Shams, El-Deen A: Bone marrow changes in asbestos. Med Lavoro 65 (5–6):168–173, 1974
31. Langlands AO, Maclean N, Kerr GR: Carcinoma of the male breast. Report of a series of 88 cases. Clin Radiol 27:21–25, 1976
32. Graham J, Gram R: Ovarian cancer is asbestosis. Environ Res 1:115–128, 1967
33. Winslow JD, Taylor HB: Malignant peritoneal mesothelioma. Clinicopathological analysis of twelve fatal cases. Cancer 13:127–136, 1960
34. Roberts GH, Irvine RW: Peritoneal mesothelioma: A report of four cases. Br J Surg 57:645–650, 1970
35. Henderson WJ, Joslin CAF, Turnbull AC, et al: Talc and cancer of the ovary and cervix. Obstet Gynaecol Br Commonw 78:266–272, 1971

SECTION 7
HYPERTROPHIC PULMONARY OSTEOARTHROPATHY

Hypertrophic pulmonary osteoarthropathy (HPOA) is a syndrome of thoracic disease accompanied by (1) digital clubbing, (2) periosteal new bone formation and synovitis in the extremities, and (3) nonpitting swelling of the soft tissues at the ends of the long bones. Digital clubbing is invariably present and is a less severe manifestation. Earlier statements that the soft tissue changes of clubbing are not of the same etiology as the bony changes[1,2] are no longer widely accepted.

Asbestosis has been defined by the presence of three or more of five standardized clinical abnormalities, including dyspnea, rales, finger clubbing, reduced vital capacity, and characteristic radiographic shadows.[3] Finger clubbing and the skeletal changes of HPOA may be due to asbestos-related bronchogenic carcinoma and pleural mesothelioma in addition to the pulmonary fibrosis of asbestosis.

Digital clubbing without any bony changes is seen in a wide variety of thoracic and extrathoracic disease (see Fig. 2-96). These include benign and malignant pleural and parenchymal tumors, cyanotic heart disease, chronic obstructive and inflammatory lung disease, diffuse interstitial pulmonary fibrosis of many etiologies, biliary cirrhosis, ulcerative colitis, regional enteritis, subacute bacterial endocarditis, and idiopathic steatorrhea. Moreover, digital clubbing alone may be a familial disease or may be associated with bone changes in thyroid acropachy, leukemic acropachy, and pachydermoperiostosis.[4,5,9]

The full syndrome, digitial clubbing and skeletal changes, has been reported in the following thoracic abnormalities: chronic sepsis of lung and pleura; benign and malignant pleural tumors; primary carcinoma of the bronchus, thymus, and thyroid; metastases to pleura and lung; achalasia; benign and malignant esophageal tumors; Hodgkin's disease; and occasionally, cyanotic heart disease. Extrathoracic causes are known.

An unusual feature is the association between HPOA and fibrous tumors of the lung and pleura. Although 80 percent of patients with HPOA have primary bronchogenic tumors, the overall incidence of HPOA in primary bronchogenic tumors is only about 12 percent.[4,5,9] Fibrous tumors of the lung

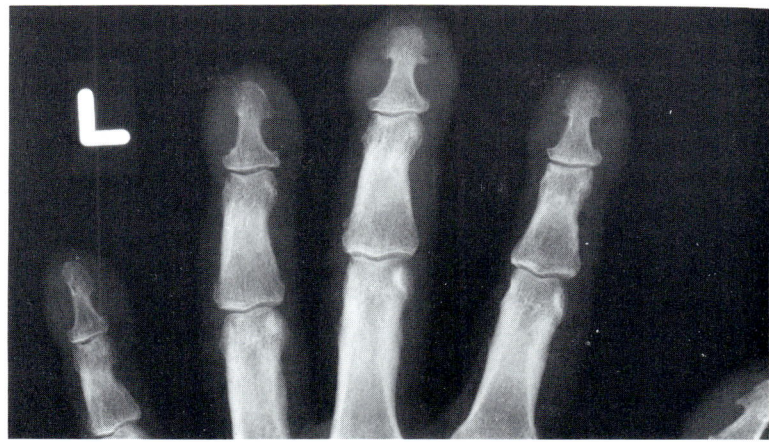

Fig. 2-96. *Digital clubbing in an asbestos worker with pulmonary fibrosis. A rapid increase in clubbing, especially when painful, may indicate development of an associated bronchial carcinoma.*

and visceral pleura, fibroma, fibrosarcoma, and benign and malignant mesothelioma have an incidence of HPOA of between 50 and 67 percent, and metastatic osteosarcoma, fibrosarcoma, and leiomyosarcoma, which have a predominantly fibrous tissue stroma, have a similar high incidence. The reason is unknown.[6]

CLINICAL FEATURES

HPOA usually manifests itself after the underlying disease has been present for some time. Rarely is it the first clue to the disease. Its severity may diminish during treatment of the underlying disease[7] and increase with recurrence. Treatment with adrenergic blocking drugs reduce pain and limb hypervascularity.[8] The clubbing associated with asbestos-induced pulmonary fibrosis is slow to develop and painless; if it is associated with bronchogenic carcinoma or mesothelioma, it may develop more rapidly and be more painful. Clubbing without periostitis is usually painless; if periostitis is present, pain usually, but not invariably, occurs. An adjacent synovitis may cause arthralgia. In descending frequency the distal radius and ulna, tibia and fibula, femur, metacarpals and metatarsals, and proximal and middle phalanges are involved. The terminal phalanges are usually spared (see Fig. 2-97).

The incidence of digital clubbing in industrial surveys of asbestos workers

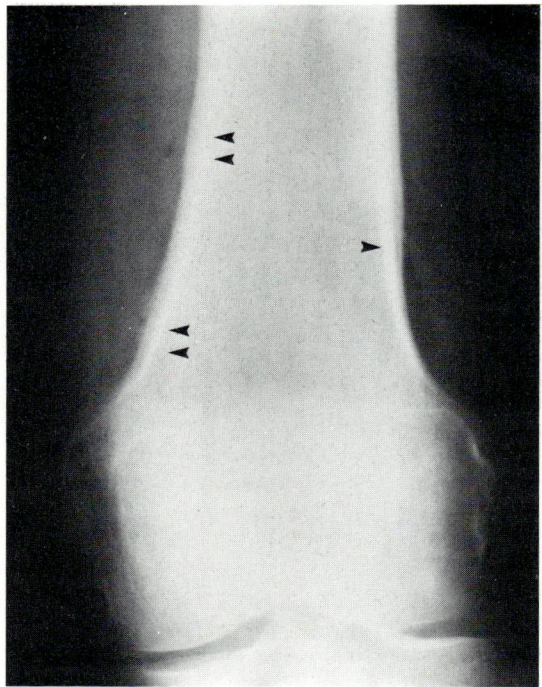

Fig. 2-97. *Left femur in an asbestos worker with severe pulmonary fibrosis who had bilateral HPOA. Tibia and fibula were also involved. Lateral femoral border (single arrow) shows a lucent line between diaphysis and periosteal lamellae; laterally the new bone is wavy and has been incorporated into the shaft. Note sparing of the bone end.*

is variable. Using measurements derived from casts of the hyponychial angle of both index fingers, clubbing was present in 4 percent of Belfast insulation workers; using clinical assessment only, the percentage was approximately double.[10,20] Clubbing usually precedes the periostitis by several months, but occasionally the two may develop together.

PATHOLOGICAL FEATURES

The affected soft tissues show proliferation, edema, and increased vascularity. The overgrowth of vascular connective tissue precedes periosteal new bone formation. The increase in blood flow is related to an overgrowth of connective tissue and not to periostitis.[4,5,9] Periosteal new bone that is laid down becomes incorporated into the shaft; the rate of formation of endosteal bone is increased. The mechanism of lamellated periosteal reaction in areas of venous stasis, a form of hypervascularity, has been studied in dogs.[11] It appears that the most superficial subperiosteal lamella produces perpendicular buds of bone that elevate the periosteum. The inner osteogenic layer of periosteum then forms a new superficial lamella beneath the elevated periosteum. This new superficial layer is connected to the next deeper layer by bony buds or bridges. The process continues by new bud formations, periosteal elevation, and further lamella formation. When the sequence is rapid and filling in appositional bone formation lags behind, the lamella become radiographically visible.

Rarely, there may be sterile joint effusions that may be recurrent. Synovial biopsy shows some synovial cell hypertrophy without inflammatory cells in the effusion.

PATHOPHYSIOLOGY

There are three main theories concerning the etiology of HPOA: neuronal, hormonal, and vascular.

Neuronal

Flavell suggested a neurogenic theory.[12] A reflex originates either in the diseased lung or in the adjacent pleura. The afferent limb is thought to be either the vagus or possibly the intercostal nerve. The distal limb is unknown. It may be the sympathetic nervous system. Thoracic or cervical vagotomy, mediastinal dissection which damages the vagus, and adrenergic blocking drugs which reduce sympathetic activity reduce blood flow in affected hands and lessen pain but cause no discernible improvement in bony changes, which may actually worsen despite reduction of pain. Because of double innervation of the lung, unilateral denervation may result in bilateral relief. Transaction of the intercostal nerves may also be followed by regression of the arthropathy.[13] Since involved organs are all served by the ninth or tenth cranial nerves, a reflex arc appears to be a reasonable hypothesis.[14]

Hormonal

An etiologic role has been postulated for estrogens, growth hormone, and vasoactive substances. Increased estrogen levels were seen in some patients with HPOA and bronchogenic carcinoma.[15] The level decreased after removal of the tumor, but estrogens were not found in the tumor itself. The blood levels could be due to increased adrenal excretion or abnormal hepatic function affecting metabolism of estrogenic precursor. The levels of estrogen tended to be higher in the presence of periostitis but not directly related to it; estrogen is unrelated to the presence or absence of digital clubbing.

The large digits of patients with clubbing, reminiscent of acromegaly, suggested a possible role for growth hormone as an etiologic agent. No proof exists that HPOA is related to increased production of growth hormone. Some malignant tumors synthesize and secrete a growth-hormone-like substance, and plasma levels may revert to normal after resection of the mass.

In a patient with squamous cell carcinoma of the cervix and adenocarcinoma of the pulmonary hilus, irradiation of the uterine cancer produced regression of hypertrophic osteoarthropathy prior to thoracotomy to obtain a tissue diagnosis of the hilar mass. This is additional evidence suggestive of a hormonal etiology.[7]

Vascular

Vasoactive substances such as 5-hydroxytryptamine and the kinins also have been incriminated. Arteriovenous shunts may allow these substances to bypass the pulmonary circulation where they are normally inactivated and exert their effect peripherally. This theory may be acceptable for digital clubbing in cyanotic heart disease but seems untenable as an explanation in other conditions associated with HPOA.

RADIOGRAPHIC FEATURES

Periosteal new bone is most pronounced in the diaphyses. In descending order of involvement are the distal radius and ulna, distal tibia and fibula, femur, metacarpals, matatarsals, and proximal and middle phalanges. Periostitis may not involve the phalanges and metacarpals even when digits are severely clubbed. In such patients the distal radius and ulna may show periostitis and should be included in the radiograph. The radiographic appearance has been classified[16] as (1) simple periosteal elevation with translucency between it and the cortex, (2) onion skin type, (3) localized small areas of periostitis, (4) long segments with wavy contour, and (5) wide cortex, a result of incorporation of periostitis in the shaft. The duration of the disease to some extent controls the radiographic appearance. Long-standing asbestos-related pulmonary fibrosis may allow incorporation of periostitic lamella to produce a wide shaft; the shorter life expectancy of patient with asbestos-related mesothelioma or bronchogenic carcinoma may allow production of shorter and narrower segments of periostitis. Synovitis is usually not detectable radiographically. Difficulties in diagnosis may arise when HPOA is the presenting clinical symptom; the etiological factor must then be found. The arthralgia usually has no radiographic signs, and if present without periostitis, it may be a problem in diagnosis. The periostitis is usually symmetrical, but when asymmetric,[17] it may be a diagnostic problem.

SCINTIGRAPHIC FEATURES

Scintigraphic features of HPOA have been the subject of many case reports.[18,19] Technetium 99m diphosphonate is commonly used. It is selectively deposited in the new periosteal lamellae either by chemisorption onto hydroxyapatite crystals or by complexing with receptors such as alkaline phosphatase. In patients with asbestos-related malignant diseases, it is important to differentiate the scintigraphic appearance of HPOA from that of metastatic disease, which is usually medullary. An associated uptake in areas of synovitis may be helpful in suggesting HPOA; the distribution of HPOA in the distal portion of limbs is unusual for metastatic disease. HPOA affecting proximal parts of the limbs is occasionally seen, however, and metastatic bronchogenic carcinoma to digits is rare but recorded. The occasional asymmetry of HPOA may cause a problem. Differentiation of metastic disease from HPOA is important in planning therapy. CT scans with appropriate manipulation of window height and width holds promise in the detection of cortical metastases.

All conditions that cause digital clubbing or generalized periostitis enter into the differential diagnosis. Periostitis in adults is seen in pachydermoperiostosis (idiopathic hypertrophic osteoarthropathy), thyroid and leukemic acropachy, vitamin A excess, collagen disease, and periarteritis nodosa.

REFERENCES

1. Skorneck AB, Ginsburg LB: Pulmonary hypertrophic osteoarthropathy (periostitis). N Engl J Med 258:1079–1082, 1958
2. Holling HE, Brodey RS, Boland HC: Pulmonary hypertrophic osteoarthropathy. Lancet 2:1269–1234, 1961
3. Murphy RLH, Ferris, BG, Burgess, WA, et al: Effects of low concentration of asbestos. Clinical, environmental, radiologic and epidemiological observations in shipyard pipe coverers and controls. N Engl J Med 285:1271–1278, 1971
4. Steinbach HL, Gold RH, Preger L: Thyroid acropachy, in The Hand in Diffuse Disease. Chicago, Year Book Publishing Co., 1975

5. Steinbach HL, Gold RH, Preger L: Pachydermoperiostitis, in The Hand in Diffuse Disease. Chicago, Year Book Publishing Co., 1975
6. Firoonzia H, Seliger G, Genieser NB, et al: Hypertrophic osteoarthropathy in pulmonary metastases. Radiology 115:269–174, 1975
7. Steinfeld AD, Munzenrider JE: The response of hypertrophic pulmonary osteoarthropathy to radiotherapy. Radiology 113:709–711, 1974
8. Reardon G, Collins, AJ, Bacon PA: The effect of adrenergic blockade. Postgrad Med J 52:170–173, 1976
9. Steinbach HL, Gold RH, Preger L: Hypertrophic osteoarthropathy, in The Hand in Diffuse Disease. Chicago, Year Book Publishing Co., 1975, pp 259–262
10. Wallace WFM, Langlands JHM: Insulations workers in Belfast. 1. Comparison of a random sample with a control population. Br J Ind Med 28:211–216, 1971
11. Volberg FM, Whalen JP, Krook L, et al: Lamellated periosteal reactions: A radiologic and histologic investigation. Am J Roentgenol Radium Ther Nucl Med 128:85–87, 1977
12. Flavell G: Reversal of pulmonary hypertrophic osteoarthropathy by vagotomy. Lancet 1:260–262, 1956
13. Goldstraw P, Walbaum PR: Hypertrophic pulmonary osteoarthropathy and its occurrence with pulmonary metastases from renal carcinoma. Thorax 31:205–211, 1976
14. Carrol KB, Doyle L: A common factor in hypertrophic osteoarthropathy. Thorax 29:262–264, 1974
15. Ginsberg J, Brown JB: Increased estrogen excretion in hypertrophic osteoarthropathy. Lancet 2:1274–1276, 1961
16. Greenfield GB, Schorsch HA, Shkolnick A: The various roentgen appearances of pulmonary hypertrophic osteoarthropathy. Am J Roentgenol Radium Ther Nucl Med 101:927–931, 1967
17. Freeman MH, Tonkin AK: Manifestation of hypertrophic pulmonary osteoarthropathy in patients with carcinoma of the lung. Radiology 120:363–365, 1976
18. Donnelly B, Johnson PM: Detection of hypertrophic pulmonary osteoarthropathy by skeletal imagine width. ^{99m}Tc-labelled diphosponate. Radiology 114:389–391, 1975
19. Terry DW, Isitman AT, Holmes RA: Radionuclide bone images in hypertrophic osteoarthropathy. Am J Roentgenol Radium Ther Nucl Med 124:571–576, 1975
20. Langlands JHM, Wallace WFM, Simpson MJC: Insulation workers in Belfast. 2. Morbidity in men still at work. Br J Ind Med 28:217–225, 1971

3
ILO U/C INTERNATIONAL CLASSIFICATION OF RADIOGRAPHS OF THE PNEUMOCONIOSES

Leslie Preger

The grading system of changes in chest radiographs of those exposed to asbestos is of use in clinical assessment, compensation adjudication, evaluation of quality of dust control in epidemiologic surveys, and identification of those individuals who have radiographic evidence of pulmonary fibrosis and therefore must be informed of the need to change occupation.

An internationally accepted system is now available, the ILO U/C 1971 system,[1] which is applicable to coal workers' pneumoconiosis (CWP), silicosis, and asbestosis. The historical development of the system is of interest. The first internationally accepted classification of the radiographic appearance of the pneumoconioses was made in 1950 in Sydney by the ILO (International Labor Organization). This was restricted to findings resulting from coal and silica, and like all later classifications, it was strictly descriptive and avoided any interpretive comments or inferences. In 1958, a meeting in Cincinnati of several interested organizations from North America and the International Union Against Cancer (WHO) decided that the patterns characteristic of asbestos exposure be added so that the system of grading would be applicable to the radiographic patterns seen in those exposed to asbestos as well as coal and silica. This became known as the U/C classification. At about the same time, the ILO realized that the ILO 1950 classification was unsuitable for asbestosis in which the typical parenchymal opacities are linear or irregularly shaped and not rounded as in coal workers' pneumoconiosis. The ILO then issued a new classification, ILO 1958 systems, in which the small rounded opacities typical of CWP continued to be graded, but other small opacities were only recorded (and not graded) using the symbols I (linear opacities) and hc (honeycomb pattern). The 1958 meeting at Cincinnati was followed by a period of years in which this North American classification, which graded both rounded and irregular (or linear) opacities, was tested and eventually published in 1968 as the UICC/C classification. Finally in 1971, the ILO reviewed and adapted the UICC/C classification, the final product being known, in deference to its antecedents, as the ILO U/C International Classification of Radiographs of the Pneumoconioses, 1971.

FUNCTION OF THE CLASSIFICATION

A comprehensive analysis using simple descriptive terms of the radiographic appearances that may follow exposure to all mineral dusts, coal, carbon, asbestos, beryllium, and silica may be made. It indicates the severity of radiographic change only. It does not attempt to deduce working capacity or degree of disability that may ensue from these changes; nor does it indicate any specific etiology. It is purely descriptive and not interpretative in the histological sense, e.g., a term such as fibrosis is not used. Its use in individual patients without correlation to history, symptoms, physical signs, and laboratory data is limited. A main use is in epidemiologic work in assessing the incidence of pneumoconiosis and the efficacy of methods of dust control. When ILO U/C classification is used, it is essential that a set of standard radiographs is available and used for comparison with the patient's film. Otherwise errors, especially in assessment of lesser degrees of parenchymal involvement, become frequent.

OUTLINE OF ILO U/C 1971 CLASSIFICATION

The full classification covers about 30 pages of small print and is obtainable from the ILO offices. Only an outline is presented here. For a more precise account the full text and accompanying set of Standard Reference Radiographs should be obtained from the International Labor Office, Occupational Safety and Health Branch CH 1211 Geneva 22, Switzerland. To use the classification, one needs to identify and record the following radiographic changes:

    Small opacities, rounded or irregular
    Large opacities, size and definition of margins

Classification of Radiographs of Pneumoconioses

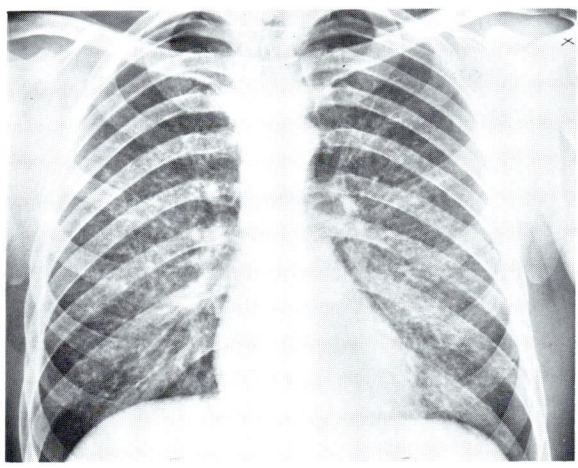

Fig. 3-1. *Small rounded opacities type p, up to 1.5 mm in diameter, profusion 3/3. These are typical of coal workers' pneumoconiosis. (CWP). (Courtesy of Medical Radiography and Photography, published by Radiography Market Division, Eastman Kodak Co.)*

Pleural thickening and calcification, site and extent
Diaphragmatic and cardiac outline—ill-defined or not

Small Rounded Opacities

Rounded opacities are typical of CWP and silicosis but not of asbestos exposure, which is characterized by irregular opacities. In some patients with asbestosis and especially in cement asbestosis, however, both types occur. They are graded for diameter: p, up to 1.5 mm (Fig. 3-1); q, 1.5–3.0 mm (Fig. 3-2); and r, 3.0–10 mm (Fig. 3-3). Their profusion may be graded as absent or very few (Category 0), few (Category 1), numerous (Category 2), or very numerous (Category 3) if the short classification is used. A more complete classification grading profusion is available using a 12-point scale developed by the National Coal Board (United Kingdom). In this system, an "I'm not sure" element is introduced. Thus, Category 2/2 indicates that the observer feels that Category 2 is warranted, while 2/1 implies probably Category 2 but could be Category 1, and 1/2 indicates probably Category 1 but could be Category 2. The spectrum of changes may therefore be described from the most severe, 3/4, to a film in which there are no small opacities, or if a few are thought to be present, they are insufficiently definite or numerous for Category 1 to be considered—this is Category 0/0. An 0/0 film may show other abnormalities

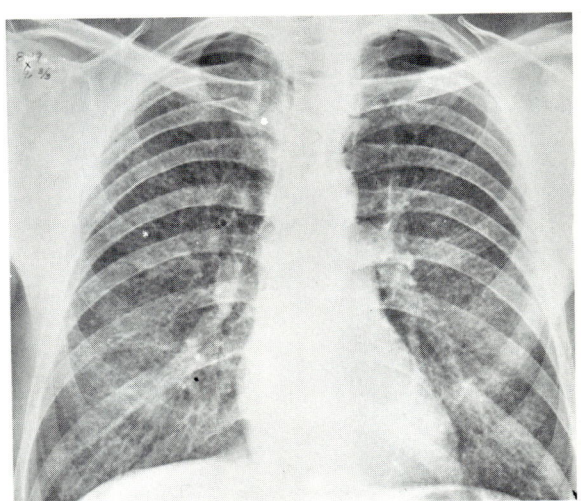

Fig. 3-2. Small rounded opacities, type q, between 1.5 and 3 mm in diameter, profusion 3/3. Typical of CWP. (Courtesy of Medical Radiography and Photography, published by Radiography Market Division, Eastman Kodak Co.)

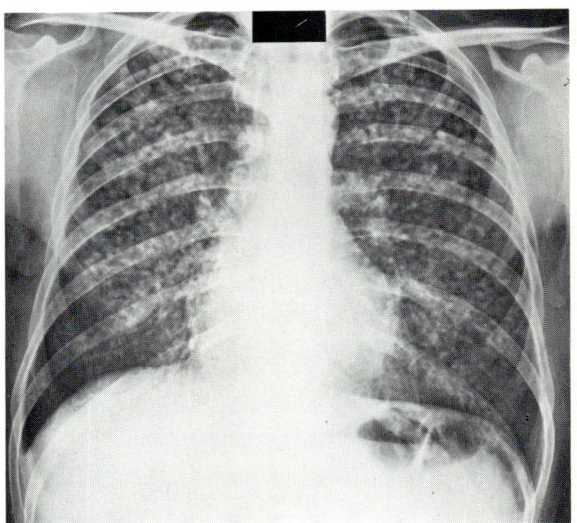

Fig. 3-3. Small rounded opacities type r, between 3 and 10 mm in diameter, profusion 3/3. These are typical of CWP. (Courtesy of Medical Radiography and Photography, published by Radiography Market Division, Eastman Kodak Co.)

Classification of Radiographs of Pneumoconioses

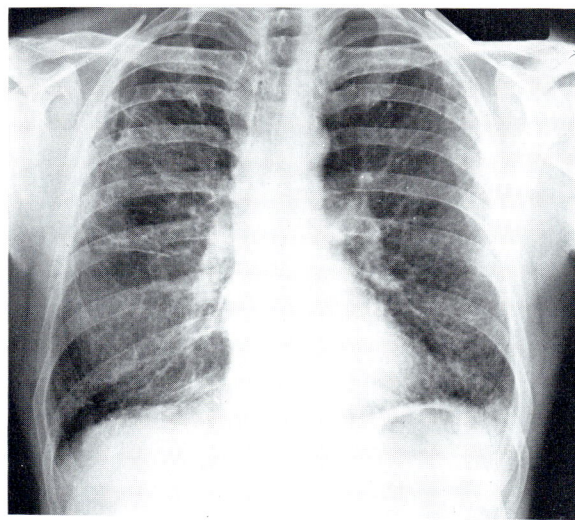

Fig. 3-4. *Fine irregular or linear opacities, type s. The profusion is 3/3, all zones of each lung are involved, and there is an ill-defined cardiac outline of severity 2. These findings are typical of asbestosis. (Courtesy of Medical Radiography and Photography, published by Radiography Market Division, Eastman Kodak Co.)*

unrelated to pneumoconiosis. To allow for this, an "exceptionally" normal film with no abnormalities irrespective of causes is classified 0/-. This appearance is usually found in young adults. In addition to profusion, the complete but not the short classification indicates zones of involvement (upper middle or lower) in each lung.

Small Irregular Opacities

Irregular small opacities are characteristic of asbestos exposure but may be seen in diatomite workers and occasionally in coal workers. Cement-asbestos workers have both rounded shadows due to silica and irregular shadows due to asbestos, in a ratio of about 1 : 4. Synonyms for the irregular shadows include honeycomb, reticular, network, linear, and blotchy. These shadows are classified by thickness only:

s = fine irregular or linear opacities (Fig. 3-4)
t = medium irregular opacities (Fig. 3-5)
u = coarse (blotchy) irregular opacities (Fig. 3-6)

Mensuration is not attempted. As with small rounded opacities, profusion is

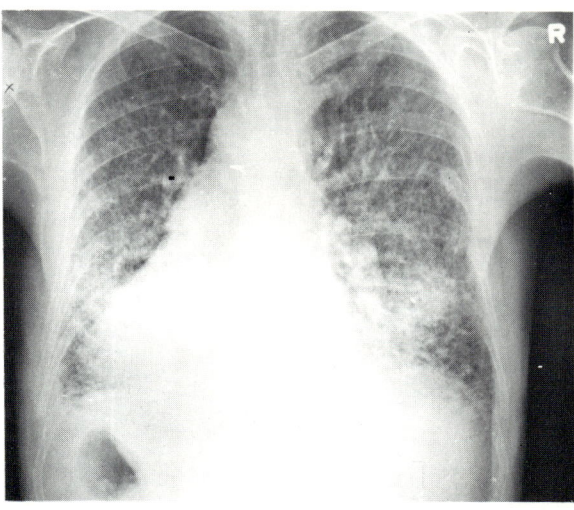

Fig. 3-5. *Medium irregular opacities, type t. The profusion is 3/3; all zones of each lung are involved. There is an ill-defined cardiac outline of severity 2, and both leaves of the diaphragm are partly obscured. Costophrenic angle is obscured (⊥), pleural thickening on the left side is graded b 1 (between 5 and 10 mm thick at widest part and not exceeding one-half of the projection of one lateral wall). There are also large opacities of type id B (ill-defined opacities the sum of whose greatest diameters exceeds 5 cm but is less than the equivalent of right upper lobe). Typical of asbestosis. (Courtesy of Medical Radiography and Photography, published by Radiography Market Division, Eastman Kodak Co.)*

graded 0-1-2-3; in Categories 2 and 3, normal lung markings are partly or completely obscured, respectively. Involvement by lung zone is also noted; each lung is divided into three zones—upper, middle, and lower. Figures 3-4, 3-5, and 3-6 illustrate small rounded opacities typical of CWP so that comparison may be made with Figures 3-1, 3-2, and 3-3, which illustrate small irregular opacities typical of asbestos exposure. The small rounded opacities are classified pqr (see page 229).

Large Opacities

Large opacities are rarely seen in asbestos workers. Their presence should suggest exposure to silica, as in cement asbestosis and some South African asbestos miners; or development of an asbestos-related malignancy or some unrelated cause. They may be single or multiple and are graded according to size and number:

Classification of Radiographs of Pneumoconioses 233

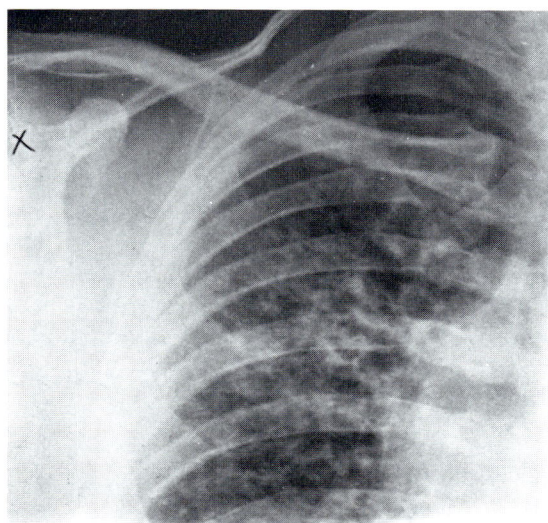

Fig. 3-6. *Small, irregular, coarse, blotchy opacities type u, profusion 3/3. These are typical of asbestosis. (Courtesy of Medical Radiography and Photography, published by Radiography Market Division, Eastman Kodak Co.)*

Category A   Single opacity, 1–5 cm diameter, or several opacities, each greater than 1 cm, but the sum of the diameters is not greater than 5 cm.

Category B   One or more opacities larger or more numerous than Category A, whose combined area does not exceed the equivalent of the right upper lobe.

Category C   One or more opacities whose combined area exceeds the equivalent of the right upper lobe.

In addition, sharpness of margin is described as "wd" and "id," well-defined and ill-defined, respectively.

Pleural Thickening

This is assessed according to width, extent, and site. Width is graded a, b, and c.

Grade a   Less than 5 mm thick at widest point
Grade b   Between 5 and 10 mm thick at widest point
Grade c   10 mm or greater at widest point

Extent is graded by adding the vertical extent on both sides:

    Grade 0   Absent or less than Grade 1
    Grade 1   Total length does not exceed one-half of lateral chest wall
    Grade 2   Greater extent than Grade 1

Costophrenic angle blunting alone is recorded separately because it has varying etiologies. Uncalcified pleural plaques are recorded with the symbol "pq."

Diaphragm Outline

Ill-definition due to plaques is recorded if more than one-third of one leaf of the diaphragm is involved.

Cardiac Outline

Ill-definition of either border due to adjacent mediastinal pleural plaques or superimposition of anterior or posterior parietal pleural plaques or parenchymal disease is graded by extent. Involved lengths are added.

    Grade 0   Absent or less than one-third length of left cardiac border
    Grade 1   Between one-third and two thirds
    Grade 2   Between two-thirds and whole
    Grade 3   More than whole

Pericardial fat pads are excluded from the grading.

Pleural Calcification

This is graded by extent; unilateral or bilateral involvement is indicated because unilateral plaques may be due to trauma or infection.

    Grade 0   No pleural calcification
    Grade 1   Single or multiple areas, total greatest extent, 2 cm or less
    Grade 2   Single or multiple areas, total greatest extent, 2–10 cm
    Grade 3   Single or multiple areas, total greatest extent, more than 10 cm

Pleural Effusions

The symbol "ef" is used to record pleural effusion.

INTERPRETIVE PROBLEMS

Any radiographic classification system must be easy to use so that large numbers of radiographs may be read quickly and contain criteria sufficiently clear to detection to keep interobserver and intraobserver error at a minimum. Ease of use is shown by the Quebec survey[3] using a system essentially the same as that of the ILO U/C classification in which 300 to 500 films could be read accurately by one reader in one day. The misreading rate (intraobserver variation) for the various radiographic changes in this series is given as:

Assessment of grade of pleural thickening	3.2%
Assessment of grade of pleural calcification	0.7%
Assessment of profuse small irregular opacities	3.9%
Assessment of large opacities	0.9%

Interobserver variation was greater; it is known from other studies that individuals are reasonably consistent in repetitive observations but that a proportion will consistently "see" more or less detail than the majority. The interobserver differences in the above series were as follows:

Assessment of grade of pleural thickening	13%
Assessment of grade of pleural calcification	6%
Assessment of profusion of small irregular opacities	18%
Assessment of large opacities	12%

For more statistical information, Rossiter's article may be consulted.[3] The use of computers to assess radiographs of patients with pneumoconiosis is as yet not great. Preliminary studies[4,5] are encouraging, although computer assessment is less specific than that of trained observers. A current problem is that blood vessels seen end-on appear to the computer not too dissimilar from rounded opacities of pneumoconiosis. An advantage of computer evaluation of radiography of pneumoconiosis is the elimination of intraobserver and interobserver variations. A particular problem in interobserver disagreement is whether opacities are rounded or irregular;[6] less disagreement is present on diameter or thickness of opacities. Nevertheless, the ILO U/C 1971 classification is considered of great practical use in epidemiologic surveys of industrial hygiene standards.[7]

In epidemiological surveys it is more important to assess correctly the profusion of small opacities than the type. Both rounded and irregular opacities may coexist in asbestos workers. A separate assessment of the profusion of each type is needed in addition to an assessment of the combined profusion. To determine the subtypes of rounded or irregular opacities, the dominant type is selected. If a film shows a few p and many q opacities, the scoring is done as if all the opacities were q. If a film shows that a few p, many q, a few s, and many t opacities are present, scoring is done separately for q and t and in addition a combined profusion score is made.

The ILO U/C classification may be modified in the near future. It has been suggested that each lung zone—upper, middle, lower, left, and right—be assessed separately for degree of profusion. Currently, the zonal position of opacities is noted, but profusion is averaged out between the six zones. For averaging purposes, minimal variations of profusion are ignored. If there is a major discrepancy between zones, the lesser zones involved are excluded from the averaging process.

There are additional difficulties in the use of the ILO U/C classification. A well-defined opacity may be irregular in shape and misclassified because its irregularity is ill-defined. Excessive collagenisation may falsely suggest calcified granulomata.

There are 20 additional symbols whose use is suggested. These are listed in Table 3-1. Rules for use of these symbols are not included with the ILO U/C classification, and there is scope for interobserver error. Thus, ax (coalescence of small rounded pneumocomiotic opacities) is rarely used since it would offset the value of the pqr classification. Eggsehell calcification of hilar or mediastinal lymph node(s) is not defined but is usually used when two or more nodes are involved, one of the nodes is at least 1 cm in diameter, and the calcification involves the whole of the periphery of at least one node. The uncalcified pleural plaque symbol (pq) is used when pleural thickening is present, even when a plaque-like shape is not apparent. The symbols tba (tuberculosis, probably active) and tbu (tuberculosis, activity uncertain) are to be used, although assessment of activity is usually based on clinical and microbiological data.

In trials, when consecutive radiographs are assessed on twin viewing boxes, there is a tendency to grade the film on the right-hand viewer with a greater degree of profusion since it is assumed to be the later film.

The accurate use of the ILO U/C classification entails serious study and, ideally, a period of apprenticeship. Examinations in reader proficiency are held from time to time in the United States under the auspices of the Department of Health, Education and Welfare, National Institute for Occupational Health and Safety, in conjunction with the American College of Radiology.

A word of caution is indicated in the assessment of asbestos pneumoconiosis. The extent of pleural or parenchymal change has a variable relation to the amount of dust in the lung or the intensity or duration of exposure. Given a certain minimal exposure, plaques may develop inexorably and are not always dose related, and the extent of irregular opacities beyond a certain

Table 3-1
ILO U/C Classification Symbols

ax—	Coalescence of small rounded pneumoconiotic opacities	hi—	enlargement of hilar or mediastinal lymph nodes
bu—	bullae	ho—	honeycomb lung
ca—	cancer of lung or pleura	k—	septal (Kerley) lines
cn—	calcification in small pneumoconiotic opacities	od—	other significant disease. This includes disease not related to dust exposure, e.g., surgical or traumatic damage to chest walls, bronchiectasis, etc.
co—	abnormality of cardiac size or shape		
cp—	cor pulmonale		
cv—	cavity	pq—	pleural plaque (uncalcified)
di—	marked distortion of the intrathoracic organs	px—	pneumothorax
ef—	effusion	rl—	rheumatoid pneumoconiosis (Caplan's syndrome)
em—	marked emphysema	tba—	tuberculosis, probably active
es—	eggshell calcification of hilar or mediastinal lymph nodes	tbu—	tuberculosis, activity uncertain

minimal grade may well be a function of immunologic response in an individual. This is discussed more fully in Chapter 2, Section 2.

REFERENCES

1. ILO U/C 1971 International Classification of Radiographs of the Pneumoconioses, International Labor Office, Geneva, 1972
2. ILO U/C 1971 International Classification of Radiographs of the Pneumoconioses. Med Radiogr Photogr 48:3, 1972. Jacobson G, Lainhart WS (eds), Eastman Kodak Co., Rochester New York
3. Rossiter CE: Initial repeatability trials of the UICC/Cincinnati Classification of the Radiographic Appearance of Pneumoconiosis. Br J Ind Med 29:407–419, 1972
4. Jagoe JR, Paton KA: Reading chest radiographs for pneumoconiosis by computer. Br J Ind Med 32:267–272, 1975
5. Fox AJ: Classification of radiological appearance and the derivation of a numerical score. Br J Ind Med 32:273–282, 1975
6. Liddell FDK: Radiological assessment of small pneumoconiotic opacities. Br J Ind Med 34:85–94, 1977
7. Bohlig H: Probleme und Erfahrungen mit der EDV-Gerechten Rontgenbefundung von Pneumouconiosen. Problems and Experiences with Computerized Coding of Radiological Findings in Pneumoconioses. Radiologe 17:2–8, 1977

4
THE INDUSTRIAL MEDICAL OFFICER AND CORPORATE RESPONSIBILITY

Paul Kotin

Like their colleagues in other fields of medicine, industrial medical officers are faced with a number of changes in society and the environment that affect their responsibilities and their relationship with their patients. Among these changes are the following:

1. The changing character of the environment
2. The changing character of the population
3. The changing character of the problems
4. The changing character of health responsibility

The environment obviously plays a predominant role in man's health, but rapid technological change, the accumulation of contaminants and waste products, the increasing population and per capita consumption, and the progressive concentration of people in urban centers have greatly magnified the threats to health and complicated the problems of health care. Current hazards are increasingly microchemical rather than microbiological, and while the principles used so successfully in the control of infectious disease have some degree of application to the current situation, a new set of guidelines and criteria for evaluating the hazards must be evolved. Chemical agents for which toxicity has been demonstrated at high concentrations exist in microquantities in all compartments of our environment—air, water, food, and consumer products—with potentially hazardous effects. While a variety of chemical agents has always been present in the several compartments of the environment, it is only in the recent past that virtually all agents—metals, organic compounds, etc.—have assaulted man from several sources simultaneously, so that the quantification of a chemical in a single environmental site as a basis for assessing a potential hazard is of limited use and validity. New to the environment, however, are the ever-increasing numbers of synthetic agents. These polymeric substances synthesized from organic molecules vary in chemical and physical properties, in survival in the environment, and in anatomic and metabolic fate within the body. Most important, there has been very little in the evolutionary sense in the way of adaptive accommodation to them through the eons of time.

The population is also changing, not only in numbers but also in its characteristics. Many, many people are now alive as a result of the therapy they have received. This therapy, which is salvaging people with diseases that were fatal 30 or 40 years ago, is obtained at a cost: depletion of physiological reserve. This has, in turn, created a growing segment of the population with lowered susceptibility to the adverse effects of environmental agents. For example, the maintenance of life in the presence of significantly decreased cardiorespiratory reserve or hepatorenal function through the use of pharmacologic agents is well known; the corollary, though, is the reduced efficiency of the detoxification mechanisms in patients with hepatic or renal disease and the increased susceptibility of tissues and organs with parenchymal damage to continuing injury.

An aspect of the changing character of the population that has received too little attention is its increased mobility. Mobility in terms of our current patterns of life in the United States means spanning oceans or countries in a matter of hours. Again, in the absence of evolutionary adaptation, physiological equilibrium and the ability of a tissue or an organ to withstand injury are significantly attenuated when biological time clocks have been manipulated.

We come now to the changing character of the problems; some of the factors to be considered are as follows:

1. Health hazards associated with long-term exposure to environmental agents present at concentrations below those producing rapid adverse reaction;
2. Combined effects of environmental agents from multiple sources interacting with one another and with man;
3. The complex nature of cause-and-effect relationships;
4. Public concern over the quality of health as distinguished from ill health.

In the microbiological era, most infectious diseases had an incubation period that was reasonably predictable. It was short; either recovery or death ensued. For the most part, recovery was tantamount to restoration to the predisease state. Health hazards today, however, are associated with long-term exposure.

The problem of the combination of effects, as well as the interaction of environmental agents, is also one of complexity. It is difficult to investigate the additive, synergistic, or inhibitory effects of two agents; for more than two agents the task is enormous. Nevertheless, there can be no effective resolution of the problems of the role of environmental agents as disease determinants without some understanding of the combinations of interactional effects.

The complex nature of cause-and-effect relationships is obvious. When a disease takes 30 or 40 years to develop, the long latent period not only tends to obscure the cause-and-effect relationship but also tends to subject it to modification. If diseases develop over such a span of years, they are being modified just by the exigencies of life.

What about the changing character of health responsibility? The relevant factors are as follows:

1. Need for criteria and standards to ensure that we have an environment of high quality;
2. Need for a scientific basis for these criteria and standards;
3. Need for fundamental information on which to base predictive criteria;
4. Assessment of problems associated with interactions of multiple agents in man;
5. Recognition of the effects of environmental agents on man's behavior;
6. Need for scientific basis for determining benefits and risks in relation to control measures.

Criteria and standards must have a scientifically valid basis. A completely uncontaminated environment is impossible. What is really needed is to know how much contamination man can be exposed to safely. It is reasonable to suppose that there is a threshold of safety for most environmental agents, since man, being an efficient machine, has overcome many insults from his environment. In discussing threshold, one must of course consider its corollary—dose–response. Next is the need for predictive criteria. We have gone from one crisis to another and have been confronted with adverse effects after they have done some environmental harm. With fundamental knowledge of the interactions between stimuli and biological systems, techniques for predicting adverse effects could be devised.

What do all these changes mean to the industrial medical officer? First, the scope of industrial medicine has expanded to the broader category of occupational health. The industrial medical officer today is responsible for more than providing treatment for occupational injuries or illnesses, advising on suitable work placement, and undertaking general health education programs for employees. The industrial medical officer is also responsible for identifying occupational hazards and advising on their control, which means a complete knowledge of how substances in the work place will be handled, how processes operate, and what exposures may be likely.

Second, other disciplines must be incorporated in the development of a comprehensive medical program. These disciplines include biostatistics and epidemiology in order to:

1. Establish and maintain uniform procedures for collection, storage, and retrieval of employee vital data, including preemployment and periodic examinations;
2. Implement regular audits of employee health records at all sites to detect developing problems at an early stage;
3. Analyze mortality and morbidity data and test hypotheses of causes of disease and death.

In addition, industrial hygiene and toxicology programs are crucial in providing the base data necessary for recommended control measures and for the analysis of potential health hazards.

In the asbestos industry, industrial medical officers must deal with a number of issues in responding to their expanded responsibilities in the prevention of occupational health problems. These issues are as follows:

1. Does the principle of dose–response apply to the interaction and effect of asbestos on animals, including man?
2. Is there a level of exposure at which no adverse effect can be demonstrated? To determine this, three factors must be carefully considered: (a) whether exposure history is accurate, (b) whether an adequate time period has elapsed, and (c) whether the surveillance of workers and medical evaluation are competently accomplished.
3. Are the engineering and technological measures adequate to ensure environmental control of asbestos concentrations, with full recognition that employee protection by personal devices such as respirators is a transient solution and an interim measure?
4. Are there measures of worker surveillance and evaluation that can provide a basis for regulatory criteria as well as enhance our ability to identify the exquisitely susceptible employee so that prompt, appropriate steps for employee protection can be taken?
5. Will workers, through their own efforts and those of their representatives, enter into a partnership with management to ensure an acceptable work environment?

In responding to these issues, the industrial medical officer as a member of management as well as a physician has the following responsibilities:

1. To participate in the support of research and other efforts to accumulate data that will contribute to the establishment of meaningful criteria, standards, work processes and practices, and consumer product characteristics that will reduce the hazard or risk incidental to exposure.
2. To utilize all available and technologically feasible engineering controls and to upgrade them as technological advances are made.
3. To practice good industrial hygiene, including accurate and regular monitoring of the work place, appropriate use of adequate personnel protection equipment, and good housekeeping.
4. To develop educational programs and revise them when necessary to familiarize employees and consumers with the hazards that may exist and the work practices, procedures, and even personal habits that may minimize or eliminate the hazards.
5. To use the standards established by regulatory agencies, not as end points, but essentially as way stations to further reduction of hazards. The existence of a regulatory standard indicates that an agent or practice is considered potentially hazardous by responsible judgments. Industry should not be satisfied with the acceptance of standards as end points even by the employees themselves, should it be shown that an employee, for whatever reason, is willing to accept a hazard. Employee acquiescence does not relieve industry of efforts to do better.
6. To require worker surveillance and evaluation through techniques whose benefits and limitations are clearly understood. All such techniques should be based on scientific understanding, not on expediency or pressure. Industry has the obligation to use diagnostic and screening procedures that are valid and reliable. "Screening" is here defined as "identification of persons (workers) at potential high risk, through the presence of stigmata of exposure and pathophysiological or pathological abnormalities, in order to decrease impact on morbidity and mortality." "Diagnostic" is defined as "leading to the identification of disease." For test procedures on the leading edge of diagnosis, a distinction should be made between those monitoring methods of documented value and those still in the research state. For example, sputum cytology is still in the research state with respect to its usefulness as a screening tool, yet the existence of high-risk populations such as asbestos workers provides an excellent opportunity to assess the potential of sputum cytology as a screening procedure. Industry should enthusiastically participate in such research efforts.
7. To ensure responsible use of asbestos through ongoing surveillance of the

material. The environmental train must be followed, with recognition of the universal "warranty" responsibility of industry. This responsibility can be met by (a) agreements with purchasers of asbestos fiber and asbestos products to ensure both the purchaser's capability for safe use and, where necessary, the education of the customer by the producer to facilitate full compliance with all regulations; (b) labeling directions for safe product use in a manner similar to those used for industrial chemicals or products such as explosives or for such consumer materials as aspirin, pesticides, and caustics and bleaches; and (c) special labeling when indicated or required, e.g., the use of descriptive terms such as "lung irritant," "skin irritant," or "potential cancer hazard." In other words, producers must concern themselves with "end uses" and the user. Inasmuch as asbestos-related disease is the result of the inhalation of excessive amounts of asbestos fiber, a major concern and effort must be that of eliminating or reducing to acceptable levels the likelihood of asbestos fibers becoming airborne. Each product must be examined and a decision made as to the benefit/risk of the product. Where the end product does not lock in the fibers to eliminate the possibility of these fibers becoming airborne or where it is impractical to control the end-use application of the product in creating asbestos-containing dust, the products should be discontinued (e.g., spackling and joint cement, asbestos in fireplace logs, and so on).

8. To facilitate communication, cooperation, and collaboration between management and the worker. The adversary relationship cannot be nor should it be eliminated, but productive cooperation can flourish in an adversary condition to the extent that effort and energies are not dissipated in distrust, antagonism, and hostility. Consultation and joint efforts toward resolution of specific differences and crises are necessary, as well as joint involvement in responding to recommendations of regulatory agencies. Of greater importance are joint efforts such as management–union committees which offer a real vehicle for educational activities for workers and for clearinghouse functions for occupational hazards. Industry should not be held totally responsible for assaults on health and safety to which it has only been a partial and not necessarily the cardinal contributor. Personal habits (cigarette smoking and excess alcohol ingestion) are frequently codeterminants in the ultimate eventuation of some of the disease states classically described in texts on occupational health. Thus, joint efforts with unions and workers are important in order to eliminate, for example, the contribution of cigarette smoking to bronchogenic cancer through the enforcement of no-smoking policies or to censure unacceptable work practices.

Although the objective of industrial medical officers is no different than that of physicians in other areas of medicine, their role is a special one by virtue of the fact that (1) industry has the front-line responsibility for the locale where the potential for harm exists, and (2) except for government, industry has more resources than anyone else to approach and ameliorate problems. The task facing industry is to reeducate itself, to recruit competent and committed staff, and to work with government, labor, and academia in anticipating problems in occupational health and in responding to them. The cooperation and collaboration of all these components in ensuring a work environment acceptable to the worker, the employer, the consumer, and the general public is vital; otherwise, progress will be halting.

5

MEDICOLEGAL ASPECTS

Jack Werchick

This chapter is intended to apprise the reader of the legal problems that may be encountered in performing radiological examinations of asbestos-related disease, with some illustrations of how to avoid involvement in litigation and some discussion of the applicable law. Although the chapter is directed to radiologists, the basic principles of law would apply equally to physicians practicing in other fields of medicine.

BASIC RIGHTS AND DUTIES

Every person is bound to refrain from injuring the person or property of another or infringing upon any of his rights and would be responsible for any injury caused to another by his want of ordinary care or skill. The measure of damages for the breach of such obligations is the amount that will compensate for all the detriment caused as a result. In a recent California case, a pathologist failed to recognize a malignant melanoma in the tissue submitted, and the correct diagnosis was delayed for 2 years until metastases were discovered in chest radiographs taken for a complaint of chest pain. The pathologist claimed that an earlier diagnosis would have made no difference, but the patient sued successfully and was awarded damages because of the emotional stress caused by the uncertainty of whether longer survival would have resulted from wider excision of tissue or other forms of therapy that may have been tried. However, negligence on the part of a radiologist, or his assistant, is of no legal consequence unless it causes damage or injury to the patient. Negligent failure to diagnose metastatic adenocarcinoma would probably make no difference in the survival time of the patient and might be considered negligence without injury. Thus, if a missed or incorrect diagnosis made no difference in the survival time, suffering, disability, or treatment of the patient, the errant physician may incur no liability. In the case of a patient with a mesothelioma, where the pathologist incorrectly interpreted the biopsy to be fibrous tissue as a result of which no definitive surgery was done, the court held that no damage resulted from the incorrect diagnosis, since there was no known life-extending treatment for mesothelioma.

STANDARD OF CARE REQUIRED

Negligence is conduct that is not reasonable and prudent under the circumstances of a given case. Professional negligence or malpractice is essentially nothing more than conduct by a person in the practice of his profession (such as physicians, attorneys, architects, engineers, or others who have special knowledge and training in a given field of endeavor) that falls below the usual standards of performance in that profession. Negligence does not require malice or intent to injure, since a physician with the very best intentions would nonetheless be liable for injury negligently caused. A radiologist owes to his patient the duty to have the degree of learning and skill ordinarily possessed by radiologists in good standing and to use the degree of care ordinarily exercised by reputable radiologists under similar circumstances. He is not negligent simply because his efforts prove unsuccessful; it is possible for a physician to err in judgment or to be unsuccessful in his diagnosis or treatment without being negligent. If a radiologist possesses the requisite education, training, and skill and exercises the requisite degree of care, he would not be held liable for a diagnosis that later turned out to be incorrect. Thus, in the case of a patient with complaints of chest pain where routine films are negative initially and when repeated in 4 months, but special films later show cancer, no liability would attach if such diagnostic conduct was within the practice of standard care.

If there is more than one approved method of diagnosis or treatment and none of them is used exclusively by all practitioners of good standing, a radiologist is not negligent if he selects one of the approved methods that later turns out to be a wrong choice. This is true even if the method selected has the approval of only a minority of the radiologists, as long as it constitutes a respectable minority and is not still in the experimental stage.

Recent surveys indicate that many physicians order extra x-ray examinations as a defense against malpractice suits. The first obligation of any physician is to his patient, so the answer to medical questions should not be influenced by the fear of litigation, i.e., so-called "defensive medicine." If there is no valid medical reason for a given procedure, there is no valid legal reason for it. The law does not mandate how to meet or treat any particular condition but requires only that the physician meet the applicable standard of care.

EXPERT OPINION REQUIRED

The standard of professional learning, skill, and care required in a given instance may be determined only from the opinions of physicians who are qualified as experts as to the standard applicable in the particular situation unless the facts concerning it are matters that are common knowledge. This concept and rule is frequently unknown to, or misunderstood by, many physicians, who incorrectly declare that "there is no standard of care applicable to the particular problem—it is a matter of my judgment." While the applicable standard required in any given situation may not be found in a medical journal or book under the label "standard of care," it is created and exists under the description, "good medical or surgical practice." The exercise of the physician's best judgment does not excuse injury caused by substandard conduct. It requires that the radiologist, in undertaking service to a patient, have the required education, training, and experience and exercise the necessary care and skill in the diagnosis or treatment of a patient; "his best judgment" is no substitute for good medicine. An inadequately trained physician can exercise "his best judgment" for his level of training and still not meet the requirement of "good medicine." Sometimes, experts accepted by the court as qualified to provide information on the subject differ as to the standard that should have been followed, creating a conflict in the evidence. Jurors generally resolve such conflict by applying the information provided by the expert witness who had the most impressive qualifications and who impressed the jurors as being the most reliable authority.

THE LOCALITY RULE

The "locality rule" formerly required that the patient's physician need have only the training and skill, and exercise only the degree of care, possessed and exercised by the other physicians in his community. It would thus have been a defense to show that the general quality of medical practice in the community was poor, thereby establishing a lower standard geographically in suits against doctors. With modern facilities for communication and travel and the availability of continuing education through medical journals, seminars, refresher courses, and other meetings, however, the modern physician—even in remote areas—has the means of keeping up to date in knowledge, facilities, and equipment in his practice or referring the patient to a specialist or specialized institution, so the reason for the "locality rule" is rapidly disappearing along with the rule itself. Thus, asbestos plaques that may require oblique views of the chest for diagnosis in New York will also require oblique views in a rural community. Differences in standard of care required may still exist, however, based on absence of highly specialized or sophisticated equipment or personnel, as between a remote rural area and a large, urban teaching center. Such difference might be applicable in emergency situations but not in elective procedures with no urgency involved.

OBTAINING HISTORY

It is the responsibility of the physician to ask his patient questions designed to elicit the necessary history, since the patient is not expected to know what information is pertinent and what is not. A physician performing a checkup of a patient should ascertain the patient's employment and, if appropriate, determine whether the patient has been exposed to toxic or carcinogenic agents such as dust or asbestos fibers in his work or daily activities. Failure to do so might render the physician liable for failure to initiate diagnostic procedures that might lead to the discovery of lung lesions. Thus the examining physician may need to know which jobs expose workers to asbestos, since a painter may not use it but may work next to a carpenter sawing fiberboard. The clinician who learns that the patient's long-time employment involved exposure to asbestos fibers and who fails to order x-ray examination of the chest or to refer the patient to a specialist might be held liable for any damage caused the patient by such omission. If a physician follows the practice of obtaining history directly from the patient, he should be wary of delegating the history-taking function to a nonexpert assistant.

If the radiologist suspects prior exposure of the patient to asbestos fibers and no such information was supplied by the referring physician, a dilemma occurs. If he questions the patient and thereby frightens him with a resulting emotional or coronary disease reaction, he may be held liable for not consulting the referring physician before directing such questions to the patient. If he does not question the patient and is unable to reach the physician, delay or postponement of the studies may occur. It would be safer to risk the delay unless an emergency existed.

Frequently, x-ray examination orders state only "PA and lateral chest" with no clinical information, even though the order form contains the printed designation of "clinical information/data" before a blank space. Such an order would require the radiologist to provide the x-rays requested and no other unless he or his assistant become aware of a condition requiring additional or different examination or investigation. For example, if the x-ray shows "fine nodulations," such findings must not only be reported to the referring physician but should also be accompanied by an adequate explanation that will cause the referring physician to follow this finding with the appropriate investigative procedures to identify the cause.

A radiologist working in an area where asbestos-related or dust-caused diseases were common would be required to have greater familiarity with the signs of such disease than would one working in an area where such conditions were rarely found, although the latter may be held to the higher standard if a better-qualified consultation was readily available. Furthermore, the radiologist in the area where asbestos-related or dust-caused diseases abounded would be required to know fiber types that would be important in recognizing final radiographic appearances if the patient had been exposed to only a single type (e.g. asbestos mining), whereas it would not be important to know the fiber type if the patient was exposed to commercial asbestos that may have any combination of fibers.

THE REFERRING PHYSICIAN

A radiologist may be held responsible for injuries to a patient resulting from his failure to consult with the patient's prior or referring physician where such consultation is required by the applicable standard of care. Thus, if the referring physician requests the radiologist to perform a coronary arteriogram on a patient whose condition contraindicates such procedure, the radiologist would probably be held responsible for injuries occurring to the patient because of the study if such contraindication would be apparent to a qualified radiologist. Furthermore, if the radiologist undertakes such invasive study with inadequate skill or experience in a community where cardiologists customarily perform such studies, he would probably be held liable for injuries caused to the patient because of his lack of skill. Likewise, where a radiologist is asked to conduct studies to help establish or rule out a diagnosis of asbestos-related disease in a patient who has been x-rayed previously, the radiologist should request and compare prior films and reports.

The main problem between radiologists and their referring physicians is knowledge and communication. Orders hastily stated to a nurse or secretary sometimes result in the wrong studies being done. In other situations, the lack of knowledge about the significance of the patient's complaints or signs found on examination will result in ordering the wrong x-ray studies. The radiologist probably would not be charged with negligence in such situations unless the condition of the patient becomes known to the radiologist as one requiring more or different roentgenographic study. This may present another problem, because radiologists are sometimes accused of performing excessive or more expensive studies for monetary motives. The welfare of the patient must be paramount nevertheless, and a jury will rarely blame such a radiologist if he is competent, careful, and conscientious; this is, however, an area where complete and accurate record keeping could be crucial in supporting the decision to perform additional studies.

A radiologist who receives a referred patient from a nonspecialist may not, without risk of incurring liability, undertake or perform dangerous diagnostic procedures solely based on the fact that the referring physician requests it. The specialist will be held to a higher standard of care than the nonspecialist and must request that the referring physician obtain adequate determination as to whether or not the requested procedure is medically indicated. Thus, if a general practitioner requests a radiologist to perform a bronchogram on a patient with suspected asbestos-related disease, most radiologists would probably accede to the request, since the study is a minimal risk procedure and chances of complication or injury to the patient are remote. If a general practitioner requested a percutaneous needle biopsy be done on his patient, however, a radiologist could be held liable if it were contraindicated and injury resulted. On the other hand, if these studies were requested by a board-certified internist, the radiologist would probably be free of liability where he relied upon the opinion of the internist, even if it were later discovered that the study was contraindicated and injury resulted to the patient by its performance. Of course, if the contraindications were obvious and apparent to the radiologist, he should not be excused from responsibility if he performed the procedure.

When a referring physician orders x-ray radiographs that are inadequate to establish the diagnosis, e.g., PA and lateral views when oblique views are necessary, it is the duty of the radiologist to so inform the referring physician as soon as this becomes apparent. This should be done even in the face of the risk that the radiologist may be accused of "creating unwarranted business." Thus, if the physician has ordered posteroanterior and lateral chest films and, when these are performed, the result is ambiguous in such a way that computed tomography examination seems to be necessary, this should be reported to the referring physician with adequate explanation of the reasons for such recommendation.

THE RADIOLOGIST'S REPORT

A radiologist's report must be stated in terminology ordinarily used in such circumstances, avoiding ambiguity and terms with very restricted meanings familiar only to specialists. He would be liable if such disapproved language caused the referring physician to advise the patient incorrectly, thereby causing injury. The report should be based on the assumption that the physician to whom it is to be sent has the general knowledge of practitioners in his field of practice on the subject in question but should not assume that he has any special, additional knowledge about it. Simplification and clarity should not offend anyone, while ambiguity or very technical terminology may cause problems.

If the procedure ordered and done raised a suspicion of cancer that could not be ruled out in those studies, the report should state this. This should be done whether the report is dictated for the benefit of a general practitioner or a chest specialist. Even in cases where the radiologist has extensive experience with the particular referring physician, it probably would be safer for the radiologist to adopt a practice of including warnings in reports to all physicians to avoid liability if one of his referring specialists misses such a diagnosis. If a radiologist assumes that the referring physician has greater knowledge about a particular subject than he actually possesses, he may be liable for any damage caused the patient by such erroneous assumption if the standard in such situation required a simpler report. The same would apply where the report is incomplete, omitting some crucial information, and obviously where it is incorrect, with resulting injury to the patient.

The law does not require a superhuman performance from physicians. For example, in cases in which pulmonary fibrosis is diagnosed, the cause may be attributed to asbestos and also to other diseases such as rheumatoid arthritis or some immunologic disorder. If history, examinations, investigative procedures, etc. provide information to identify the most likely cause, it should be stated as a probability, not as an absolute. Where such identification is not feasible with the available information and studies, that fact should be reported. Thus, if pulmonary fibrosis is found in an ex-asbestos worker, the probability of it being due to asbestos should be reported with a statement that other factors may be responsible.

Other possible areas of radiologist liability for misreporting should be avoided. For example, a radiologist would probably be liable if he reported that a lesion was located on the anterior end of the patient's eleventh rib, resulting in surgery in which part of the rib was removed and found to be normal, and it was later discovered that the lesion was on the tenth rib. Failure to recognize and report thickening of the pleura, fine reticular markings in the lower lung fields, or bilateral pleural calcifications as possible indications of one of the pneumoconioses may impose liability on the radiologist.

DEGREE OF PROOF REQUIRED

In workers' compensation hearings, administrative hearings and civil trials, where the question of *causation* may be determinative of whether or not the claimant receives compensation benefits for a given condition, the physician is prohibited from guessing or speculating about any issue, particularly the connection between a worker's job environment and his disease. Some physicians go too far and refuse to express opinions, citing the inexactness of medical science and the resulting inability to "guarantee" the accuracy of the opinion. This attitude creates unnecessary problems in the administration of the particular system—whether judicial or administrative—since all that is required for proof is that the physician deal in probabilities. For example, it would be quite appropriate to state that "based on the available information and data, the most probable cause (selecting from all the reasonable medical possibilities) is 'A' or cause 'B'." Expressed as an opinion, with reasonable reasons supporting it, it is entirely proper and acceptable when offered by a properly qualified expert witness.

THE PHYSICIAN–PATIENT RELATIONSHIP

Usually a limited relationship is created between a radiologist and a patient who is sent to him for diagnostic studies by a clinician who either requests specific studies or, by description of the significant part of the history or complaints, suggests the general area of inquiry. The only responsibility the radiologist has is to perform (or have performed by his assistant) the x-ray examinations indicated by that information competently and carefully and to interpret and report them correctly. Some courts have held that in such situations the "usual" doctor–patient relationship was not created and the radiologist owed only the duty not to injure the patient and to perform, read, and report the x-ray examinations correctly. However, in at least one case, a radiologist told the patient that the films showed a little infection in the lungs when actually the patient had silicosis which went untreated until permanent damage resulted; the court held the radiologist responsible.

In a recent California case, the physician employed by an asbestos manufacturing company was held liable to the patient when he reported to the employer that triennial x-rays taken of an employee repeatedly showed indications of developing pneumoconiosis, but no one disclosed that finding to the patient or to his personal physician, with the result that nothing was done about those findings. An expert testified that, given such findings, the standard of care required that the physician report it to someone who would see to it that the patient was removed from the dust or fiber atmosphere.

A Texas court ruled against an employee in a suit against her employer's regularly employed physician for failing to discover from chest radiographs taken during a preemployment examination that she had a far-advanced pulmonary disease. The court there determined that the examination was solely for the employer's benefit and that no physician–patient relationship was created. But most courts have ruled that since the relationship of physician and patient is one of trust and confidence, it imposes upon the physician a fiduciary duty to reveal to the patient that which in his best interest he should know.

In an Iowa case, the court ruled that the radiologist was under no duty to report to the patient his "impression" of appendicitis from x-ray films because other tests by the clinician ruled out appendicitis and indicated that another disease process was causing the symptoms. A Maryland court, however, exonerated a radiologist from liability but held a physician employed by the plaintiff's employer for the purpose of conducting an annual chest x-ray examination of its employees—although not thereby placed in a physician–patient relationship—nevertheless liable where the radiographs revealed that the employee had silicosis. The referring physician was liable for concealing this finding, but the radiologist was not, since his duty was only to report it to the clinician who had ordered the radiographs.

When a clinician sends a patient to a radiologist for chest radiographs and positive findings of fibrotic disease of the lungs are made, the radiologist should report the findings to the referring physician and not discuss it with the patient. If the patient asks the radiologist about the findings, the radiologist probably would incur no liability if he directs the patient's inquiry to the referring physician. He should not, under any circumstance, misrepresent or falsify the findings. If he does discuss the condition with the patient, he risks potential liability if he fails to take into consideration the patient's emotional condition such that disclosure further damages him, especially if the referring physician would not have disclosed the finding directly to the patient.

The nature and extent of disclosure that is required of a physician depends on the duty he owes and to whom he owes it. For example, if he is employed by an employer exclusively for the purpose of informing him of the fitness of employees for the particular jobs to be performed, the physician would generally only be required to report that information to the employer. Circumstance may create other concomitant duties, however, as in the case of an employee who has a work-incurred, compensatory disease, such as an asbestos-related disease, where most courts would require that protective measures be taken for the employee's welfare and impose liability on employer and physician alike for injury occurring to the employee because of the failure of someone to protect him.

Some states follow the common law rule (which is codified in California) that a physician learning of a patient with a communicable disease shall promptly report it to the appropriate health official. Thus, if a radiologist learned from his films that a given patient had a highly infectious condition (e.g. tuberculosis or other communicable disease), he should take care in reporting his findings to the referring physician to inquire whether the communicable disease was reported if required by law in that state. A recent California case held that a hospital that failed to report a communicable disease might be held liable to a person who contracted such disease from a former patient of the hospital.

Radiologists have been sued for injuries to patients caused by allergic reaction to contrast material. The courts do not generally impose liability merely for the use of such material if the patient has had no previous experience with that drug, since it is difficult, if not impossible, to determine such sensitivity in advance. Liability has been imposed when the reaction occurred early in the use of the material and when the radiologist then failed to discontinue its use with that patient, as well as in cases where the physician was unprepared for such allergic reaction and failed to treat it promptly when it occurred. In the use of an iodized oil in bronchography where the patient began to sneeze repeatedly and showed other signs of sensitivity and the use of iodized material was not discontinued, the radiologist would probably be liable for injury caused as a result.

LIABILITY OF RADIOLOGIST FOR ACTS OF OTHERS

A radiologist is liable for the negligent acts of his assistant or employee when performed as part of the radiologist's services. This is true regardless of whether the assistant or employee is another physician, technician, nurse, aid, or other worker, so long as the radiologist is in control because of his employer status or his authority in the circumstance. A radiologist who practices in a hospital may be held responsible for the actions of a hospital employee or another physician regardless of who employs or pays the assistant (physician, nurse, technician, etc.) if, while engaged in any such work, that assistant is under the direction of the radiologist so as to become his temporary agent. In this type of situation, any negligence on the part of such assistant, occurring while he is under such direction of the radiologist, is chargeable to the radiologist. He would also be liable for any injury caused by the incompetence of an assistant whether he was aware of the incompetence or not, under the rule of respondeat superior.

When physicians are partners in the practice of medicine, each member of the partnership is responsible for the acts of the others within the scope of the partnership. However, a physician who refers his patient to another for consultation, x-ray examination, surgery, or to take over the patient's care is not liable for the acts of the one he sent the patient to unless such referral or change was not indicated *and* resulted in foreseeable injury to the patient because of lack of competency or care by the receiving physician.

Where two radiologists are concurrently participating in services to a patient and one sees the other commit a negligent act, such as misreading an x-ray film with potentially serious consequences, he must call that error to the attention of the second radiologist to avoid liability of both. If the erring physician repeats such conduct, it would be the other physician's duty to report him to the appropriate hospital committee.

Radiologists and pathologists who frequently have contracts with hospitals in which they practice—and are independent contractors by reason of the provisions of that contract—sometimes under extraordinary circumstances may be held to be the "ostensible agent" of the hospital if the hospital intentionally, or by want of ordinary care, causes a third person to believe that the radiologist is the employee or agent of the hospital. Ostensible agency may occur when the hospital appears to exercise control over the radiologist, as in cases in which the radiologist must accept all patients needing x-rays, works in the hospital using hospital facilities and equipment, must be on duty at times specified, and sometimes even bills through the hospital. The hospital, as well as the "ostensible agent," could be held liable for the negligence of the radiologist in such cases.

INFORMED CONSENT

It is a basic principle of law that every man is the master of his own body, entitled to do with it as he will. Thus, when a procedure inherently involves a known risk of death or serious bodily harm, the question arises of whether the physician must disclose such risk to the patient or not. In some states, the physician is required to do so only if a reasonably prudent physician would do so under the same circumstances, having in mind the possibility of emotional trauma and possible consequence that such disclosure could have. In other states, the law requires the physician to disclose to his patient the possibility of such outcome, explaining it in terms that the patient will understand, including all relevant information sufficient to enable the patient to make an informed decision of which risk he wishes to take—the risk of undergoing the procedure or the risk of the consequences of not having the procedure done. The physician is not required to so inform his patient if the patient has indicated that he does not want to know about the potential hazards of the procedure or where the procedure is very simple and the danger very remote. Thus, in cases of asbestos-induced disease, if intervention such as bronchoscopy, lung biopsy, thoracotomy, or laparotomy may be needed to confirm the diagnosis, this possibility, with the potential risks clearly described, would have to be explained to the patient in states requiring complete disclosure. In some instances, it may be the function of the clinician to provide the explanation; in others, it may be the radiologist or surgeon who should do it—especially when the clinician is not knowledgeable on the subject or requests that the radiologist do so. But *someone* must do it or *both* may be held liable.

The rule of informed consent applies to the prescription of drugs that may have dangerous side effects as well as to performance of invasive radiological studies, surgery, or any investigation or treatment with such risks. Evidence that the physician has so informed the patient may be admitted by the patient, by the statement of the physician who informed the patient, by a statement to that effect signed by the patient, or by entry into the office record or hospital chart by the physician. Consent forms obtained in hospitals for surgery and other procedures usually do not apply to "informed consent," since they only grant permission to perform the procedure. Some medical groups and organizations have produced informed consent forms for various procedures for use by their members, with extensive details about the risks and hazards involved.

NEGLIGENT WORSENING OF A PREEXISTING CONDITION

A rule of law frequently misunderstood by physicians is the law pertaining to preexisting conditions. A patient who has a disease or disability at the time he is subjected to negligent conduct is not entitled to recover damages for the preexisting condition but is entitled to damages for any aggravation or worsening of the condition or its effects caused by such negligence. This is true even if the preexisting condition made him more susceptible to such worsening effects than a healthy person would have been and even if a healthy person would not have suffered any injury from such conduct. The damages in such cases are only for the worsening and its effects.

If negligent conduct by a physician or hospital employee causes an infection to a patient, the patient is entitled to be compensated for the infection and its effects. If the infection lowers the patient's resistance to disease and he sustains other complications, the negligent party is liable for the complications and their effect on the patient. Similarly, if a patient with asymptomatic degenerative arthritis was negligently permitted to fall out of bed and sustain injuries that exacerbated the arthritis and caused pain and disability, the negligent party would be liable for the worsening effects. In the case of a workman who was permitted to return to work in an asbestos plant after lung lesions suggesting asbestos-related disease were found, the negligent physician would be liable, not for the original condition he found, but only for the worsening effects caused by subsequent exposure to asbestos.

CONFIDENTIAL COMMUNICATION

The information that a radiologist obtains about a patient's physical or mental condition is privileged against disclosure by the radiologist to any third parties unless authorized by the patient, or required in the care or treatment of the patient by another physician, or ordered by a court, or the privilege is somehow waived by the patients, or where the examination by the radiologist in the first place was for the patient's employer or insurance company. The radiologist is otherwise required by law to protect and claim the privilege on behalf of the patient. Where radiographs are taken on behalf of the employer to determine the employee's fitness for his job and the employer orders and pays for the examination, no approval is needed from the employee to authorize disclosure of the findings to the employer.

If a guest is injured in a hotel and its insurance company agrees to pay medical expense and damages, a radiologist's report may be sent to the insurance company without further approval of the guest. An Ohio court, among many others, has ruled that the physician need obtain no consent for such transmittal and that he need not even disclose the contents of his report to the patient. In spite of the rulings of some courts obviating the need for consent from the patient for such disclosure, cautious physicians nevertheless obtain the signature of the patient on a form authorizing such disclosure.

California and some other states authorize physicians and other providers of health services to disclose or send copies of their records to attorneys when authorized to do so by written consent of the patient.

STATUTE OF LIMITATIONS

The statute of limitations operates to prevent the prosecution of stale claims. This restriction upon the filing of lawsuits varies from state to state as well as in the federal courts. This rule has in some cases caused the permanent dismissal of some lawsuits, while in others, the court has declined to apply this drastic result. The last day on which such a lawsuit may be filed is the time specified in the law of the state in which the negligent injury occurred (2 years in actions against the federal government); some states allow 1 year from the date of the negligent injury, and some allow up to 6 years. Failure to file within that time outlaws the lawsuit, terminating the potential liability of the wrongdoer.

In medical malpractice cases the rule is different than it is in automobile accident cases because the patient is sometimes unaware of negligent conduct by his physician or of injury due to medical care. Under the law in most states, the time for commencing a lawsuit by filing a complaint is extended until the patient discovers the negligence. California generally imposes a 3-year limitation on late discovery; Florida allows 2 years, as does Indiana; New York allows 2 years and 6 months from the negligent act or the last treatment (if continuous); other states vary. Almost all states permit later filing in cases of fraudulent concealment of the negligent conduct and in cases of foreign bodies left in the patient during surgery.

Asbestos-related disease may develop many years following exposure, and its recognition may be long delayed. Although this may present a problem in worker's compensation cases in identifying the source or single cause of the condition, it presents a different problem to radiologists to whom the worker is sent for "checkup" examination or in seeking to identify the cause of symptoms. The limitations on filing a lawsuit against a radiologist in such situations would, in most states, be 1 year from the negligent act (missing a recognizable diagnosis or misreading a radiograph) or 2, 3, or 4 years from the late discovery of such negligent conduct, depending on which state law applied.

Thus, a worker seeking compensation for a disease he claims was caused by his having worked during World War II in an asbestos environment would be faced with the problem of obtaining medical evidence to establish the relationship between such employment and his diseased condition. This might well be impossible, especially if, during that interval, the patient were a heavy smoker or developed other chest disease such as a pulmonary sarcoid that simulated asbestos-related disease or coexisted with it. As indicated above, proof based on the physician's opinion as to the most probable cause, or the percentage of disability attributable to the asbestos-related condition, would be necessary. In some cases, such distribution of causation might be possible; in others, it might not. Absent such evidence such a claim would almost inevitably fail.

HOW TO AVOID MALPRACTICE

Although this is not an absolute or comprehensive list of standards to observe in the practice of radiology, the following checklist should aid in reducing the hazard of inadvertant substandard conduct:

1. Do not exceed your training and experience.
2. Consult where necessary.
3. Do not exceed the needs of the patient's condition.
4. Do not accept more patients than you and your associates can handle competently.
5. Keep adequate and accurate records.
6. When explaining a problem, do it honestly and accurately.
7. Adopt and follow a fee schedule that is proper for the community and work involved.
8. Employ competent employees and supervise or instruct as necessary.
9. Devote the necessary time to each phase of your work.
10. Require and practice orderliness and systematic routine in your offices, examining rooms, among your personnel, etc.
11. Maintain your facilities and equipment in good condition.
12. Keep up to date in your knowledge in your field of practice.
13. Avoid telephone diagnosis and treatment as much as possible.

INDEX

Page numbers in *italics* refer to figures; page numbers followed by t refer to tables.

Air pollution, 5, 174, 210
Airborne fibers, 3, 4, 5, 6–7
Airway function measurement, 11
Alcohol intake, 174
Allergic reactions, 256; *see also* Immune response
Alveolar exudate, 82–83
Alveolitis, cryptogenic fibrosing, 88, 89
Amosite, 7, 8, *37*, 78, 85, 86, 89, 122, 124, 135, 185, 189, 190t, 211
Amphiboles, 86, 88, 123, 124, 211
Ankylosing spondylitis, 89
Anthophyllite, 7, 8, 32, *37*, 42, *43*, 78, 84, 85, 86, 121, 124, 186, 189, 190t, 205, 210, 217
Antigens
  HLA-B12, 24, 87
  HLA-B27, 87, 89
  HLA-BW5, 24, 87
  HLA-W27, 24, 178
Antinuclear antibodies, 17, 24, 25, 87
Aorta, in pulmonary mesothelioma, 163
Arsenic, 174
Aryl hydrocarbon hydroxylase, 174, 175, 185
Asbestos bodies; *see* Ferruginous bodies
Asbestos cement, 4, 8, 210
Asbestos dust-control measures, 1, 6, 7, 8, 12, 122–123

Asbestos dust (fiber) levels, 6–7, 11
  pulmonary fibrosis and, 87–88
Asbestos exposure, 1–6
  dose estimation, 6
  dose-response relationship, 6–7, 101
  dose-time relation, 29, 41–42, 123–124, 187–189t, 188t
  duration of, 6, 7
  environmental, 5–6, 42, *43*, *44*
  heavy, 6, 7t
  by ingestion, 206, 210
  latency period, 6
  minimum, 12, 14–15
  1930–50 period, 6
  nonoccupational, 5, 122, 206, 210
  objective evidence, 8–10
  occupational, 3t–4, 7t, 42, 121–123, 127, 206
  threshold effect, 8
Asbestos exposure history, 1, 2, 6, 7
Asbestos fiber distribution, 83
Asbestos fiber type, 35, 36–*37*, 42
  lung carcinogenesis and, 189–190t
  mesothelioma and, 78, 124, 189
  pulmonary fibrosis and, 84, 85, 86–87
Asbestos ingestion, 206, 210
Asbestos milling, 3–4
Asbestos mining, 3, 121
Asbestos production, 1

Asbestos products, 4t
  handling, 5, 122, 127
Asbestos-related disease, 1–2; see also specific diagnoses
  extrathoracic, 205–219, 206t
  follow-up examinations, 11–12
  screening examinations, 10
Asbestos type, 7–8
  carcinogenesis and, 8
Asbestos utilization, 1, 2
Asbestos warts, 205
Asbestosis, 16–19
  biopsy in, 18
  blood groups and, 24
  clinical findings, 10–11
  diagnosis, 10–12, 17
  immune response, 23–25
  lymphocytes in, 25
  management, 19
  physical examination, 17
  pulmonary function tests, 11, 12, 13, 17
  radiography in, 10, 11, 12, 17
  symptoms, 17
Australia, 86, 122, 189
Azygous vein, 166

Benign asbestos effusion, 113–119, 134, 137, 139
Beryllium disease, 18
Beverage filtration, 210
Biological time clocks, 240
Blacks
  lung cancer in, 178
  lung volumes of, 11
Blood groups, 24, 211
Breast cancer, 216–217
Bronchogenic carcinoma; see Lung cancer
Busulphan, 174

Canada, 20, 84, 121, 187, 210
Caplan's syndrome, 89–90, 97, 99, 123
  radiography in, 99
Carcinogenesis
  chemical factors, 190
  trace elements and, 190
Carcinogens, lung, 174, 175t
Cardiac tamponade, 142
  extensive mesothelioma and, 137

Cellular immunity, 25; see also Immune response
Cement asbestosis, 90, 97, 99–101, 100t; see also Asbestos cement
  radiography in, 99–101, 100t
Cermik disease, 44
Chemical toxins, 239–240
Chrysotile, 5, 7, 8, 20, 36, 37, 42, 44, 78, 84, 85, 86, 88, 90, 101, 121, 122, 124, 185, 186, 187, 188t, 189, 190t, 206, 210, 211
Cigarette smoking, 11, 12, 14, 17, 19, 137, 213
  lung cancer and, 174, 175t, 185–187, 186, 190
Clothing, asbestos-laden, 5, 89
Coal workers' pneumoconiosis, 19
Collagen disease, 17, 18, 25
Colonic cancer, 212, 214
Communicable disease, 256
Computed tomography, 50–55, 51–54
  in lung cancer, 102, 104, 193, 196, 198–200, 199
  in pleural mesothelioma, 167–170, 168–169
  in pleural plaques, 108
  in pleural (visceral) thickening, 108
  in pulmonary fibrosis, 102–108, 105–107
  pulmonary vascular bed and, 108
  technology, 102n, 104
Confidential communication, 259
Conjugal asbestosis, 44
Constrictive pericarditis, 130–131, 137, 138, 141–142
Construction industry, 4
Cor pulmonale, 17, 113
Corporate responsibility, 239–245
Crocidolite, 7, 8, 37, 78, 84, 85, 86, 90, 101, 102, 122, 124, 185, 187, 189, 190t, 211
Cryptogenic fibrosing alveolitis, 88, 89
Cyprus, 42
Czechoslovakia, 5, 12

Detoxification mechanisms, 240
Diaphragmatic plaques, in pleural mesothelioma, 159, 163

Digital clubbing, 17, 114, 138, 220, 221–222, 224
"Dog with lice and fleas" syndrome, 108

Echocardiography
 in mesothelioma, 130–131, 141–142, 167
Environmental factor, 239–240, 241; see also Asbestos exposure
 multiple agent interaction and, 240–241
Epidemiology
 of gastrointestinal cancer, 207t–209t
 of lung cancer, 176–177t
 of mesothelioma, 121–123
 of pleural plaques, 41–45
Esophageal carcinoma, 131, 163, 212, 213
Exhaust gases, 174
Expert opinion, 249

Ferruginous bodies, 5, 8–9, 17, 18, 83
 autopsy findings, 9–10
 in gastrointestinal cancer, 211–212
 lung cancer and, 174, 182, 184t
 with pleural plaques, 35–36, 42
Fibrosing alveolitis, cryptogenic, 88, 89
Filtration, beverage, 210
Finland, 8, 32, 42, 78, 121, 205

Gastric cancer, 212
Gastrointestinal cancer, 23, 86, 205–212
 asbestos source, 206, 210
 dose-response relationship in, 6
 epidemiology, 207t–209t
 ferruginous bodies and, 211–212
 mucosal barrier and, 211
 pathogens in, 210–211
 pathology, 211–212
 radiography in, 212
 research, 205, 206, 210–211, 215
Germany, 5
Glucose-6-phosphate dehydrogenase deficiency, 123
Granuloma, 82, 83

Health responsibility, 241
Hemopoietic system malignancy, 215–216
Histiocytosis-X, 94
Hormonal factor, in hypertrophic pulmonary osteoarthritis, 223–224
Hospital liability, 257
Household contacts, 5, 44, 89, 122
Humoral immunity, 25; see also Immune response
Hyalinosis complicata, 14, 45, 46t
 mesothelioma differentiation, 15
Hyalinosis simplex, 15, 45, 46t
Hyaluronic acid, 21
Hydrocarbons, 174–175, 190
Hydropneumothorax, 153
Hypertrophic pulmonary osteoarthritis, 95, 220–226
 clinical features, 221–222
 hormonal theory, 223–224
 neurogenic theory, 223
 pathological features, 222–223
 pathophysiology, 223–224
 radiography in, 224–225
 scintigraphic features, 225
 vascular theory, 224

Iceland, 5
ILO U/C International Classification, 10, 227–238
 on cardiac outline, 234
 development of, 227–228
 on diaphragm outline, 234
 function of, 228
 interpretative problems, 235–238
 on large opacities, 232–233
 outline, 228–234
 on pleural calcification, 234
 on pleural effusion, 234
 on pleural thickening, 233–234
 on pulmonary effusion, 113
 on pulmonary fibrosis, 93–94, 108
 on small irregular opacities, 231–232, 233
 on small rounded opacities, 229–231, 230
 symbols, 236, 237t

Immune response, 23–25
  in lung cancer, 174, 175, 178
  in mesothelioma, 123
  in pleural plaques, 24, 37, 40
  in pulmonary fibrosis, 87, 88, 89
Immunoelectrophoretic patterns, 25
Immunoglobulins, 25
Immunosuppressive therapy, 174
Industrial medical officer, 239–245
  responsibilities, 241–244
Informed consent, 257–258
Insulation, 4, 121–122
Interferon, 24
Interstitial fibrosis, 16–17, 18
  idiopathic diffuse, 18
Italy, 20

Japan, 210, 211

Klinefelter's syndrome, 217

Laryngeal cancer, 213–214
Leukemia, 174
Lipid pneumonia, 18–19
Lobular thickening, in pleural mesothelioma, 152–153, *154–157*
Lung biopsy
  in asbestosis, 18
  in lung cancer, 178, 181
  transbronchial, 18
Lung cancer, 19, 174–204
  adenocarcinoma, 178, *179*t, *180*t, 181t, 182, 184t, *192, 193, 194*
  asbestos type and, 8, 189–190t
  biopsy in, 178, 181
  cigarette smoking and, 174, 175t, 185–187, *186*, 190
  computed tomography in, 102, 104
  cytology, 116, 139
  dose-response relationship in, 6
  epidemiology of, 176t–177t
  exposure dose-time relationship in, 187–189t, 188t
  ferruginous bodies in, 174, 182, 184t
  fibrosis and, 102, *103*, 104
  histologic type, 178, 179t, 180t, 181t, 184t
  immune response and, 174, 175, 178
  location, 181–182t, *183*
  mesothelioma differentiation, 200
  metastases, *198–199*
  oat cell, 178, 179t, 181t, 184t
  pleural effusion and, 113, 119
  pleural plaques and, 13–14, 45, 185, *193–196, 194–195, 197*
  pleural plaques masking, 75
  pulmonary fibrosis and, 175, 178, 182, *183, 184*t, 185, 191–*193, 192*
  squamous cell, 179t, 181t, 184t, *195*
Lung cancer radiography, 102, *103*, 191–200
  computed tomography, 193, 196, 198–200, *199*
  mesothelioma differentiation, 200
  pleural plaques and, 193–*196, 194–195, 197*
  pulmonary fibrosis and, 191–*193, 192*
Lung carcinogens, 174, 175t
Lymph node involvement, in mesothelioma extension, 132, 155
Lymphocytes, 25; see also Immune response

Macrophages, in pulmonary fibrosis pathogenesis, 83–87
Magnesium, 85
Malpractice, 248; see also Medicolegal problems
  suit avoidance, 261
Medicolegal problems
  basic rights and duties factor, 247–248
  communication factor, 251–252
  confidential communication and, 259
  contraindications and, 251–252
  damages, 247–248
  diagnostic error and, 247–248
  employee-employer relations and, 254–256
  expert opinion and, 249
  findings disclosure and, 254–256
  history factor, 250–251
  informed consent and, 257–258
  invasive procedures and, 251, 252

liability for the acts of others, 256–257
locality rule, 249–250
negligence, 247–248, 252
negligent worsening of preexisting condition and, 258–259
patient-physician relationship and, 254–256
proof required factor, 254
radiologist's report and, 253–254, 255
referring physician role in, 251–252
standard of care required and, 248–249, 255
statute of limitations and, 260–261
unnecessary examinations and, 248–249, 252
Mesothelioma; see also Peritoneal mesothelioma; Pleural mesothelioma
  asbestos type and, 8, 78, 124, 189
  benign fibrous, 135
  cell origin, 135
  cocarcinogens and, 124
  cytology, 116, 139, 141
  diagnostic procedure efficacy in, 139, 141t
  epidemiology, 121–123
  exposure and, 2, 5
  exposure dose-time factor in, 123–124
  histochemical techniques for, 136
  histological classification, 135
  histological diagnosis, 135–136
  household contacts and, 122
  hyalinosis complicata differentiation, 15
  immune response and, 123
  incidence, 121–123
  latent period, 122–123
  lung cancer differentiation, 200
  microscopic features, 135–136
  mortality statistics, 121, 122, 187
  natural history, 124–134
  nonasbestos-related, 122
  occupational exposure and, 121–123 127
  ovarian carcinoma differentiation, 127
  pathogenesis, 123–124
  pathology, 124–134
  pleural effusion and, 16, 113, 114, 116, *117*, 119
  pleural-peritoneal ratio, 127t
  pleural plaques and, 13–14, 45, 78
  pulmonary fibrosis and, 136
  site, 124, *125–126*, 127
  technetium 99m scintigram of, *143–147*
  treatment, 142
Mexican Americans, 178
Myeleran, 174

Negligence, 247–248, 252, 258–259
Neurogenic factor, in hypertrophic pulmonary osteoarthritis, 223
Nuclear scanning, in pulmonary fibrosis, 109

Occupational environment evaluation, 12, 14–15
Occupational health, 241–242
Occupational history, 2–4, 5–6
Osteoarthritis; see Hypertrophic pulmonary osteoarthritis
Ovarian carcinoma, 217
  mesothelioma differentiation, 127

Paint, 5, 44
Paraplegia, in extensive mesothelioma, 131–*132*
Pericardial effusion, 163, 167
Pericardial mesothelioma, 124, *125–126*, 163, 166–167
Peritoneal mesothelioma, 22–23, 124, 127t, *128*, 134
  clinical features, 138–139
  diagnosis, 23
  extension of, 134
  pleural plaques and, 78
  pulmonary fibrosis and, 102, 161
  radiography in, 170
  symptoms, 22
  therapy, 23
Physician-patient relationship, 254–256
Physiological reserve, 240
Pleural adhesions, 52, 63, 66–67

Pleural biopsy
  in pleural mesothelioma, 21–22
  tumor spread and, 22
Pleural cyst, 157
Pleural effusion, 16, 113–120
  clinical features, 113–115
  diagnosis, 16
  etiology, 114–115
  lung cancer and, 113, 119
  mesothelioma and, 16, 113, 114, 116, *117*, 119, 133–134, 142, 146, 147t, *148–150*
  pathology, 116, 118
  pleural plaques and, 116, *117*, 118–119
  pleural plaques masking in, 75, *76–77*
  pleural (visceral, parietal) thickening in, 116, *117*, 118, 119
  pulmonary fibrosis and, 113, 114, 116, 118, 119
  symptoms, 16
Pleural effusion radiography, *114, 115,* 116, *117,* 118–119
  ILO U/C classification, 113
Pleural fluid analysis, 115, 116
Pleural lipoma, *155*
Pleural mesothelioma, 19–22, 89, 124, *125–126,* 127t, *128,* 130–134
  above diaphragm extension, 161, 163, 166–167, 170
  age factor, 136–137
  asbestos exposure and, 20
  below diaphragm extension, 170
  benign malignant differentiation, 152–153, *156*
  biopsy in, 21–22
  clinical features, 136–138
  decortication and, 127, *129,* 137
  diagnosis, 20–21
  diaphragmatic plaques and, *159, 163*
  differential diagnosis, 21
  extension of, 130–134, *131, 132, 133,* 137–138, *139–141,* 155, *158, 160–161, 162,* 163, 166–167, 170
  hilar adenopathy in, 155
  histology, 20–21
  hydropneumothorax in, 153

incidence, 136
life expectancy and, 22
lobular thickening in, 152–153, *154–157*
lymph node involvement, 155
physical examination, 20
pleural effusion and, 133–134, 142, 146, 147t, *148–150*
pleural plaques and, 78, 128, 129t, *130,* 150–151, 159, *164, 165*
pleural (parietal, visceral) thickening and, *150–151*
pneumothorax with, 127, *129,* 152, 153, *155*
postmortem diagnosis, 21
pulmonary fibrosis and, 102, 161, *166*
pulmonary function tests in, 20
satellite lung lesions, 155, *158–159*
symptoms, 19–20, 137t
therapy, 22
Pleural mesothelioma radiography, 20, 143, 146–170
  aortic wall involvement, 163
  azygous vein in, 166
  cardiac silhouette in, 163, 166
  computed tomography, 167–170, *168–169*
  diaphragmatic plaques, *159, 163*
  hilar adenopathy, 155
  hydropneumothorax, 153
  lobular thickening, 152–153
    differentiation, 153, *154–157*
  mesothelioma extension, *160–161, 162,* 163, 166–167, 170
  pericardial effusion, 163, 167
  pericardial mesothelioma and, 163, 166–167
  pleural effusions, 142, 146, 147t, *148–150*
  pleural plaques, 159, *164, 165*
  pleural (parietal, visceral) thickening, *150–151,* 161, 163, 166–167, *168–169,* 170
  pulmonary fibrosis, 161, *166*
  satellite lung lesions, 155, *158–159*
  signs in, 143
  solitary mass, 153, *157*

Index

Pleural plaques, 12–15, 17, 29–81
  asbestos particles in, 35–36, 37
  biopsy, 13
  calcification, 31–35, 32, 33, 34, 45, 68, 70–74, 72–73
  clinical manifestations, 45–46t
  diaphragmatic, 32, 35, 36, 56, 58–59, 67, 71, 72–73
  environmental exposure and, 42, 43, 44
  epidemiology, 41–45
  exposure dose-response factor, 6, 42
  exposure dose-time factor, 29, 41–42
  extension, 29–30
  ferruginous bodies in, 35–36, 42
  fiber transport and, 36–37, 39
  fiber type and, 42
  follow-up examination, 14–15
  gross appearance, 13, 30–31
  histology, 13, 14, 15
  immune response and, 24, 37, 40
  location, 29–30, 36, 38, 39
  lung cancer and, 13–14, 45, 185, 193–196, 194–195, 197
  masking lung cancer, 75
  masking pleural effusion, 75, 76–77
  mediastinal, 70–71
  with mesothelioma, 13–14, 45, 78, 128, 129t, 130, 150–151, 159, 164, 165
  microscopic appearance, 31–35
  from occupational exposure, 42
  pathogenesis, 36–39, 38, 40, 41
  peripheral location, 70
  with pleural effusion, 116, 117, 118–119
  with pulmonary fibrosis, 45, 90, 92, 93, 108
  risk factor, 13–14
  in sarcoidosis, 108, 109
  talc, 71, 74
  in unexposed groups, 44–45
  unilateral, 67–68, 69
Pleural plaques radiography, 13, 46–78
  calcified plaque detection, 68, 70–74, 72–73
  chest wall shadows differentiation, 63, 65, 66–67
  computed tomography, 50–55, 51–54, 108
  for diaphragmatic location, 56, 58–59, 67, 71, 72–73
  film size, 46
  hyaline plaque detection, 56–67
  image quality, 48–49
  kilovoltage, 46–48, 47, 49t
  lateral chest wall, 57–58, 60
  for mediastinal location, 70–71
  mesothelioma and, 78
  muscle insertion differentiation, 63, 64–65, 66–67, 68t
  oblique projections, 58–59, 61, 62, 63
  for peripheral location, 70
  plaque identification, 56–74
  pleural adhesions differentiation, 63, 66–67
  pleural effusion masking, 75, 76–77
  pleural (visceral) thickening and, 74
  pulmonary carcinoma masking, 75
  talc plaques, 71, 74
  technique, 46–55
  unilateral plaque assessment, 67–68, 69
  xerography, 49–50
Pleural plaque ultrasonography, 49
Pleural rind, exudative, 15, 16
Pleural sarcoma, 153, 154
Pleural (parietal, visceral) thickening, 74
  in pleural effusion, 116, 117, 118, 119
  in pleural mesothelioma, 150–151, 161, 163, 166–167, 168–169, 170
Pneumoconiosis, 89
  ILO U/C classification, 227–238
Pneumonia
  desquamative interstitial, 88
  lipid, 18–19
Pneumothorax, with pleural mesothelioma, 127, 129, 152, 153, 155
Population factor, 240
Population mobility, 240
PPD skin tests, 89
Pseudotumors, 152, 155, 200
Pulmonary bullae, 108

270 Index

Pulmonary carcinoma; see Lung cancer
Pulmonary diffusing capacity, 11, 17
Pulmonary fibrosis, 82–112
  alveolar exudate and, 82–83
  animal research, 84, 86
  asbestos cement exposure and, 90, 97, 99–101, *100*t
  asbestos dust (fiber) level and, 87–88
  asbestos fiber characteristics and, 84, 85, 86–87
  asbestos fiber penetrability and, 86
  clinical features, 90
  etiology, 82–83
  granuloma formation and, 82
  gross appearance, 84
  household contact and, 89
  immune response and, 24, 87, 88, 89
  inorganic dust and, 83
  lung cancer and, 102, *103*, 104, 175, 178, 182, *183*, *184*t, 185, 191–193, *192*
  macrophages and, 83, 84, 85–86, 87
  massive, 89, 98–99
  mechanical factor, 85
  mesothelioma and, 136
  microscopic appearance, 83–84
  nonasbestosis-related, 108–*109*
  nuclear scanning in, 109
  pathogenesis, 84–88
  peritoneal mesothelioma and, 102, 161
  pleural effusion and, 113, 114, 116, 118, 119
  pleural mesothelioma and, 102, 161, *166*
  pleural plaques and, 45, 90, *92*, *93*, 108
  pulmonary vascular bed and, 108
  rheumatoid arthritis and, 89
  in sarcoidosis, 108–*109*
  variants, 88–90
Pulmonary fibrosis radiography, 82, 90–109
  cardiac silhouette, 97
  computed tomography, 102–108, *105*–*107*
  densities, 93–94
  exposure-dose response factor, 101
  ground glass appearance, 98
  hairline shadows, 94, 96
  honeycombing, 94, *95*, 96–97, 101, 104
  ILO U/C classification, 93–94, 108
  in lung cancer, 102, *103*
  massive fibrosis, 98–99
  nuclear scanning, 109
  opacities, 93, 97–98
  parenchymal changes, 90, *91*, *92*, 98t
    classification, 93–94
  pleural plaques and, 90, *92*, *93*
  ring shadows, 94, *95*, 96–97, 104
  septal lines, 94, 96
  suboptimal, 98
  variants, 98–101
Pulmonary function tests, 45
  in asbestosis, 11, 12, 13, 17
  in pleural mesothelioma, 20

Quebec, 42, 78, 121, 186, 188t

Race factor, 178
Radiography; see also specific techniques and diagnoses
  in asbestosis, 10–11, 12, 17
  in Caplan's syndrome, 99
  in cement asbestosis, 99–101, *100*t
  contrast in, 48–49
  edge enhancement, 49
  in gastrointestinal cancer, 212
  in hypertrophic pulmonary osteoarthritis, 224–225
  ILO U/C classification, 227–228
  image quality, 48–49
  kilovoltage, 46–48, *47*, 49t
  in lung cancer, 102, *103*, 191–200
  in mesothelioma, 20, 142, *143*–*147*, 146–170
  in peritoneal mesothelioma, 170
  in pleural effusion, *114*, *115*, 116, *117*, 118–119
  in pleural mesothelioma, 20, *143*–*147*, 146–170
  in pleural plaques, 13, 46–78
  in pulmonary fibrosis, 82, 90–109
Radiologist's report, 253–254, 255
Radon, 174
Residential area factor, 5

Rheumatoid factor, 17, 24, 25, 115
Rheumatoid arthritis, 89
Rhodesia, 32, 84
Rice, talc-treated, 210

Sacrospinalis muscle, 59
Sarcoidosis, 18, 108–109, 178, 182, 185
Scleroderma, 178, 182
Semispinalis muscle, 59
Shipyard employment, 4, 13, 45, 121, 122, 123, 185
Silicosis, 19, 83, 87
South Africa, 5, 78, 86, 89, 93, 121, 122, 189
Soviet Union, 121
Statute of limitations, 260–261
Superior vena cava syndrome, 133
Systemic sclerosis, 178, 182

T-cells, 25, 178; see also Immune response
Talc, 44, 71, 210, 211, 217
Talc plaques, 71, 74

Talcosis, 71
Technetium 99m scintigram
   in hypertrophic pulmonary osteoarthritis, 225
   in mesothelioma, 143–147
Teratogenesis, 206
Trace elements, 86, 190
Turkey, 5, 44

Ultrasonography, 49
United Kingdom, 5, 42, 122, 123, 178, 188t, 210

Vascular factor, in hypertrophic pulmonary osteoarthritis, 224
Vena cava involvement, in extensive mesothelioma, 132–133, 163
Viral infection, 24
Vitamin A, 174

Warts, asbestos, 205
Water supply, 5, 206, 210

Xerography, 49–50